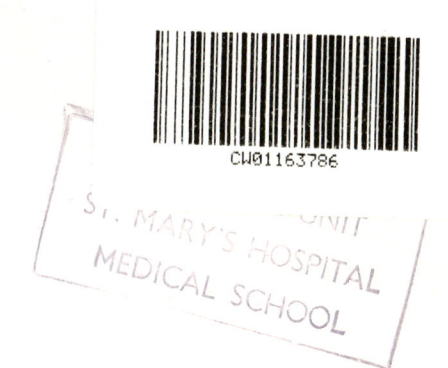

Butterworths International Medical Reviews

Pediatrics 1

Hematology and Oncology

Butterworths International Medical Reviews

Pediatrics 1

Editorial Board
G. C. Arneil
F. C. Battaglia
R. D. H. Boyd
J. K. Lloyd
J. Metcoff
A. D. Milner
C. R. Scriver
S. Siegel
M. L. N. Willoughby

Next volume

Perinatal Medicine

Butterworths
International
Medical
Reviews

Pediatrics 1

Hematology
and Oncology

Edited by

Michael Willoughby, MD, MB BS, FRCPath
Consultant Haematologist,
Royal Hospital for Sick Children,
Glasgow, UK

and

Stuart E. Siegel MD
Head, Division of Hematology-Oncology,
Children's Hospital of Los Angeles,
Los Angeles,
California, USA

Butterworth Scientific
London Boston
Sydney Wellington Durban Toronto

All rights reserved. No part of this publication may be reproduced
or transmitted in any form or by any means, including
photocopying and recording, without the written permission of
the copyright holder, application for which should be addressed to
the Publishers. Such written permission must also be obtained
before any part of this publication is stored in a retrieval system of
any nature.

This book is sold subject to the Standard Conditions of Sale of
Net Books and may not be re-sold in the UK below the net price
given by the Publishers in their current price list.

First published 1982

©Butterworth & Co (Publishers) Ltd. 1982

British Library Cataloguing in Publication Data

Pediatrics.—(Butterworths international medical
  reviews, ISSN 0260-0099)
  1.
  1. Pediatrics — Periodicals
618.92′0005   RJI

ISBN 0-407-02308-9

Photoset by Butterworths Litho Preparation Department
Printed and bound in England by Robert Hartnoll Ltd., Bodmin, Cornwall

Preface

In this volume we have tried to select slightly more than a dozen key topics which are critical to current and evolving practice within the field of paediatric haematology and oncology. Our primary objective has been to bring together those topics which most consistently occupy the attention of those involved in this challenging exciting field.

To achieve this end we have been privileged to be able to draw upon the experience of internationally acknowledged experts in each of the selected fields, these being drawn from both sides of the Atlantic. We are grateful that such inevitably busy people could find the time to write these chapters. This has placed a considerable burden upon them but it was necessary if we were to have the first-hand opinions of those close to the 'grass roots' of their subjects.

In particular, we are especially appreciative that the Chairman of the US Children's Cancer Study Group, Dr Denman Hammond, could find time to describe paediatric tumors where combined modality of therapy improves survival. Closely related to this is Dorothy Pearson's chapter concerning problems and limitations in the practice of radiotherapy in paediatric oncology. Dr Pearson is actively involved with both the UK Children's Cancer Study Group and the MR Childhood Leukemia Studies. Dr Tim Eden, also associated with both of these UK groups, updates his information on testicular involvement in acute lymphocytic leukaemia in the chapter on extramedullary leukaemia. One of the most important and previously neglected areas in our overall management has been the psychosocial aspects of paediatric haematology-oncology, reviewed here by Drs Jonathan Kellerman and James Varni, who work closely with the Therapy Team at the Childrens Hospital of Los Angeles. Moving from the family unit to the leukaemic cell membrane, but related to long-term prognosis, we were fortunate to procure a succinct chapter on the significance of immunologic cell surface markers in childhood ALL from the Boston Group of Dr James Garvin and Stephan Sallan.

In addition to the psychosocial aspects, two other chapters span the fields of paediatric oncology and non-malignant haematology. These are the contributions of Stephan Ladisch on histiocytosis, who pinpoints our current conceptual dilemma concerning this group of disorders, and also the chapter from the Leyden bone marrow transplant team, by Professor Dooren and Dr Jacques Vossen. They review the increasingly broad applications of marrow transplantation across the field of paediatrics including not only leukaemia and aplastic anaemia, but also immunodeficiency syndromes, Marble-Bone disease, hereditary metabolic disorders and possibly, in the future, thalassaemia major and Blackfan-Diamond syndrome.

In the day-to-day practice of paediatric haematology, the two haemorrhagic disorders, idiopathic thrombocytopenic purpura and haemophilia, share a major time-consuming set of clinical problems. New concepts are clarifying the well-known disease of ITP and Margaret Karpatkin's current review is timely. Home therapy has transformed the lives of patients with severe haemophilia or Christmas disease. Jack Lazerson was an innovator of this therapeutic approach and we are fortunate to have his mature evaluation 10 years after its initiation.

A uniquely paediatric compartment of haematology lies in the neonatal field and early manifestations of hereditary blood disorders. Greater understanding of physiological changes in oxygen transport and binding to fetal erythrocytes in the neonatal period has emerged from studies by Dr Oski's group of co-workers in Syracuse. His colleague, James Stockman, has written a comprehensive review of changes in oxygen transport and delivery in relation to neonatal erythropoiesis. From Great Britain we have an equally important discussion of the present status of antenatal diagnosis of thalassaemia and haemoglobinopathies by Bernadette Modell, and of haemophilia and Christmas disease by Reuben Mibashan in a joint chapter.

Although the potential for correction of the basic molecular defect in thalassaemia by genetic engineering is currently the subject of intense investigation, the major clinical challenge of these diseases remains the problem of chronic iron overload. The recent advances in iron chelation therapy using desferroxamine, as well as new agents of potential value are discussed in the chapter by Dr Jorge Ortega, Director of the Hemoglobinopathy Program at the Childrens Hospital of Los Angeles.

Haematology, and oncology also, begin and end with cellular proliferation; and so does our book, with a fundamental review of the contribution of myeloid and erythroid stem-cell culture techniques to our increased understanding of erythropoietic changes and blood disorders in childhood, by one of Europe's leading investigators in this field, Cesare Peschle.

We hope that this collection of articles will be both explanatory and stimulating to those who, like us, are engaged in clinical practice and research within this growing branch of paediatrics.

Michael Willoughby
Stuart Siegel

List of Contributors

Leonard J. Dooren, MD
Professor of Pediatrics, Department of Pediatrics, University Hospital, Leiden, The Netherlands

Osborn B. Eden, MB, MRCP
Consultant Haematologist, Department of Pediatric Haematology, Royal Hospital for Sick Children, Edinburgh, UK

James H. Garvin, Jr, PhD, MD
Clinical Fellow, Division of Pediatric Oncology, Sidney Farber Cancer Institute; Fellow in Medicine, Division of Hematology and Oncology, Children's Hospital Medical Center; and Research Fellow, Department of Pediatrics, Harvard Medical School, Boston, Mass., USA

Denman Hammond, MD
Professor of Pediatrics, University of Southern California; and Chairman, Children's Cancer Study Group, University of Southern California School of Medicine and Comprehensive Cancer Center, Los Angeles, Calif., USA

Margaret Karpatkin, MD
Professor of Pediatrics, Director of Pediatric Hematology and Oncology, New York University Medical School, New York, NY, USA

Jonathan Kellerman, PhD
Associate Clinical Professor of Pediatrics, University of Southern California School of Medicine and Consultant to Hematology–Oncology, Children's Hospital of Los Angeles, Calif., USA

Stephan Ladisch, MD
Assistant Professor of Pediatrics, Division of Hematology/Oncology, University of California at Los Angeles School of Medicine, Los Angeles, Calif., USA

Jack Lazerson, MD
Professor of Pediatrics and Pathology, Division of Hematology-Oncology, Department of Pediatrics, University of California at Davis, Sacramento, Calif., USA

Reuben S. Mibashan, MD, FRCP
Senior Lecturer and Honorary Consultant, Department of Haematology and Haemophilia Centre, King's College Hospital Medical School, London, UK

Bernadette Modell, MD
Consultant in Perinatal Medicine, Department of Obstetrics and Gynaecology, Faculty of Clinical Sciences, University College, London, UK

Jorge A. Ortega, MD
Professor of Pediatrics, Division of Hematology-Oncology, Children's Hospital of Los Angeles, Calif., USA

Dorothy Pearson, MB, ChB, DMRT, FRCR
Consultant Radiotherapist and Oncologist, Christie Hospital and Holt Radium Institute, Withington, Manchester, UK

C. Peschle, MD
Research Director, Laboratorio Patologia non Infettiva, Istituto Superiore di Sanità, Rome, Italy

Stephen E. Sallan, MD
Clinical Director, Division of Pediatric Oncology, Sidney Farber Cancer Institute and Division of Hematology and Oncology, Children's Hospital Medical Center; and Associate Professor, Department of Pediatrics, Harvard Medical School, Boston, Mass., USA

James A. Stockman, III, MD
Professor of Pediatrics, State University of New York, Upstate Medical Center, Syracuse, NY, USA

James W. Varni, PhD
Assistant Clinical Professor of Pediatrics, University of Southern California School of Medicine and Codirector, Behavioral Pediatrics Program, Orthopaedic Hospital, Los Angeles, Calif., USA

Jaak Vossen, MD
Professor of Pediatric Immunology, Department of Pediatrics, University Hospital, Leiden, The Netherlands

Contents

1 Multidisciplinary management of childhood cancers: a model for the future   1
  Denman Hammond

2 Psychosocial aspects of pediatric hematology-oncology   14
  Jonathan Kellerman and James W. Varni

3 Radiotherapy in paediatric oncology   30
  Dorothy Pearson

4 Extramedullary leukaemia   47
  Osborn B. Eden

5 Significance of immunologic cell surface markers in childhood acute lymphoblastic leukaemia   80
  James H. Garvin, Jr and Stephen E. Sallan

6 Histiocytosis   95
  Stephan Ladisch

7 Potential of bone marrow and fetal tissue transplantation in paediatrics   110
  Jaak Vossen and Leonard J. Dooren

8 Antenatal diagnosis of inherited haematological disease   162
  Bernadette Modell and Reuben S. Mibashan

9 Neonatal erythropoiesis: changes in oxygen transport and delivery   196
  James A. Stockman, III

10 Thrombocytopenic purpura: current immunological and clinical aspects   224
  Margaret Karpatkin

11 Clinical consequences and management of chronic iron overload   236
    Jorge A. Ortega

12 Home therapy in hemophilia and Christmas disease   248
    Jack Lazerson

13 Hemopoietic stem and progenitor cells: recent advances and physiopathologic relevance   263
    C. Peschle

Index   297

1
Multidisciplinary management of childhood cancers: a model for the future
Denman Hammond

One of the most gratifying accomplishments in the history of cancer therapy has been the development of successful therapy for and the increasing cure rate of many of the cancers of infants and children. However, the best known treatment results yet achieved are not being obtained by all who treat children with cancer. The best results are being achieved by institutions which have developed effective teamwork among the specialists with all the relevant expertise and skills needed for the diagnosis, treatment and clinical investigation of cancer.

The 'state of the art' of pediatric cancer therapy today has resulted from the conduct of many clinical trials by many investigators at numerous institutions. The advances of the past two decades have not resulted from 'breakthroughs'. They are the outcome of sophisticated analyses of data painstakingly obtained by carefully planned clinical research and the application of these findings in successive generations of clinical trials, which in turn are designed to seek additional knowledge from the answers to questions carefully designed into trials of still newer treatments.

THE TEAM MANAGEMENT OF CANCERS OF CHILDREN

One of the major achievements that has contributed very significantly to the successful treatment of the cancers of children is that in many countries there has been almost total reorientation of the manner in which pediatric patients are managed. Children with cancer are not commonly diagnosed and treated by pediatricians or family physicians. They are usually referred to the nearest major pediatric medical institution where there are available teams of specialists, including physicians, biomedical scientists, nurses, technologists, and others, which include the variety of skills required for a complete diagnosis and the development of a treatment plan optimized for each patient. Since cancer is uncommon among children, it is only in large pediatric institutions that such expertise in multidisciplinary pediatric cancer management is available.

It was a finding of major importance when the effectiveness of post-operative chemotherapy for tumors thought to be surgically completely resected, was found to improve the outcome achieved by surgery alone. Once it was demonstrated in large controlled studies[1,4] that chemotherapy given following surgical removal resulted in a longer disease-free period and produced a survival advantage, surgeons were anxious to collaborate with chemotherapists and radiation therapists. The era of combined modality therapy inevitably followed. Multi-institution cooperative groups, which developed multi-modality clinical trials, fostered and accelerated the development of multidisciplinary management at principal pediatric institutions. The Childrens Cancer Study Group initiated committees of pediatric surgeons, radiation therapists and pathologists in 1969. Specialists in all therapeutic disciplines began to participate in designing trials, preparing protocols and conducting clinical studies. Soon, it became a requirement for membership that an applicant insitution have in-depth expertise in each of these and other disciplines. The transition of multi-institution cooperative groups from clinical trials of chemotherapy only to multi-modality, multidisciplinary therapeutic investigations of pediatric cancers was underway.

The present management of the cancers of children provides a model for the management of an increasing variety of the cancers of adults. Many adult cancer patients are managed, not by multidisciplinary teams, but by one consultant after another, often with months or years intervening. It is a good time to review the past two decades of progress, change and accomplishment in the successful treatment and cure of many of the cancers of children, in order to identify the lessons that can be learned and insure their broad application where appropriate.

DIFFERENCES BETWEEN THE CANCERS OF CHILDREN AND ADULTS

The principal cancers of infants and children differ significantly from those of adults. The most common cancers of children are the leukemias and lymphomas which total about 50 percent. Cancers of the central and sympathetic nervous system comprise about 25 percent and the remainder are mainly sarcomas of kidney, muscle and bone. Pediatric cancers usually are not carcinomas and do not involve epithelial tissues. For this reason they are not superficial cancers, nor do they exfoliate, and afford little opportunity for early diagnosis. They are usually deep-seated and commonly have spread beyond the primary site by the time of diagnosis. Thus, the remarkable improvements in cure rates for cancers of children represent therapeutic successes rather than better detection.

The principal cancers of children not only differ from those of adults with respect to the organ system involved, the histology and clinical stage at diagnosis, but are characterized by other factors which are important prognostic variables. These include the age at diagnosis, the site of involvement, the histological or cytological subclassification and the surgical findings and accomplishments at operation. Therapy has been successfully tailored to the expected outcome, particularly by use of less aggressive therapy, for example, the elimination of radiation or chemotherapy for subgroups with very favorable prognosis. On the other hand children facing a poor prognosis with conventional therapy can be identified at the time of diagnosis, so new therapeutic strategies can be employed at the outset, rather than after a period of cancer progression during ineffective treatment.

RESPONSIVENESS OF CHILDHOOD CANCERS TO MULTI-MODALITY TREATMENT

The response to treatment of many of the cancers of children is much more favorable than that of adult cancers. *Figure 1.1* illustrates the improvement in two year survival of the major cancers of children between 1940 and the present. Extirpative surgery was the only treatment widely employed in 1940. This was followed historically by post-operative radiation therapy, and later by use of single chemotherapeutic agents. Later, combinations of several active single agents were found to be much more effective. Multiple agents were combined that had different therapeutic mechanisms of action and did not produce additive toxic effects. In 1940, when surgery was the only therapeutic modality available, the two year survival ranged from 0 to 20 percent. By 1960, radiation therapy began to be widely used in this country in treating the solid tumors of children, and by 1970 multiple

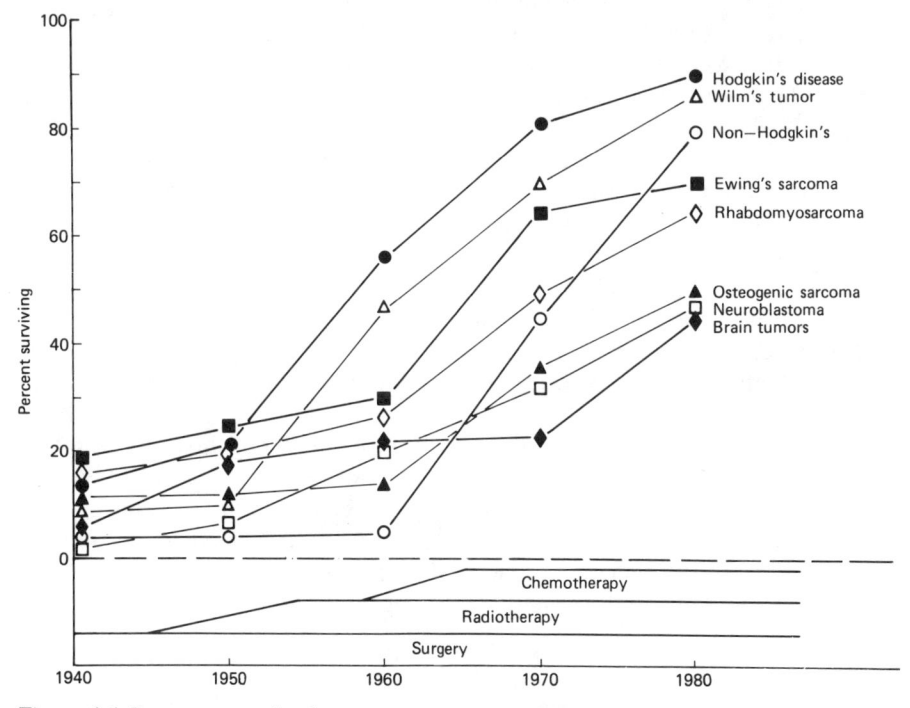

Figure 1.1 Improvement in the two year survival of children with solid tumors. Data from multiple sources are shown relating to the chronology of the widespread application of the principal modes of therapy. Many qualitative refinements in each therapy occurred during the time periods indicated. (From Hammond[2], courtesy of the Publishers, *Cancer: Achievements, Challenges and Prospects for the 1980s*)

agent chemotherapy was widely applied. Multidisciplinary treatment planning at the time of diagnosis became the customary mode of pediatric cancer management only during the last decade. The two year survival now ranges from 80 to 95 percent for several tumors, while a few have improved only to about 40 percent. The long term results of treatment of bone tumours, neuroblastoma and brain tumors are still relatively poor.

Some of the important milestones in the history of these gratifying advances are listed below and deserve emphasis, since they are applicable to some pediatric tumors that have not yet yielded to therapy and also to many cancers of adults.

(1) Extirpative surgery
(2) Post operative radiation therapy
(3) Activity of *single* chemotherapeutic agents
(4) Effective *combinations* of active agents
(5) Effectiveness of chemotherapy for surgically 'resected' tumors
(6) Combined modality therapy
(7) Development of multidiscipline therapy teams at principal pediatric institutions
(8) Development and refinement of systems of staging
(9) New principles of surgical management
(10) New principles of radiation therapy
(11) Identification of additional factors influencing outcome
(12) Design of therapy for subgroups stratified according to factors influencing prognosis
(13) Less aggressive therapy for subgroups with good prognosis
(14) Different therapeutic strategies for subgroups with poor prognosis
(15) Widespread application of new technologies by various cancer control interventions
  (a) Development of networks for professional education
  (b) Increasing availability of pediatric oncology consultants
  (c) Increasing referral of patients to principal pediatric centers for multidisciplinary evaluation, treatment planning and management

They illustrate the importance of multidisciplinary team management to establish the tissue diagnosis and pathologic subtype, the complete staging and the development of a treatment plan based upon the probable contribution and appropriate sequence of each therapeutic modality. As a result of such teamwork at major pediatric institutions the principles of surgical management and radiation therapy for pediatric tumors have undergone major changes in the last two decades.

CHANGES IN SURGICAL MANAGEMENT

Significant changes in the surgical management of tumors of children which have occurred are the following.

(1) Debulking of unresectable tumors
(2) Assessment of chemotherapy effect on tumor
(3) Fewer radical extirpative procedures
(4) Limb salvage and prostheses
(5) Second look surgery following chemotherapy and radiotherapy
(6) Resections of metastases
(7) Regional node dissections
(8) Interstitial endocurie therapy
(9) Two-team surgical approach for dumbbell lesions
(10) Preoperative multidisciplinary treatment planning

In former years, if a surgeon could not remove a tumor, the operation was terminated leaving the tumor intact. Today, the surgeon attempts to remove as much tumor tissue as is feasible so systemic therapies can be more effective. Current studies are designed to assess the effect on the tumor specimen removed at surgery of the chemotherapy given preoperatively. Pathologists can evaluate differences in the effectiveness of chemotherapy at the tumor level and obtain information which is useful in guiding subsequent therapy. There are fewer radical extirpative surgical procedures. For tumors that are chemotherapy and radiation therapy responsive, radical debilitating surgical procedures are much less common. In such patients, chemotherapy and radiation therapy can be combined following less radical surgery and produce very good outcome. There has been increasing incidence of limb salvage with insertion of prostheses for bone tumors. Surgeons now can avoid debilitating surgery, particularly on a child who might have alternative therapy that will enable a much more satisfactory lifestyle.

'Second look' operations are performed following courses of chemotherapy and radiation therapy for certain tumors, in order to assess the completeness of an apparently complete clinical remission, and also to remove residual tumor that might be present, once the patient appears to have had a maximum response from systemic therapies. It has become commonplace for surgeons to operate to remove metastases, even when multiple. New approaches to regional node dissection have become important because of new knowledge about the routes of tumor spread.

Interstitial endocurie therapy is now finding a place in pediatric cancer management. Interstitial implantation may be peformed at surgery for incompletely resectable tumors and can be combined with external beam therapy to provide optimal tumor dosimetry. Two-team approaches are being employed more commonly for surgery of lesions that involve more than one anatomical space, for example, a neuroblastoma that involves both the abdomen and the chest or extends from the abdomen into the spinal canal. A neurosurgical team and an abdominal surgical team can coordinate their separate operative approaches when such situations are identified in advance.

CHANGES IN RADIATION THERAPY OF TUMORS OF CHILDREN

Even since 1960, when radiation therapy was widely used for the treatment of the solid tumors of children, the following important changes have taken place.

(1) Transition from orthovoltage to megavoltage
(2) Increased use of radiotherapy simulators
(3) Increased use of patient molds
(4) Improved tumor imaging techniques
(5) Precision of tumor geometry and dosimetry
(6) Tumoricidal therapy to tumor
(7) Maximum sparing of normal tissues
(8) Refinements in total body and hemibody irradiation
(9) Determination of minimal effective dose
(10) Coordination and sequencing with other therapies

New tumor imaging techniques, such as computerized tomographic scanning and positron emission tomography now give even greater precision of tumor localization and geometry. Therefore, important qualitative differences have occurred in the radiation therapy given children today compared to only a few years ago.

It is necessary, particularly for patients with favorable prognosis, to reduce or eliminate radiation therapy when feasible. Patients with the most favorable stages of Wilms' tumor and rhabdomyosarcoma are not helped by radiation therapy[1,4]. Thus, a widely used standard therapy has been eliminated for selected patients who do not need it. The proper sequencing of radiation therapy, surgery and chemotherapy is being investigated. The administration of chemotherapy and/or radiation therapy prior to surgery was pioneered for children's tumors over ten years ago. It is no longer necessarily the best approach to operate first, since some tumors may be made operable by pre-operative chemotherapy, perhaps combined with radiation therapy. The coordination of radiation therapy and chemotherapy administered post-operatively now is much more sophisticated.

IMPROVEMENTS IN TREATMENT OF CHILDREN WITH ACUTE LYMPHOCYTIC LEUKEMIA (ALL)

Figure 1.2 illustrates the progressive improvement in survival achieved by several studies of leukemia done by the three national cooperative groups in the USA that were studying children with leukemia between 1956 and 1976. The median survival increased from approximately six months in 1956 to longer than six years for trials begun in 1972. Patients entered on studies since 1972 have not yet reached the median survival. This illustrates the continuous progress made in the development of more effective treatment.

While the effectiveness of treatment for ALL in children has improved remarkably during the past two decades, the heterogeneity among patients with this diagnosis has become increasingly apparent. Subgroups of patients can be identified at the time of diagnosis that have excellent prognosis for survival and cure with standard therapies, while other subgroups have extremely poor outcome[5,6]. The accurate identification of multiple prognostic variables has become important in order to advance our understanding of the clinical biology of leukemia, to enable

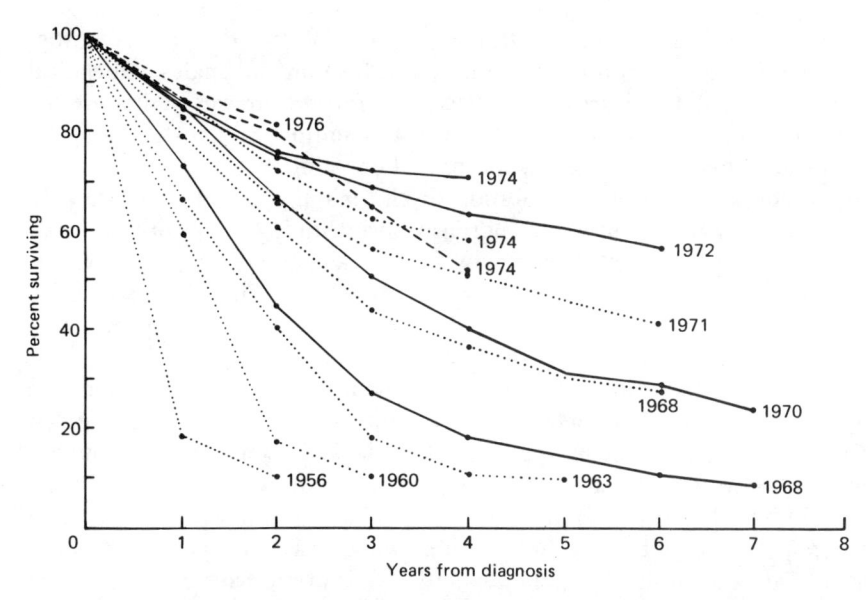

Figure 1.2 Improvement in survival of children with acute lymphocytic leukemia diagnosed between 1956 and 1976. Data from multiple studies of the Cancer and Acute Leukemia Group B, the Childrens Cancer Study Group and the Southwest Oncology Group. (From Hammond et al.[3], courtesy of the Publishers, *Cancer Research: Impact of the Cooperative Groups*)

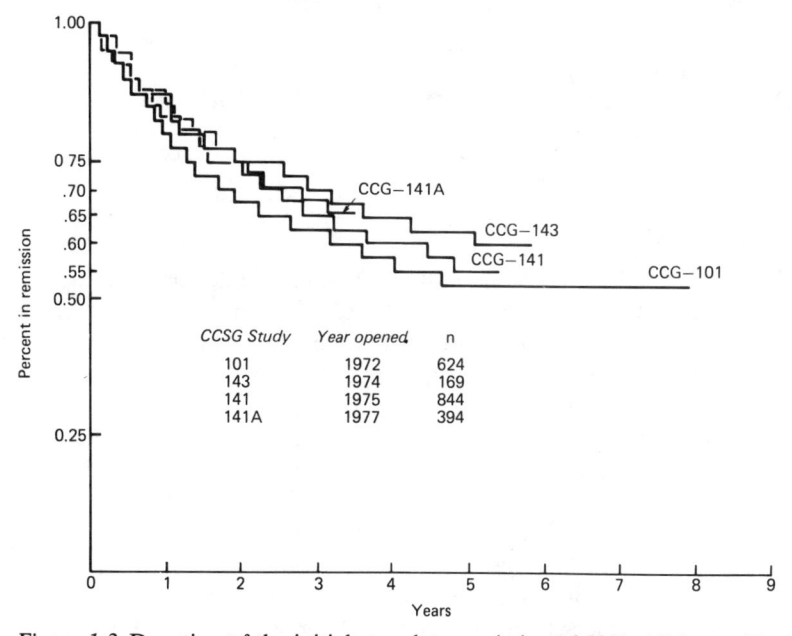

Figure 1.3 Duration of the initial complete remission of 2031 children with acute lymphocytic leukemia treated according to recent studies of the Childrens Cancer Study Group. All patients achieving complete remission were included in the analysis. (From Hammond[2], courtesy of the Publishers, *Cancer: Achievements, Challenges and Prospects for the 1980s*)

development of improved treatment strategies appropiate for the patient's prognosis and essential for the appropriate design, stratification and analysis of clinical studies. Patient populations providing specimens for preclinical studies of the biology of leukemia also must be characterized by multiple prognostic variables, lest the results of biologic tests be misinterpreted or uninterpretable.

Figure 1.3 shows curves of the duration of the initial complete remission of children with ALL managed by the Childrens Cancer Study Group on a series of four successive therapeutic trials begun between 1972 and 1977[5, 6, 8]. The therapies given and the overall study outcomes were reasonably similar. This provided a large patient population which was analyzed by stratifying patients according to a large number of clinical and laboratory variables, to determine their effect on, or their association with, outcomes such as achievement of complete remission, the duration of the initial complete remission and duration of survival. It is notable that study CCG-101, which included 624 patients who achieved complete remission, has a median duration of continuous remission of approximately eight years[8]. In the historical context, this result is the most favorable yet reported for a large unselected population of infants and children with ALL, and yet, there were subgroups of patients within the study population that would have been predicted by evaluation of specific variables to have very favorable or very poor outcomes. In study CCG-141[5] and subsequent studies, patients have been stratified prospectively to different treatment regimens on the basis of their age, initial WBC and other prognostic factors. This provided relatively homogeneous groups for study so the importance of other prognostic factors and effectiveness of treatment regimens could be detected.

PROGNOSTIC VARIABLES IN ACUTE LYMPHOCYTIC LEUKEMIA

Figure 1.4 shows the complete remission duration of a population of infants and children with ALL that are stratified according to their age at the time of diagnosis. Fewer than 20 percent of those less than one year of age at diagnosis were still in remission six years after diagnosis while 60 percent of those between one and ten years remained in continuous complete remission. Obviously, one cannot design a balanced clinical trial without taking the age of the patient into account. A small number of very poor prognosis patients entered in a comparative trial by chance can markedly influence the analysis of the trial and produce an apparent therapeutic result which is spurious.

Figure 1.5 shows the same patient population stratified according to the white blood cell count at the time of diagnosis. It has been known for years that leukemia patients with a very high WBC do not respond well to treatment. In these studies, of patients with initial WBC of 100 000 to 200 000/mm^3 at diagnosis, representing approximately 10 percent of this large group of patients, only 30 percent remained in continuous complete remission for seven years. The surprising observation is that the patients with WBC of less than 5000/mm^3 at diagnosis achieved 60 percent continuous complete remission for at least seven years. The curves show an orderly, stepwise progression in outcome simply by stratifying the population according to different levels of the white blood cell count at diagnosis.

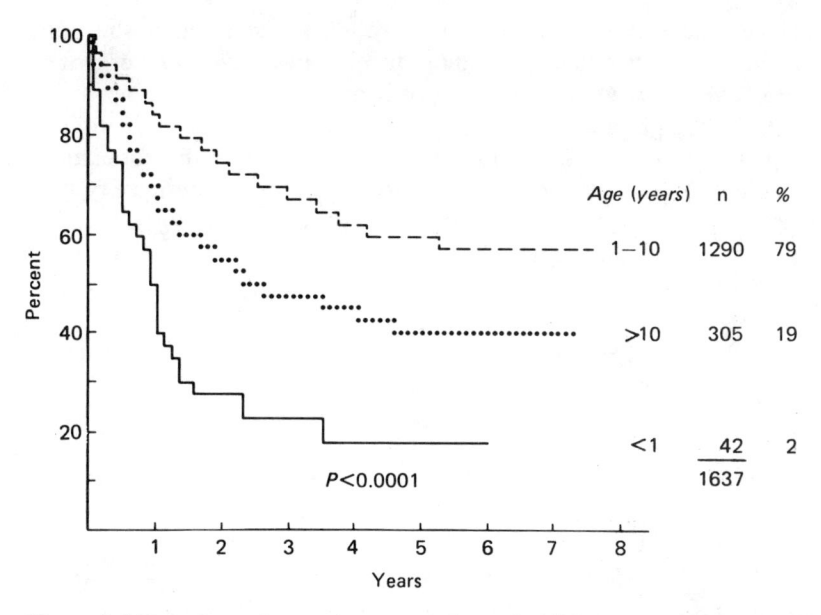

Figure 1.4 Duration of complete remission of children, stratified according to age at diagnosis of acute lymphocytic leukemia CCSG studies 101, 141, 143)

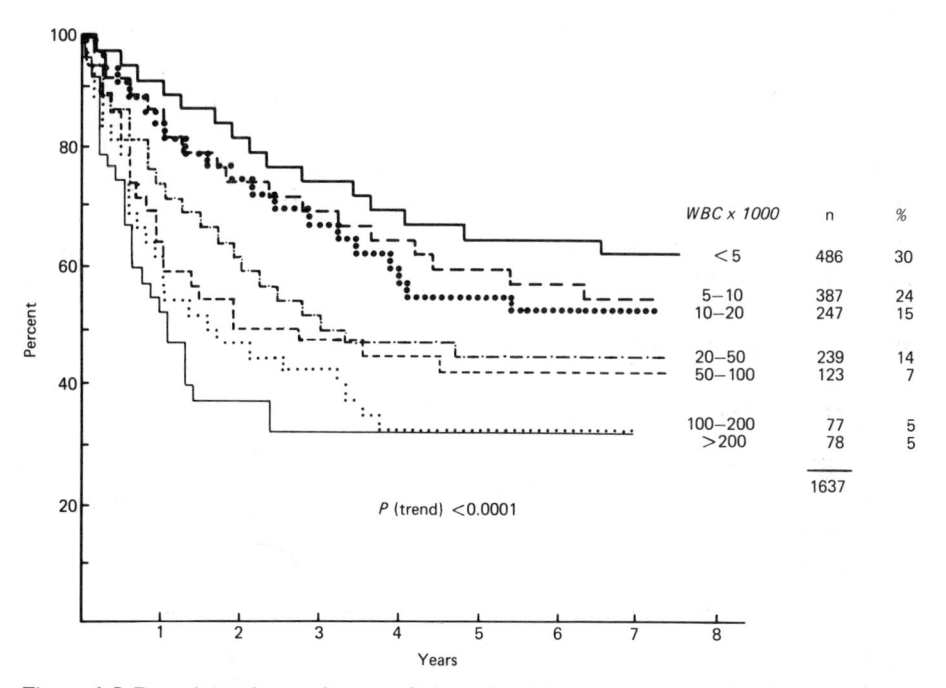

Figure 1.5 Duration of complete remission of children, stratified according to the white blood cell count at diagnosis of acute lymphocytic leukemia (CCSG studies 101, 141, 143)

Figure 1.6 shows the survival of a group of patients whose diagnostic bone marrow specimens were classified according to the French-American-British (FAB) morphologic classification of bone marrow lymphoblasts[7]. Eighty percent of patients had type L_1 lymphoblasts and this group had the best overall survival. Patients with type L_2 lymphoblasts constituted only two percent of the population, but obviously had a very poor outcome. Patients that had a preponderance of type L_1 or preponderance of type L_2 fell in between. This is another prognostic variable that must be considered in the experimental design of therapeutic trials and in selecting appropriate therapy.

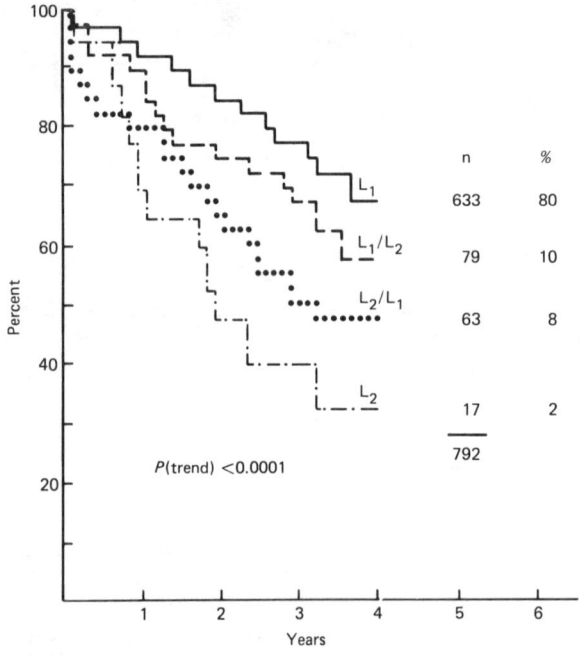

Figure 1.6 Survival duration of children with acute lymphocytic leukemia, stratified according to the morphology of lymphoblasts in the bone marrow at the time of diagnosis (*See* text for details)

From analyses to determine the strength of the association with outcome of clinical, biochemical and immunologic factors, numerous variables have been identified which show strong association with good or poor outcome when they are analyzed as independent variables (*Table 1.1*). By multivariate analysis it has been found that the initial WBC is the variable of greatest significance in predicting outcome, although many of the prognostic variables are interactive. One of the strong associations is with the initial white blood cell count. Variables which are strongly associated with the white blood cell count confer little or no additional prognostic information beyond that provided by the white blood cell count alone, while others are important predictors of outcome independent of the WBC. *Table 1.2* lists the relative prognostic contribution of several groups of variables for predicting the outcome to treatment of ALL.

Table 1.1 Clinical and laboratory variables associated with the outcome to current treatments of acute lymphocytic leukemia in children

Variable	Most favorable Value	Frequency (%)	Least favorable Value	Frequency (%)
WBC	< 5000	30	> 200 000	5
HB	< 7	44	> 10	20
Age	1–10 years	79	< 1 year	2
Blast morphology	Pure L_1	80	Pure $L_2(L_3)$	2
IgM	Normal to elevated	87	Decreased	13
Bone marrow (day 14)	Normal	68	Leukemia	9
Sex	Female	44	Male	56
Spleen size	Normal	43	Massive	15
IgG	Normal to elevated	84	Decreased	16
CNS leukemia	Absent	98	Present	2
IgA	Normal to elevated	86	Decreased	14
Cell markers	Non T, Non B	89	'T'	11
Liver size	Normal to moderately enlarged	84	Massive	16
Race	Non Black	94	Black	6
Lymph node size	Normal to moderately enlarged	93	Massive	7
Mediastinal mass	Absent	95	Present	5
Platelet count	> 150 000	18	< 150 000	82

All evaluations made at the time of diagnosis except evaluation of bone marrow after 14 days of treatment.

Table 1.2 Acute lymphocytic leukemia prognostic variables ranked according to relative importance in predicting outcome

Major	Minor
WBC at diagnosis	Node enlargement
Blast cell morphology	Cell surface antigens
Immunoglobulin levels	Race
Moderate	**Little or none**
Age	Platelet count
Sex	Mediastinal mass
Marrow response (Day 14)	Liver enlargement
CNS leukemia at diagnosis	
Hemoglobin	
Spleen enlargement	

Clinical trials must be designed to stratify patients into relatively homogeneous groups that may be necessary to obtain clear answers to the scientific questions posed by the trial. One may wish to design for a group with excellent prognosis a therapy that is less aggressive, less toxic and less likely to cause late adverse effects of treatment. New therapeutic strategies must be designed for those patients which can be identified at diagnosis as having a very unfavorable response to current therapies.

SUMMARY

During the past few decades, the results of treatment of the major cancers of children have improved dramatically. One of the principal impacts on clinical investigation of the discovery of successful chemotherapy was the impetus it provided to combine therapeutic modalities, and the subsequent development, at principal pediatric institutions, of teams of specialists that included all the relevant diagnostic and therapeutic disciplines. This model, which is now the standard mode of cancer management of children in many countries, should be applied to the management of many types of cancer of adults.

The increasing participation of surgeons, radiation therapists, pathologists and other specialties in combined therapy clinical trials for cancer has led to new approaches in the surgical and radiotherapeutic management of childhood cancers and to discoveries of previously unrecognized histological patterns of considerable prognostic importance.

Numerous clinical and laboratory evaluations of children with acute lymphocytic leukemia have been found to have strong association with outcome to current treatments and are thus important indicators of prognosis. Some of these have such a strong association with outcome that valid analyses of clinical trials cannot be done without stratifying the population under study according to important prognostic variables. Randomized, comparative clinical trials must be designed to stratify study populations according to significant predictors of outcome so relatively homogeneous populations may be compared. Some prognostic variables provide insights into the differences in biology of different types of leukemia. New therapeutic strategies must be designed which are appropriate for subgroups of patients with biological and prognostic differences.

Acknowledgements

Supported in part by grant CA-13539 to the Childrens Cancer Study Group from the Division of Cancer Treatment, National Cancer Institute, NIH, USPHS.

References

1 D'ANGIO, G. J., EVANS, A. E., BRESLOW, N. E., BECKWITH, B., BISHOP, H., FEIGL, P., GOODWIN, W., LEAPE, L. L., SINKS, L. F., SUTOW, W., TEFFT, M. and WOLFF, J. The treatment of Wilms' tumor: results of the National Wilms' Tumor Study. *Cancer*, **38**, 633–646 (1976)
2 HAMMOND, D. Progress in the study, treatment and cure of the cancers of children. In *Cancer: Achievements, Challenges and Prospects for the 1980s*, edited by Joseph H. Burchenal and Herbert F. Oettgen, 171–190. New York, Grune and Stratton, Inc. (1981)

3 HAMMOND, D., CHARD, R., D'ANGIO, G. J., VAN EYS, J., GILCHRIST, G., JONES, B., LEIKIN, S. and STARLING, K. In *Cancer Research: Impact of the Cooperative Groups*, edited by B. Hoogstraten, 1–23. New York, Masson Publishing USA, Inc. (1980)

4 MAURER, H. M., MOON, T., DONALDSON, M., FERNANDEZ, C., GEHAN, E. A., HAMMOND, D., HAYS, D. M., LAWRENCE, W., NEWTON, W., RAGAB, A., RANEY, B., SOULE, E. H., SUTOW, W. W. and TEFFT, M. The Intergroup Rhabdomyosarcoma Study – a preliminary report. *Cancer*, **40,** 2015–2026 (1977)

5 MILLER, D., LEIKIN, S., ALBO, V., VITALE, L., COCCIA, P., SATHER, H., KARON, M. and HAMMOND, D. The use of prognostic factors in improving the design and efficiency of clinical trials in childhood cancer. *Cancer Chemotherapy Reports*, **64,** 381–392 (1980)

6 MILLER, D., LEIKIN, S., ALBO, V., SATHER, H., KARON, M. and HAMMOND, D. Intensive therapy and prognostic factors in acute lymphoblastic leukemia of childhood: CCG-141. In *Hematology and Blood Transfusion*, **26,** *Modern Trends in Human Leukemia* **IV,** edited by Nath, Gallo, Graf, Mannweiler, and Winkler, 77–86. Berlin, Springer Verlag (1981)

7 MILLER, D. R., LEIKIN, S., ALBO, V., SATHER, H. and HAMMOND, D. Prognostic importance of morphology (FAB classification) in childhood acute lymphoblastic leukemia. *British Journal of Hematology*, **48,** 199–206 (1981)

8 NESBIT, M., SATHER, H., ROBISON, L., DONALDSON, M., LITTMAN, P., ORTEGA, J. and HAMMOND, D. Sanctuary therapy: a randomized trial of 724 children with previously untreated acute lymphoblastic leukemia. *Cancer Research* (in press)

2
Psychosocial aspects of pediatric hematology-oncology

Jonathan Kellerman and James W. Varni

A perusal of the early literature on psychosocial aspects of hematology-oncology reveals a substantial proportion of articles devoted to emotional aspects of death, dying and terminal care, as well as a number of anecdotal reports of psychopathology resulting from diagnosis of hematological and oncological disorders. The former studies reflect the rapidly fatal status of most forms of childhood cancer as recently as three decades ago, and the latter the relatively primitive status of the behavioral sciences in addressing those emotional issues associated with serious and chronic disease.

The past decade, however, has witnessed a significant increase of interest in psychosocial aspects of hematology-oncology. This has been due to several factors.

First, advances in medical treatment have led to a marked improvement in the survival rate for many forms of cancer and hematological disorders. Extended life expectancy has brought with it an increase in problems of adjustment encountered by surviving patients and their families[10, 12, 21, 34].

Secondly, the adoption of progressively more potent methods of treatment has led to a rise in iatrogenic problems – both organic disorders with psychological ramifications and functional reactions to treatment.

Lastly, the science known as behavioral medicine has grown rapidly. Its multidisciplinary approach, which draws from experimental and clinical psychology, medicine, biology and the social sciences, stresses observation and the experimental evaluation of outcome data and has led to the generation of clinical and research methods with clear applications in hematology-oncology.

CANCER: EXTENDED LIFE EXPECTANCY AND PROBLEMS OF ADJUSTMENT

Despite previous assertions to the contrary, the empirical data available indicate that children with cancer and their families do not develop serious psychopathological reactions to diagnosis and treatment[2, 14, 15, 19, 42, 54]. This finding is similar to those obtained with other groups of seriously ill children as well as with adults with cancer[35]. This does not imply that the diagnosis of cancer is not psychologically traumatic, but rather that the child with cancer should not be considered a psychiatric patient. He is best described as a normal child under stress for whom long-term or intensive psychiatric treatment is usually not indicated. Exceptions to this are children and families who present with a history of psychiatric or psychological disturbance that predates the diagnosis of cancer. Effective psychosocial treatment is usually short-term and aimed at helping the child and family to return to premorbid levels of functioning[12]. Owing to interactions between medical, social and psychological factors, treatment should be multidisciplinary and should stress education and preparation of patients and families. The following areas deserve special attention.

Disease-related communication

Contrary to earlier suggestions that patients and families should be shielded from knowledge of disease and treatment, a wealth of empirical findings points to the benefits of helping the child with cancer and his family understand the illness[16, 37-41]. This includes open use of the term 'cancer' as well as of specific diagnoses. Such open discussion may be avoided due to anxiety of the health professional about illness, treatment and death[51]; however a well informed patient is more likely to comply with medical regimens and to make a more positive psychological adjustment. This may be due, in part, to the fact that for children, as for most adults, there is no greater fear than fear of the unknown. The absence of accurate information is likely to bring about fantasies that provoke more anxiety than the truth. Understanding the disease and its treatment allows child and family to adjust emotionally and increases the likelihood of the child receiving emotional support from family and staff. Discussion of the disease needs to be tailored to the child's developmental level as well as to the family's belief system. Specific approaches to this have been addressed by Spinetta[41]. It should be noted that extreme care must be taken in offering prognostic information to children and families. Because of the high individual variability of response to cancer treatment, a precise prognosis is generally inappropriate and can create inaccurate, magical expectations in children and adults. What is beneficial is an open approach that encourages questions from child and family from the outset of treatment, soon after diagnosis, and provides accurate medical information when needed. The high level of stress immediately following diagnosis establishes a close rapport between the patient and the physician – who is seen as possessing the authority to alleviate discomfort – and such rapport is a good basis for the trust that is necessary to clinical effectiveness throughout the course of the illness.

School re-integration

It has been noted[10] that school for children is analogous to work for adults and that children who remain out of school for a time run the risk of developing adverse psychological reactions similar to those observed in unemployed adults. Cancer and its treatment pose a threat to regular school attendance for several reasons. Prolonged or frequent hospitalizations will interrupt schooling and cause the child to fall behind academically and to experience increased anxiety about returning to the classroom. Treatment-induced changes in appearance, such as alopecia, weight gain or loss, and alterations in skin pigmentation may further stigmatize the child, subject him to peer ridicule and reduce self-esteem. Furthermore, the fear of cancer may lead school personnel to discourage the child's return to school, or to overprotect or, less commonly, ridicule him. Finally, parental anxiety may lead to ambivalence regarding school attendance with subsequent lack of support for the child. Katz[10] has outlined specific measures to increase the probability of the child with cancer returning to school. These include education of parents and teacher, short-term crisis counseling, school visits by psychosocial health professionals, and provision of teaching in hospital to allow continuity of education. The author's (JK) experience has been that the vast majority of children with cancer are able to return to a regular schooling and derive positive psychological benefits as a result of this. Exceptions to this are some children with brain tumours directly affecting cognitive functioning to a degree that special schooling is appropriate. In such case, neuropsychological evaluation can be of help in specifying areas of decrement and suggesting suitable remedies.

Sibling's reactions

Because of the special attention paid to the child with cancer, brothers and sisters run the risk of being ignored or feeling otherwise neglected. Few studies have been conducted in this area, but the limited information that does exist indicates a substantial risk of psychological distress to siblings. This includes feeling of guilt, anger, fear of contagion, and jealousy and resentment over increased chores and responsibilities at home. One recent study (Koch and Kellerman unpublished observation), in which siblings of children diagnosed at least 6 months were interviewed, indicated that while major areas of family functioning had returned to normal, significant affective problems – anger, guilt, fear and sadness – persisted. These may be prevented, or at least alleviated, by encouragement of frequent visits and participation of siblings, by early counseling for parents outlining the importance of paying attention to siblings, short-term group counseling for siblings that offers them the opportunity to receive peer support, and by short-term individual sibling counseling.

Sexual functioning

One area that has not been extensively researched, but whose importance is likely to increase as more patients survive into adolescence and adulthood, is that of sexual functioning, including sexual activity and reproduction. For example, an adolescent male about to receive testicular radiation for a sarcoma may want to discuss the arguments for and against depositing sperm in a sperm bank for future use. Clearly, more research is needed into the biological and psychological aspects of sexual reproduction in patients who have received treatment for pediatric cancer.

CANCER: IATROGENIC PROBLEMS

Hospitalization and isolation

The growing trend to use chemotherapeutic agents that require careful inpatient monitoring of physiological processes will undoubtedly lead to more frequent and prolonged periods of hospitalization for children with cancer. The adverse psychological effects of placing children in hospitals are well documented in the literature.

With regard to cancer, the empirical findings concerning the psychological effects of long-term hospitalization and treatment in protective isolation[14-19] indicate that with provision of adequate psychosocial care, children can be expected to tolerate such treatment without developing serious or prolonged psychological disturbance. Specific recommendations include careful and adequate preparation of patient and family for entry and exit, psychosocial training and screening of nursing staff, freely available play therapy services for the patient, continuing counseling of parents of parents and siblings, physical construction of the unit to ensure visual access to clocks and windows (and thus minimize temporal and spatial disorientation) and implementation of a daily, structured routine for waking, eating, engaging in activities, and sleeping.

In general, the most effective means of reducing psychological distress due to hospitalization is adjustment of the hospital environment, taking into account the empirical findings of the science of child development. These extend beyond the area of pediatric hematology-oncology.

Central nervous system prophylaxis

One major approach that has resulted in increased survival of children with acute leukemia has been the prophylactic treatment of the central nervous system to destroy leukemic cells which have escaped the blood–brain barrier. Recently, concern has been expressed about the possible deleterious effects of the two main modes of CNS prophylaxis – CNS irradiation and intrathecal methotrexate – on intellectual and personality functioning. Moss and Nannis[25] have reviewed the relevant literature which was divided into three general areas of research: (1) studies of structural change in the brain using histological or photographic techniques; (2) psychological studies of personality change; (3) psychometric studies of changes in the level of cognitive, intellectual and perceptual functioning. These authors note that while the literature is suggestive of iatrogenic deterioration, results are generally confounded by small sample size, lack of adequate control and inappropriate research design. Most studies are retrospective, allowing no assessment of pretreatment status. Nevertheless, these preliminary studies indicate the importance of assessing the effects of CNS prophylaxis for several reasons other than the obvious right of patients and families to understand the effects of treatment.

Firstly, careful research may discover no stable pattern of deterioration, and while acceptance of the null hypothesis does not conclusively prove absence of detriment it may reduce anxiety in nursing staff and parents. Secondly, there may be a significant variation in the degree of iatrogenic damage depending on the particular mode of prophylaxis. If these prophylactic techniques are medically equivalent, adoption of the method that produced least iatrogenic deterioration would be justified. Thirdly, specific patterns of damage, such as decrement of certain areas of perceptual functioning, may be found, and clarify specific avenues of remediation. Patterns of decrement may be related to age, sex or other factors and thus identify children who are differentially at risk for iatrogenic CNS problems. Finally, longitudinal evaluation may reveal patterns of decrement that are followed by upswings in functioning due to CNS compensation, elucidating normative responses and providing for optimal family preparation and education.

The most effective method of evaluating the effects of CNS prophylaxis is multidisciplinary in approach including radiographic techniques such as computerized axial tomography as well as neuropsychological testing of specific mental functions. Such evaluation needs to be prospective and must include baseline data obtained prior to CNS prophylaxis. Furthermore, repeated longitudinal studies are clearly indicated.

Pain and discomfort

In contrast to adult cancer, chronic debilitating pain is comparatively uncommon in children with cancer. This is due to the different malignancies seen in children. Whereas adults tend to develop carcinomas that are associated with chronic pain, the most common malignancies of childhood, the leukemias and lymphomas, are generally not accompanied by debilitating pain. Obvious exceptions are children with terminal disease or infectious states related to disease and treatment, and children with certain solid tumours.

Despite the comparative lack of debilitating chronic pain in children with cancer, their well-being and adjustment to cancer are threatened by *acute* distress due to treatment. This is generally caused by two factors: (1) anxiety and pain associated with treatment procedures such as bone marrow aspirations, lumbar punctures, venepunctures and injections of chemotherapeutic agents, and (2) nausea and emesis resulting both from chemotherapy and from anticipatory anxiety associated with treatment. While iatrogenic distress is often overlooked by health professionals as a problem of cancer its importance to patients has been shown by several studies. For example, adolescents with cancer were found to differ psycholgically from their healthy peers and from cohorts with other serious diseases primarily in terms of high levels of iatrogenic distress[54]. Similar findings have been obtained in adults[33]. A behavioural observation study of 115 children with acute leukemia revealed virtually ubiquitous distress due to bone marrow aspirations[11]. In addition to the significant suffering they inflict on the child, such iatrogenic problems are of concern to the clinician in that they increase the risk of non-compliance with medical regimens. Zeltzer[53] has presented illustrative case material in this regard.

Unfortunately, more than limited local chemical anesthesia for acute procedural distress is often not feasible because of medical risk. Nausea and emesis are commonly treated with phenothiazines. Their anti-emetic effect, however, varies widely in different patients, and they produce undesirable side-effects such as drowsiness and lethargy. While recent findings concerning the efficacy of tetrahydrocannabinol (THC) in reducing nausea and emesis in adult cancer patients[30] have been encouraging, similar patterns of individual variability of response were found. In addition, methodological limitations reduce the impact of these data[55].

Behavioural approaches appear to offer additional promise in the amelioration of several types of iatrogenic distress in children with cancer. These have the advantage of being non-intrusive as well as rapidly learned. The psychological and medical literature contains numerous references regarding the efficacy of conditioning approaches to anticipatory anxiety, including some that consider this approach the treatment of choice in many anxiety-related disorders. Such conditioning therapies typically use Pavlovian deconditioning of a learned, aversive association by replacing it with an incompatible, positive association. For example, the child who has learned to associate entering the hospital with receiving an unpleasant procedure, and who subsequently experiences psychophysiological changes (palpatation, coldness in the extremities, tachycardia, pallor, nausea, emesis, etc.) consistent with anxiety may benefit from relaxation training that teaches him to experience a sense of well-being in the presence of previously noxious stimuli. A variety of methods have been used successfully in this regard – systematic desensitization, hypnosis, biofeedback, meditation, guided imagery – and despite their apparent differences, in the authors' opinion they share several important similarities. Specifically, they all emphasize classically conditioned counter-anxious response, learning of enhanced self-control and some sort of reward for successful control. (In the case of biofeedback, reward is explicitly acknowledged and provided via mechanically obtained information about psychophysiological processes. In hypnosis and desensitization, approval is offered by the therapist contingent upon success.) These methods are also called *autogenic* (self-generated) treatments.

There is evidence that autogenic techniques have other uses besides the elimination of anticipatory anxiety. The clinical efficacy of hypnosis as an anesthetic and analgesic, for example, has been documented over several centuries[5], yet little is known about the specific psychophysiological mechanisms responsible. Because of recent advances in research strategies relevant to medicopsychological processes it has become possible to subject hypnotic and related autogenic phenomena to strict experimental testing and to translate results into the lexicon of science.

Behavioural approaches have been reported as successful in the following oncology-related areas of iatrogenic distress: relaxation training for extreme anxiety, nausea and emesis in an adult patient with lymphoma[3]; parental relaxation training and operant reinforcement for night terrors in a child of 3 years with acute lymphoblastic leukemia (ALL), with symptoms apparently secondary to anxiety related to bone marrow aspirations[13]; hypnosis for multiple problems including chronic and acute pain, nausea, emesis and insomnia in a adolescent girl with chronic myeloid leukemia (CML)[8]; hypnosis for a sample of nine adolescents with various cancers with iatrogenic nausea and for 18 adolescents with procedural distress related to bone marrow aspirations, lumbar punctures and chemotherapeutic injections[56]; operant reinforcement to institute weight gain in a girl of 6 years with post-treatment anorexia[4]; systematic desensitization to eliminate gagging and increase food intake in a woman aged 53 with conditioned food aversion following successful surgery for gastrointestinal cancer[26]; reinforcement and extinction to eliminate psychosomatic coughing and retching in two adult patients treated in protective isolation[27].

With the exception of one study[56], all of the above included one or two patients only. Thus, conclusions are limited. However, the high rate of success, combined with an already established success rate of autogenic techniques in anxiety-related disorders and pain, emphasizes the need for further investigations along these lines. Findings are encouraging with regard to anticipatory anxiety and in instances where symptoms can be directly attributed to physiological effects of disease and treatment. In addition, several of these studies indicate that autogenic treatment may be useful in establishing weight gain in children with cancer. Further controlled studies are needed to specify with components of intervention bring about symptomatic amelioration.

HEMOPHILIA

The integration of biobehavioral science and medicine, or behavioral medicine, represents a relatively recent development in the comprehensive care of hemophilia[45]. In a series of investigations at the Hemophilia Comprehensive Care Centers at the Orthopaedic Hospital, Los Angeles, Varni and associates have studied a number of behavioral-medical and psychosocial problems in hemophilia. The initial findings of this research are described below.

Pain management in hemophilia

Pain has been shown to consist of both physical and psychological components which contribute in varying degrees to perceived pain in different individuals. The perception of pain involves not only sensing painful stimuli but also behavioral and cognitive components which may intensify or lessen the pain experience[50]. Whereas acute pain in hemophilia is associated with a specific bleeding episode, chronic arthritic pain secondary to hemophilic arthropathy continues for an extended period of time[6]. Pain perception – a complex psychophysiological event – is further complicated in the hemophiliac by the existence of two forms of pain requiring different treatments[48]. More specifically, the acute pain of hemorrhage is a functional signal indicating the necessity of factor replacement therapy whereas chronic arthritic pain indicates a potentially debilitating condition which may result in impaired functioning and analgesic dependence.

Chronic arthritic pain

Varni[48, 49] reported on the self-regulation of arthritic pain perception by hemophiliacs which involved progressive muscle relaxation exercises, meditative breathing and guided imagery. The patient was instructed to imagine himself in a scene previously identified or associated with experience of warmth and arthritic pain relief. The scene was initially evoked by a detailed multisensory description by the therapist; further details of the scene were then added by the patient. Once the scene was clearly visualized by the patient, the therapist made further suggestions indicating reduction of arthritic pain and increased comfort.

In the initial investigation, preliminary findings with two hemophiliacs suggested that these self-regulation techniques may be useful in the reduction of arthritic pain[48]. The next investigation systematically extended these earlier findings to three additional hemophiliacs under improved methodological conditions, including longer baseline and follow-up assessments, and measurements of multiple subjective and medical parameters in relationship to arthritic pain[49]. Each patient was instructed in the daily use of a multidimensional pain assessment instrument. In addition, each patient's subjective evaluation of the overall impact of the intervention was determined by a comparative assessment inventory at the final follow-up session. Medical charts and pharmacy records provided data on the number of analgesics ordered, the number of hemorrhages, and the units of factor replacement needed for bleeding episodes. These records were analyzed at the completion of the investigation to determine the patient's status 6 months before self-regulation intervention and during the follow-up period (on average monthly for both pre- and post-assessments).

Analysis of the data demonstrated that self-regulation significantly reduced the number of days of perceived arthritic pain per week in all three patients, maintained over an extended follow-up assessment. Further analysis of the daily pain assessment showed that on a scale from 1(mild) to 10 (most severe pain) arthritic pain perception decreased from an average of 5.1 during baseline to 2.2 on follow-up days when arthritic pain occurred. Average bleeding pain did not change markedly from baseline to follow-up conditions (6.9 to 6.8). The patient's own evaluation of the comparative assessment inventory indicated substantial improvement in arthritic pain, mobility, sleep and general overall functioning, with no reported changes in the perception of bleeding pain. The units of factor replacement prescribed varied with number of bleeding episodes for all three patients and remained essentially unchanged during pre- and postassessment periods. Prescription of analgesic tablets decreased consistently in all patients.

The above findings suggest that these self-regulation techniques did not affect the perception of bleeding pain. Substantial decreases in reported bleeding frequency and factor replacement units would have been expected had bleeding pain perception been affected. It is essential to emphasize that these techniques are not meant to replace proper and correct medical care. Nevertheless, in the case of chronic degenerative arthropathy, where the arthritic pain, in contrast to the acute bleeding pain, exceeds its functional intent, potentially limiting normal activities and leading to analgesic dependence, these techniques represent a non-invasive and supportive component in the comprehensive management of hemophilia.

Pain and analgesia management complicated by factor VIII inhibitor

The acute pain of hemorrhage is a functional signal indicating the need for factor replacement therapy. In the hemophilic child with factor VIII inhibitor, however, the intensity of the pain exceeds its functional intent, with analgesic dependence of constant concern. Varni et al.[47] recently described a hemophiliac aged nine years with factor VIII inhibitor who at the age of 4 years, when the inhibitor developed and subsequent factor VIII replacement therapy became impossible, began to require narcotics in order to tolerate the pain of each hemorrhage. The need for analgesics increased progressively for both bleeding pain and arthritic pain in his left knee secondary to degenerative arthropathy. Since the arthritic pain eventually occurred almost daily, the requests for analgesics further increased so that the acute pain of hemorrhage required even larger doses for pain relief in spite of continued home prothrombin-complex concentrate (PCC) therapy and joint immobilization for the management of bleeding episodes. As a consequence of bleeding and arthritic pain in the lower extremities, the patient was confined to his wheelchair nearly 50 percent of the time. The inhibitor had developed 4½ years prior to the study, and during that time he had been hospitalized 16 times, for a total of 80 days. Analgesic medication for pain control had been continued at his school. His condition steadily worsened, and after a particularly severe and painful left knee hemorrhage which had not responded to home PCC therapy he was given an adult dose of meperidine and intravenous diazepam from which he obtained no pain relief.

Training in the self-regulation of pain perception consisted of techniques developed earlier[48, 49], with modifications in the guided imagery techniques to reduce the intensity of bleeding pain. The patient recorded the severity of his pain on the 10-point scale for a 2½ week baseline prior to self-regulation training. The average score for both arthritic and bleeding pain during this period was 7, indicating rather intense pain. At follow-up 1 year after the self-regulation training, the patient reported that both arthritic and bleeding pain were reduced to 2 on the scale during self-regulation. In addition to this reduced perception of pain, the patient's evaluation of the comparative assessment inventory indicated substantial improvement in arthritic and bleeding pain, mobility, sleep and general overall functioning.

During the first year of self-regulating treatment of pain, the patient required no further meperidine and substantially decreased amounts of acetaminophen (paracetamol) and codeine elixir. Significant functional improvements included improved mobility as a result of physical therapy which had increased range of motion in his arthritic left knee and quadriceps strength in comparison with his normal right knee and leg. Psychosocial activities improved, suggested by increased school attendence and fewer hospitalizations. The parents noted a distinct elevation of the child's mood, stating that he was considerably less depressed during pain episodes now that he had the skills to actively reduce his pain perception without having to depend on narcotic analgesics.

The analysis of the various parameters assessed in this study suggests a significant improvement in a number of areas. Prior to the intervention, a deteriorating cycle was evident which can schematically be represented as hemorrhage → pain → analgesics/joint immobilization → atrophy of muscles adjacent to the joints/joint deterioration → hemorrhage. Thus, as has been previously suggested, pain-induced immobilization results in muscle weakness around the joints, increasing the risk of future hemorrhaging. By interrupting this deteriorating cycle at the point of pain severity, the patient was offered the opportunity to decrease immobilization and increase therapeutic activities such as swimming, which improved the strength and range of motion in the left knee. This improved mobility in turn increased school attendance and his general level of activity. The possibility that this early intervention may have prevented or reduced the likelihood of later narcotic analgesic addiction must also be considered.

Psychosocial dysfunction in hemophilia

Although psychosocial dysfunction has been suggested, few controlled treatment studies exist. Problems in self-concept, familial relationships and perceived relationship to others outside the family, as well as maladaptive response to stress have been suggested[1]. Epidemiological research has suggested that children with chronic illness and disabilities are at risk for developing behavioral disorders as a result of their illness[28], and Yule[52] has pointed out the potential of behavioral techniques in preventing further and more severe behavioral/emotional dysfunction. From this perspective, a secondary prevention strategy would be directed toward the early identification of risk factors in the hemophilic child and his family[45]. This early identification of a behavioral disorder and subsequent behavioral treatment may reasonably be expected to contribute to the child's later adjustment.

Behavioral disorders

The behavioral approach in the modification of behavioral disorders consists of training the child's parents, and teachers when indicated, in behavioral management techniques, and teaching the older child self-control skills. Recently, Varni[43] reported a case investigation designed to assess the effectiveness of behavioral techniques in reducing persistent behavior problems and encouraging age-appropriate behavior both at home and in school of a child aged 4½ years with severe classical hemophilia. At the time of referral, the child was living in a foster home because of chronic parental neglect in his hemophilia care. His hemophilia status was further complicated by a high titer factor VIII antibody, resulting in numerous hospitalizations and intensive outpatient medical care. Inappropriate behavior in the home consisted of non-compliance, temper tantrums, threatening language, answering back and aggression toward his peers. Problems at school were identified as not following directions, physically disturbing others, not staying in his seat, talking inappropriately, not paying attention, and others which interfered with successful participation in the classroom. The home intervention consisted of a point system for the daily contingency management of behavior, with appropriate behavior meriting plus points which could be exchanged for previously agreed preferred activities from a reinforcement list. Inappropriate behavior resulted in a loss of points and privileges. A home-based contingency system was developed for the school intervention whereby the teacher completed a daily checklist of classroom behaviors which were treated by the foster parents in the same manner as the home behaviors. The behavioral program resulted in clinically significant improvement in both the home and school, which was still evident at follow-up after 12 months in the home and 7 months in the school.

Disease-related chronic insomnia

Whereas in hemophilic children the stress and anxiety which may be associated with their illness may be observed as a behavioral disorder, adolescent and young adult hemophiliacs exhibit qualitatively different responses to their potentially life-threatening condition. Chronic insomnia is such a stress reaction. A recent report by Solomon et al.[36] delineated the many contraindications of sleep-inducing medications for chronic insomnia, while emphasizing the therapeutic potential of psychosocial and behavioral interventions. Varni[44] reported a patient with chronic insomnia as a secondary emotional reaction to hemophilia-related anxiety. Because of the development of an inhibitor, treatment of this patient's bleeding episodes with factor VIII replacement was not possible, further complicating his medical care. Additional medical complications included severe hemophilic arthropathy, hypertension, obesity and borderline adult onset diabetes. The patient gave a history of chronic insomnia which had been aggravated 1 year previously when his older hemophilic brother died as a result of a severe internal hemorrhage. Also at that time, the patient's antibody titer was found to be higher than before, resulting in even greater feelings of his own vulnerability. At the time of referral, the patient reported that these factors resulted in his constant worrying at bedtime about the potential consequences of severe hemorrhage.

During the initial session, four areas were identified for assessment: (1) total number of hours of uninterrupted sleep per night averaged to the half hour; (2) daily tension rating on a scale from 1 (relaxed) to 10 (most stressed); (3) number of days per week in which bleeding was evident; (4) bleeding pain intensity on a scale from 1 (mild) to 10 (most severe). A checklist was developed for the daily monitoring of these parameters by the patient himself. After an analysis of the information provided by the initial evaluation and a 3-week self-monitoring baseline, three areas were selected for intervention: (1) pre-sleep and daily tension;

(2) pre-sleep intrusive cognitions, and (3) sleep incompatible activities while in bed. Training in the self-regulation of insomnia and chronic tension consisted of four parts: (1) a 25-step progressive muscle relaxation; (2) meditative breathing; (3) cognitive refocusing involving a detailed multisensory image of a previously experienced pleasant scene; (4) stimulus control techniques, i.e. delaying bedtime until very sleepy, using the bed only for sleeping (no television viewing or reading), getting out of bed within 15 minutes if unable to sleep (for an activity such as reading) and returning to bed only when very sleepy; no daytime naps. This self-regulatory treatment significantly increased the daily number of hours of uninterrupted sleep and decreased the daily tension ratings. This improvement in uninterrupted sleep was maintained over 27 weeks, even when the bleeding frequency and pain intensity were quite high. Daily tension ratings varied with the frequency of bleeding episodes but were substantially lower than during baseline. Chronic insomnia and tension alone can result in debilitation and impaired physical and psychological functioning. If combined with the patient's numerous physical problems in addition to hemophilia, including hypertension, obesity and borderline adult onset diabetes, they might well lead to further heart disease. While the patient's status remains precarious, the control of these two potent pathogenetic variables (chronic tension and severe insomnia) further suggests the potential effectiveness of behavioral techniques in the reduction of stress and anxiety reactions secondary to hemophilia.

Therapeutic adherence in hemophilia factor replacement therapy

Hemophilia treatment centers in the USA have increasingly included the home care program as an essential component of comprehensive care. The stimulus for the development of the home care program came with the recognition of the advantages of prompt factor replacement therapy for each bleeding episode in an attempt to minimize or prevent the crippling effects of internal hemorrhaging[6]. The home care program provides training in factor replacement techniques for hemophiliacs, their parents and family members[31]. Of significance, adherence to correct factor replacement techniques is an essential but previously uninvestigated component in the hemophilia home care program.

Review of the literature indicates that the teaching method used by the clinician may influence adherence by improving the patient's comprehension and memory of the regimen[6]. The information should be provided, in verbal and written form, in discrete quantities over time and organized into specific categories. Some initial encouraging results have been reported with patients on short-term therapeutic regimens for acute illness, but results with chronic disorders have not yet been systematically investigated.

Adherence to treatment regimens represents a continuous problem, with estimates of non-compliance ranging from 4 to 92 percent and averaging over 35 percent[23]. Greater non-compliance has been associated with long-term and complex regimens[7, 22]. Behavioral techniques have been proposed to facilitate therapeutic adherence to medical regimens[24]. Recently, Sergis-Deavenport and Varni[32] studied the potential of behavioral techniques in the teaching of, and the therapeutic adherence to, correct factor replacement procedure in the hemophilia home care program. The authors combined the teaching methods described above with the behavioral techniques of modeling, observational learning and behavioral rehearsal with positive and corrective feedback. Factor replacement techniques were divided into three categories: (1) reconstitution – double-ended needle technique (20 steps identified), and needle and syringe technique (31 steps identified); (2) syringe preparation – filtering technique (20 steps identified); (3) infusion – venepuncture and injection technique (36 steps indentified). These steps were incorporated into an assessment which provided a checklist for the correct steps for factor replacement therapy. Average interobserver agreement on the instrument was 93 percent, indicating that it was a reliable method for assessing the designated factor replacement techniques.

The treatment group consisted of the parents of five hemophilic children who had no previous experience in factor replacement therapy. The parents of seven hemophiliacs who had been on the home care program for an average of 5 years were also tested on the assessment instrument during their annual evaluation. The main percentage of correct performance of the treatment group increased from 15 percent prior to the intervention to 92 percent during training, with correct adherence maintained at 97 percent over long-term follow up. In contrast, the control group averaged only 65 percent adherence to correct replacement techniques. These findings indicate that adherence to correct factor replacement procedures should be assessed regularly and that behavioral techniques may be useful in enhancing therapeutic adherence to the hemophilia home care program.

References

1 AGEL, D. P. and MATTSSON, A. Psychological complications of hemophilia. In *Hemophilia in Children*, edited by M. W. Hilgartner. Littleton, Publishing Sciences Group (1976)

2 BEDELL, J. R., GIORDANI, B., ARMOUR, J. L., TAVORMINA, J. and BOLL, T. Life stress and the psychological and medical adjustment of chronically ill children. *Journal of Psychosomatic Research*, **21**, 237 (1977)

3 BURISH, T. G. and LYLES, J. N. Effectiveness of relaxation training in reducing the aversiveness of chemotherapy in the treatment of cancer. *Journal of Behavior Therapy and Experimental Psychiatry*, **19**, 357–361 (1979)

4 CAIRNS, G. F. and ALTMAN, K. Behavioral treatment of cancer-related anorexia. *Journal of Behavior Therapy and Experimental Psychiatry*, **10**, 353–356 (1979)

5 DASH, J. Hypnosis for symptom amelioration. In *Psychological Aspects of Childhood Cancer*, edited by J. Kellerman. Springfield, Illinois, Charles C. Thomas (1980)

6 DIETRICH, S. L. Medical management of hemophilia. In *Comprehensive Management of Hemophilia*, edited by D. Boone. Philadelphia, F. A. Davis (1976)

7 DUNBAR, J. M. and AGRAS, W. S. Compliance with medical instructions. In *Comprehensive Handbook of Behavioral Medicine*, edited by J. M. Ferguson and C. B. Taylor. New York, Spectrum Publications (1980)

8 ELLENBERG, L., KELLERMAN, J., DASH, J., HIGGINS, G. and ZELTZER, L. Use of hypnosis for multiple symptoms in an adolescent girl with leukemia. *Journal of Adolescent Health Care*, **1**, 132–136 (1980)

9 KAGEN-GOODHEART, L. Re-entry: living with childhood cancer. *American Journal of Orthopsychiatry*, **47**, 651–658 (1977)

10 KATZ, E. R. Illness impact and social reintegration. In *Psychological Aspects of Childhood Cancer*, edited by J. Kellerman. Springfield, Illinois, Charles C. Thomas (1980)

11 KATZ, E. R., KELLERMAN, J. and SIEGEL, S. E. Behavioral distress in children with leukemia undergoing bone marrow aspirations. *Journal of Consulting and Clinical Psychology*, **48**, 356–365 (1980)

12 KELLERMAN, J. Psychological intervention in pediatric cancer: a look toward the future. *International Conference of Psychology and Medicine*, University of Swansea, Wales (1979)

13 KELLERMAN, J. Behavioral treatment of pavor nocturnus in a child with acute leukemia. *Journal of Nervous and Mental Disease*, **167**, 182–185 (1979)

14 KELLERMAN, J., RIGLER, D., SIEGEL, S. E., McCUE, K., POSPISIL, J. and UNO, R. Psychological evaluation and management of pediatric oncology patients in protected environments. *Medical and Pediatric Oncology*, **2**, 353–360 (1976)

15 KELLERMAN, J., RIGLER, D., SIEGEL, S. E., McCUE, K., POSPISIL, J. and UNO, R. Pediatric cancer patients in reverse isolation utilizing protected environments. *Journal of Pediatric Psychology*, **1**, 21–25 (1976)

16 KELLERMAN, J., RIGLER, D., SIEGEL, S. E. and KATZ, E. Disease-related communication and depression in pediatric cancer patients. *Journal of Pediatric Psychology*, **2**, 52–53 (1977)

17 KELLERMAN, J., RIGLER, D. and SIEGEL, S. E. The psychological effects of isolating patients in protected environments. *American Journal of Psychiatry*, **134**, 563–565 (1977)

18 KELLERMAN, J., RIGLER, D. and SIEGEL, S. E. Psychological response of children to reverse isolation in a protected environment. *Journal of Behavioral Medicine*, **2**, 263–274 (1979)

19 KELLERMAN, J., ZELTZER, L., ELLENBERG, L., DASH, J. and RIGLER, D. Psychological effects of illness in adolescence: anxiety, self-esteem and the perception of control (1). *Journal of Pediatrics*, **97**, 126–131 (1980)

20 KELLERMAN, J., ZELTZER, L., ELLENBERG, L. and DASH, J. (unpublished observations)

21 LANSKY, S. B., LOWMAN, J. T., VATS, T. and GYULAY, J. School phobia in children with malignant neoplasms. *American Journal of Disease of Children*, **129**, 42–46 (1975)

22 LITT, I. F. and CUSKEY, W. R. Compliance with medical regimens during adolescence. *Pediatric Clinics of North America*, **27**, 3–15 (1980)

23 MARSTON, M. V. Compliance with medical regimens: a review of the literature. *Nursing Research*, **19**, 312–323 (1970)

24 MASEK, B. J. and JANKEL, W. R. Therapeutic adherence. In *Behavioral Pediatrics: Research and Practice*, edited by D. C. Russo and J. W. Varni. New York, Plenum Press (in press)

25 MOSS, H. A. and NANNIS, E. D. Psychological effects of central nervous system treatment on children with acute lymphocytic leukemia. In *Psychological Aspects*

of Childhood Cancer, edited by J. Kellerman. Springfield, Illinois, Charles C. Thomas (1980)

26 REDD, W. H. *In vivo* desensitization in the treatment of chronic emesis following gastrointestinal surgery. *Behavior Therapy*, **11**, 421–427 (1980)

27 REDD, W. H. Stimulus control and extinction of psychosomatic symptoms in cancer patients in protective isolation. *Journal of Consulting and Clinical Psychology*, **48**, 448–455 (1980)

28 RUTTER, M., TIZARD, J. and WHITEMORE, K. (Editors) *Education, Health and Behavior*. London, Longsmens (1970)

29 RUTTER, M. and GRAHAM, P. Psychiatric aspects of intellectual and educational retardation. In *Education, Health and Behavior*, edited by M. Rutter, J. Tizard and K. Whitemore. London, Longsmens (1970)

30 SALLAN, S. E., CRONIN, C., ZELEN, M. and ZINBERG, N. E. Antiemetics in patients receiving chemotherapy for cancer. A randomized comparison of delta-9-tetrahydrocannabinol and prochlorderazine. *New England Journal of Medicine*, **302**, 135–138 (1980)

31 SERGIS, E. and HILGARTNER, M. W. Hemophilia. *American Journal of Nursing*, **72**, 2011–2017 (1972)

32 SERGIS-DEAVENPORT, E. and VARNI, J. W. (Unpublished observation)

33 SCHULTZ, L. S. Classical (pavlovian) conditioning of nausea and vomiting in cancer chemotherapy. *Abstracts of American Society of Clinical Oncology*, **21**, 381. Abstract no. C244 (1980)

34 SIEGEL, S. E. The current outlook of childhood cancer: the medical background. In *Psychological Aspects of Childhood Cancer*, edited by J. Kellerman. Springfield, Illinois, Charles C. Thomas (1980)

35 SILBERFARB, P. M., PHILIBERT, D. and LEVINE, P. M. Psychosocial aspects of neoplastic disease: affective and cognitive effects of chemotherapy in cancer patients II. *American Journal of Psychiatry*, **137**, 597–601 (1980)

36 SOLOMON, F., WHITE, C. C., PARRON, D. L. and MENDELSON, W. B. Sleeping pills, insomnia, and medical practice. *New England Journal of Medicine*, **300**, 803–808 (1979)

37 SPINETTA, J. J. The dying child's awareness of death: a review. *Psychological Bulletin*, **81**, 256–260 (1974)

38 SPINETTA, J. J., RIGLER, D. and KARON, M. Anxiety in the dying child. *Pediatrics*, **52**, 841–845 (1973)

39 SPINETTA, J. J. and MALONEY, J. L. Death anxiety in the outpatient leukemic child. *Pediatrics*, **56**, 1035–1037 (1975)

40 SPINETTA, J. J. and MALONEY J. L. The child with cancer: patterns of communication and denial. *Journal of Consulting and Clinical Psychology*, **46**, 1540–1541 (1978)

41 SPINETTA, J. J. Disease-related communication: how to tell. In *Psychological Aspects of Childhood Cancer*, edited by J. Kellerman. Springfield, Illinois Charles C. Thomas (1980)

42 TAVORMINA, J., KASTNER, L, S., SLATER, P. M. and WATT, S. L. Chronically ill children: a psychologically and emotionally deviant population? *Journal of Abnormal Child Psychology*, **4**, 99–110 (1976)

43 VARNI, J. W. Behavior therapy in the management of home and school behavior problems with a 4½-year-old hemophilic child. *Journal of Pediatric Psychology*, **5,** 17–23 (1980)

44 VARNI, J. W. Behavioral treatment of disease-related chronic insomnia in a hemophiliac. *Journal of Behavior Therapy and Experimental Psychiatry*, **11,** 143–145 (1980)

45 VARNI, J. W. and RUSSO, D. C. Behavioral medicine approach to health care: hemophilia as an exemplary model. In *Handbood of Psychological Factors in Health Care*, edited by M. Jospe, J. E. Nieberding and B. D. Cohen. Massachusetts, Lexington Books (1980)

46 VARNI, J. W., KATZ, E. R. and DASH, J. Behavioral and neurochemical aspects of pediatric pain management. In *Behavioral Pediatrics: Research and Practice*, edited by D. C. Russo and J. W. Varni. New York, Plenum Press (1982)

47 VARNI, J. W., GILBERT, A. and DIETRICH, S. L. Behavioral medicine in pain and analgesia management for the hemophilic child with Factor VIII inhibitor. *Pain*, **11,** 121–126 (1981)

48 VARNI, J. W. Behavioral medicine in hemophilia arthritic pain management. *Archives of Physical Medicine and Rehabilitation*, **62,** 183–187 (1981)

49 VARNI, J. W. Self-regulation techniques in the management of chronic arthritic pain in hemophilia. *Behavior Therapy*, **12,** 185–194 (1981)

50 VARNI, J. W., BESSMAN, C. A., RUSSO, D. C. and CATALDO, M. F. Behavioral management of chronic pain in children: case study. *Archives of Physical Medicine and Rehabilitation*, **61,** 375–379 (1980)

51 VERNICK, J. and KARON, M. Who's afraid of death on a leukemia ward? *American Journal of Diseases of Children*, **109,** 393–397 (1965)

52 YULE, W. The potential of behavioral treatment in preventing later childhood difficulties. *Behavioral Analysis and Modification*, **2,** 19–31 (1977)

53 ZELTZER, L. The adolescent with cancer. In *Psychological Aspects of Childhood Cancer*, edited by J. Kellerman. Springfield, Charles C. Thomas (1980)

54 ZELTZER, L., KELLERMAN, J., ELLENBERG, L., DASH, J. and RIGLER, D. Psychological effects of illness in adolescence: crucial issues and coping styles. *Journal of Pediatrics*, **97,** 132–138 (1980)

55 ZELTZER, L., BARBOUR, J., LeBARON, S. and KELLERMAN, J. Delta-9-tetrahydrocannabinol (THC) as an anti-emetic. *New England Journal of Medicine*, **302,** 1364 (1980)

56 ZELTZER, L., KELLERMAN, J., ELLENBERG, L. and DASH, J. (Unpublished observation)

3
Radiotherapy in paediatric oncology
Dorothy Pearson

Radiation therapy, in combination with surgery and chemotherapy, is the basis of the present management of children with malignant disease. Today it is important that radiation therapy should be carefully applied and that the radiation therapist should understand the considerable interaction which takes place between radiation and cytotoxic drugs. In this chapter the author discusses the problems that arise in giving radiotherapy to children, the complications that may arise and the factors which limit its use.

PROBLEMS

Radiotherapists usually gain most of their experience from treating adults, and whilst their expertise is perfected in the adult field, it is important that they recognise the differences which have to be taken into account when they come to treat children. These are discussed under three main headings.

Differences in tissue sensitivity

The basic action of radiation is to cause cellular damage and death, and the cells most likely to be adversely affected are those which are actively growing and dividing. In adults the great majority of normal tissues are only dividing at a slow rate for normal 'wear and tear' replacement, and are therefore usually less sensitive than the tumours being treated, so that the Therapeutic Ratio is in favour of successful therapy. However, even in adults there are certain tissues or organs which are more sensitive than others, such as the marrow and gonads in the reproductive years. In children, particularly in the very young, all normal tissue is growing more actively and is therefore more likely to sustain damage which may alter normal growth and development. The tissues most at risk are the brain and lens of the eye in very young children, particularly under the age of 2 years, and bone and cartilage throughout childhood until growth has ceased. It also seems likely that there is a greater risk of damage which will interfere with endocrine function when endocrine glands are irradiated, though the different glands have differing sensitivity. It is important to remember that the effects of this increased tissue sensitivity and subsequent damage may not be apparent in the immediate posttreatment period and will only become so as development in the broadest terms takes place. These complications are discussed later in the chapter. However, these differences in sensitivity must be taken into account when planning therapy so that they may be either avoided or minimized, but not to the extent that eradication of the tumour is compromised.

Practical problems of delivering radiation therapy to a child

Radiation therapy for the radical treatment of patients with cancer is usually given on a daily basis for 5 days a week over several weeks, although other fractionations are sometimes used. On each occasion the radiation fields must be accurately reproducible. This requires not only skill on the part of the technical staff involved, but also co-operation from the patient, the most important aspect of which is the ability to remain in one position for several minutes. This is particularly important when the radiation fields are small or when careful shielding of certain sensitive structures such as the eye is employed. Obviously these aspects of radiation therapy may be more difficult to achieve in children than in adults, particularly in the very young child. There are, however, several ways in which this can be achieved.

Handling of the children

Achieving accurate radiotherapy in children does not depend on the use of unnatural devices for keeping them in the correct position, but is the result of patient care and handling by all staff involved. In planning and prescribing radiotherapy, the radiotherapist and radiographers must be prepared to take longer than they would for an adult. It is always preferable to explain to any patient what is likely to happen, and whilst very young children may not fully understand, it is possible to explain enough for them to accept the procedures necessary for treatment preparation. If devices for beam direction or other special techniques have to be made, great patience is required of the mould room staff. It often helps to make the procedure something of a game; for instance it is not a waste of mould room time to produce a device for a toy as well as the child (*Figure 3.1*). When the child attends for actual exposure, success is again mostly achieved by patience and a gaining of the child's trust by the radiographer. When several children are being treated, it helps to have them all in the department at the same time so that they can see one another being treated; children feel safer with other children. The author believes that accurate radiotherapy is more easily achieved in departments treating several children at any one time than in those where a solitary child is

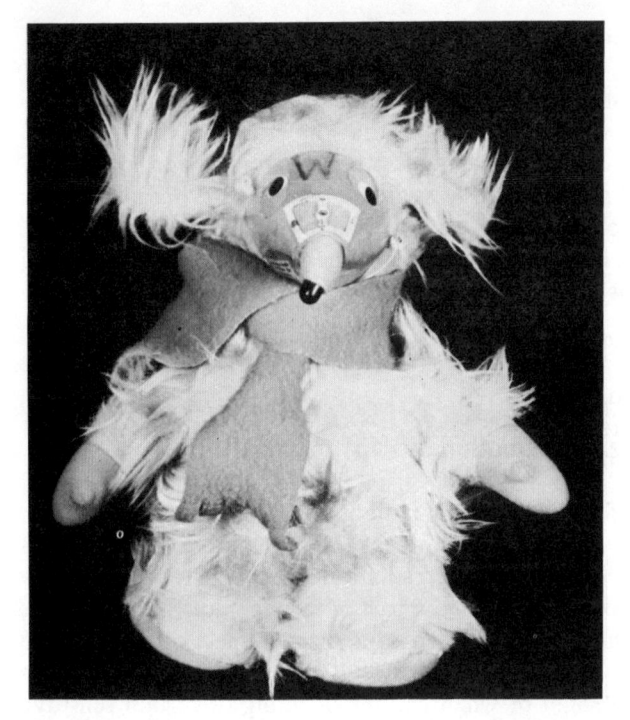

Figure 3.1 Beam direction shell made for a child's toy

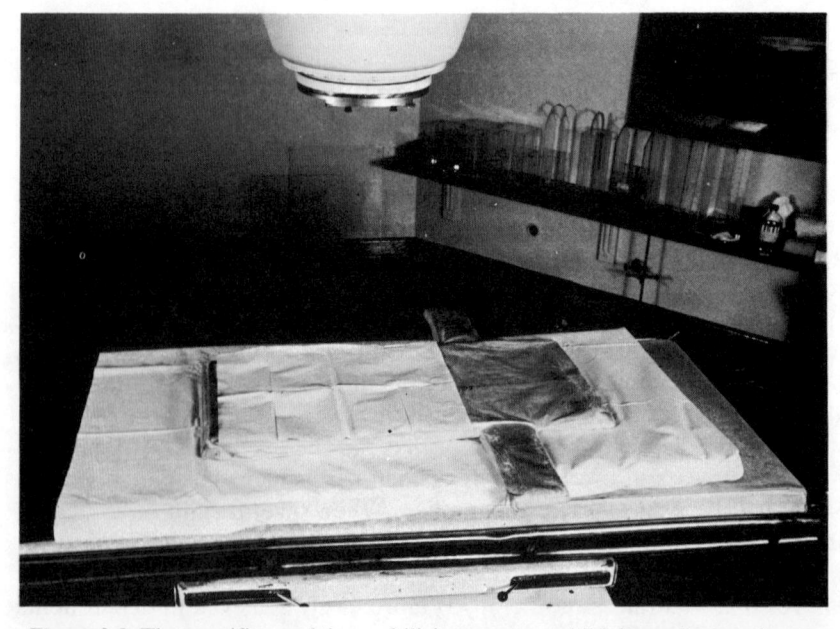

Figure 3.2 The crucifix used for stabilizing a young child for radiation therapy

occasionally treated. It is also more successful, even in large departments, performed by one small group of radiotherapists treating all the children whatever their tumours.

Restraining devices

Although most children over the age of 3 years can be persuaded to lie still for treatment, there are certain restraining devices which may be used to make sure they do not fall off the couch or, particularly for the younger child, to help keep them still.

For most children it is reasonable to place sandbags on each side to hold them in place on the couch. Soft crepe bandages may be used to tie the child to the couch or keep limbs out of the way. Children under 1 year old are probably safer on a padded board cross or crucifix, (*Figure 3.2*). Soft crepe bandages hold the child in position and prevent him rolling off the couch, which may be quite high for some techniques.

Sedatives and anaesthetics

For very fractious children, where it is obviously going to be difficult to keep them still, it may be necessary to give some sedation for the first few treatments. The author considers that trimeprazine (Vallergan) and diazepam (Valium) are the most useful drugs. It is her experience that after a few treatments when the child has observed that there is no pain, many then settle very well and do not require further sedation. Some centres use ketamine, but this can have unpleasant side-effects and preferably is used only with full anaesthetic standby. It is therefore no more convenient than general anaesthesia. In the author's experience, it is rare for children to need full general anaesthesia and, in a department treating many children, is considered to be a failure on the part of radiotherapists and radiographers in their handling of the children, if performed frequently.

Interaction of radiation and chemotherapy

Paediatric oncology is really the only field in which there has been a considerable increase in the use of chemotherapy throughout the whole period of management of the patient. Radiotherapy is often now given after initial chemotherapy. Since this change, immediate differences in radiation reactions in normal tissue have been noticed. The first reported were the enhanced skin reactions observed when actinomycin D (dactinomycin) was given simultaneously with radiation[4]. Also 'recall' reactions have been reported with later courses of the drug given long after the radiation was completed. Before the use of chemotherapy the tolerance of certain organs such as the lungs, kidneys and liver was well established, but since chemotherapy has been used, both acute and chronic damage of these organs has occurred at doses below those previously considered to be safe. Although most of the clinical evidence for this enhancement has been described for actinomycin D, other drugs also interact and produce enhanced damage at certain sites. The author has seen radiation pneumonitis at a dose of 20 Gy (2000 rad) in 5 weeks in patients having either vincristine or actinomycin D. This is radiobiologically equivalent to 15 Gy (1500 rad) in 2 weeks, previously considered to be well below tolerance. It seems likely that with enhancement a 30 per cent reduction in dose is necessary. Equally, the radiotherapist and chemotherapist must be aware that certain specific toxic effects of the drugs used may occur at lower doses of the drug when radiation is also given. This is the case particularly in the cardiotoxicity of adriamycin which occurs at lower doses when chest radiation is given.

These problems mean that the child must be monitored carefully both during and in the few months following radiation therapy, and the radiotherapist and chemotherapist must note any adverse reactions to combined treatment and be prepared to alter schedules and doses where necessary. It would be helpful if radiobiological research could define the drug and radiation schedules which would be both safe and effective, but the reproduction of the clinical situation in animal experiments is difficult.

In Manchester it has been shown that the degree of enhancement is related to the time between drug administration and radiation[6]. It would appear that if actinomycin D is given some time before radiation there is little or no enhancement, but if given at the same time, the same radiation doses produce a greater effect. Undoubtedly this problem will be gradually overcome as more information becomes available from both research and increasing clinical experience. Fortunately it would appear that where cytotoxic agents and radiotherapy do work together, the radiation dose needed to be curative can be less, because the enhancement in tumour tissue appears to be even greater than in normal tissue. For example, the cure of chest metastases from Wilms' tumour with radiation alone, using dosages of 20 Gy (2000 rads) in 3 weeks was about 14 per cent, whereas using cytotoxic drugs such as actinomycin D and vincristine plus 12–15 Gy (1200–1500 rads) of radiation the cure rate was raised to 50 per cent.

SEQUELAE OF TREATMENT

Rather than just comment on the complications of radiation – a word which suggests that something has not been quite right – the author prefers to discuss the effects of radiation, first those in the immediate period during and for a few weeks and months following radiation, and secondly those effects which have only been noted and documented many years after radiation, as development is taking place.

Immediate reactions

Any radiation treatment, except those at very low doses, will produce a reaction. It is important that all clinicians, not just radiotherapists, should know what these effects are and when they are likely to occur after the start of radiation treatment. With the modern combinations of chemotherapy and radiation, and particularly where radiation may be given later in the management, there is a greater chance that infections may occur. These mimic the symptoms of radiation reaction and delay diagnosis. The time of appearance of symptoms after the start of radiation treatment can be helpful in making the correct assessment. It would seem reasonable, therefore, to describe the common reactions and their time of appearance.

The problems which may arise in the first few days of treatment are confined to those techniques which either include a large part of the body, e.g. the whole CNS and mantles, or include the abdomen or head, causing nausea and even vomiting a few hours after the first treatment. This is usually controllable with anti-emetics and indeed, as treatment continues, becomes less of a problem. Some leukaemia patients having prophylactic cranial radiation may also develop a headache on the first day. The smaller volume techniques, which are not so commonly used in children, usually produce no symptoms at this time.

The reaction begins to appear about 10 days after the beginning of treatment, where visible, showing first as an increased redness on skin or mucosa within the treated volume. Over the next 7–10 days this reaction increases, the severity being dependent on the dose. As most children are given relatively large-field therapy, the skin reaction rarely goes beyond the erythema stage, though in small fields receiving a higher dose it will progress through the pigmentation stage to dry desquamation. Moist desquamation occurs very rarely, the reaction is maximal 3–3½ weeks after the start of radiation, healing taking a further 3–4 weeks. Mucosal reaction is best seen in the oropharynx, reaching maximum at the same time, and characterized by early appearance of small ulcerated areas which then coalesce so that the whole irradiated area shows as an ulcerated mucosa with fibrin formation. It must be remembered that this type of reaction is also likely to occur in other mucosa (such as the gut when abdomen is irradiated) and that it is not visible but will produce symptoms. The likely symptoms of the various mucosal reactions are the following.

Oropharyngeal reactions

These produce difficulty in swallowing and hoarseness may develop if the larynx is included. The appearance, particularly when separate ulcers are present, may be confused with fungal infection, and in children treated with chemotherapy and radiotherapy both reaction and infection may be present. However, if mouth ulceration occurs early in radiation treatment it is due to either fungal infection or previously used drugs. Management during this reaction has several objectives. First, to reduce the discomfort as much as possible, helped by bland mouth washes which keep the mouth clean, and which should be given many times daily and always after food. Secondly, the presence of any infections should be identified, swabs being taken to establish the presence of fungal infection particularly, so that treatment can be instigated. Thirdly, painful and difficult swallowing can be helped, particularly in older children, by the sipping of aspirin or paracetamol mucilage half an hour before food is due, which usually allows a soft diet to be tolerated. During this time the child's nutrition may be difficult to maintain. Fluid intake is most important and all should be recorded on a fluid balance chart. Fortified drinks may be given to increase calorie intake. Fortunately, the acute phase lasts for only 10 days approximately and as improvement occurs appetite and nutrition return to normal. Finally, in patients in whom the parotids have been irradiated, a dry mouth may persist after the acute reaction has settled and is best dealt with by taking drinks with food, and continuing mouth washes.

Bowel reactions

These are the other main important reactions of mucosa in children, commonly following radiation to the abdomen. The symptoms are an increase in bowel action, with a watery diarrhoea, appearing 2½–3½ weeks after the start of treatment. The severity varies between individuals and is usually a small-bowel reaction. Drugs which reduce motility, e.g. propantheline, diphenoxylate (Lomotil) and the opiates are useful. There has been some evidence to suggest that a gluten-free diet during radiation therapy to the abdomen will reduce the reaction. It seems to be helpful even if only introduced when symptoms appear in the more severe cases. Unfortunately, as with all radiation reactions, the effect on different patients can vary greatly, so that until the diet is tested by a clinical trial the true benefit cannot be assessed.

General effects

Even when the abdomen is not being treated and there is no local interference with eating, appetite is reduced in the later weeks of radiation treatment and is only recovered weeks after treatment is completed. This is not a marked effect with small fields, but is commonly present in all large-field treatment. Fluid intake must be carefully monitored and a regular check of the child's weight should be made. Calorie intake should be maintained.

Marrow depression

In all large-field treatment a proportion of the marrow is irradiated, although less than would be the case in adults. This produces marrow depression which results in blood count changes. All children having this type of radiation should undergo bi-weekly blood counts, including haemoglobin and red cell levels, total and differential white cell counts, and platelet counts. Those first affected are the white cell and platelet counts. As with other reactions the changes are gradual, the counts being gradually depressed, the lowest levels being seen between 2½–3½ weeks from the start of treatment. Even with continuing treatment, recovery often takes place so that treatment can be completed. If the total white cell count decreases to 3000/mm^3 and platelets to 100 000/mm^3, daily counts should be arranged and treatment modified in the light of further changes. The recommended levels at which it is necessary to modify treatment is a total white cell count of 2000/mm^3 and a platelet count of 75 000/mm^3. The management during this phase is helped by an experienced radiotherapist who has learnt when it is safe to continue treatment even at levels below those quoted. Other factors which may be taken into account are an imminent, planned break or the near completion of treatment, when it may be reasonable to take slight risks and continue meanwhile.

The reactions described above are all independent of chemotherapy. All show recovery towards the normal state soon after radiation ceases, the child usually improving quickly in the first week, but then more slowly; usually with complete recovery by 6–8 weeks from the end of therapy.

Interaction with chemotherapy

The addition of chemotherapy to management, particularly those drugs such as actinomycin D which produce enhancement, may change the pattern described in that the reactions may start earlier, be more severe if the radiation dose is kept the same, and last longer. There may also be a reappearance of a healing or healed radiation reaction when further courses of the drug are given in the maintenance period. These differences have already been discussed in the present-day problems of radiotherapy in children, but the author would like to enlarge a little on the interaction relating to three specific organs, namely the liver, lungs and kidneys, as all the three produce early warning signs a short time after irradiation. In the latter two organs, the author's experience of these changes has meant that alterations have been made to prevent these complications. However, the liver, because of its close anatomical relationship to the right kidney, has to be included in the radiation field when this kidney is being treated, and it is difficult to shield large portions without shielding the tumour.

Liver damage

This has occurred mainly in the treatment of right-sided Wilms' tumour. It seemed likely from previous experience that the liver would tolerate 30 Gy (3000 rad) in 4 weeks. Since the use of either actinomycin D or vincristine this dose has produced liver damage in a percentage of the patients, characterized by a greater platelet reduction towards the end of treatment, without the recovery expected towards and after completion of treatment. Mild cases may not not show any other features, but an isotope liver scan demonstrates a decrease in uptake of the isotope. More severe cases show abnormalities of liver function, hepatomegaly and in severe cases, ascites. If further actinomycin D is given shortly after irradiation, mild liver damage may become severe, so it is now the practice in right-sided tumours necessitating radiation to the liver either to omit or halve the first post-irradiation dose of actinomycin D. It is important to recognise this post-irradiation problem and limit toxicity as much as possible. Severe cases may later progress to fibrosis of the liver. Oesophageal varices due to portal hypertension have been reported years after acute liver damage.

Lungs

Acute radiation pneumonitis occurs approximately 6–8 weeks after the completion of radiation therapy. Previous experience with whole lung irradiation in children with metastatic Wilms' tumour showed that the lung tolerated 25 Gy (2500 rad) in 4 weeks, and that even at higher doses acute pneumonitis was rare although later fibrosis occurred. As mentioned previously a dose of 20 Gy (2000 rad) in 5 weeks – equivalent to 17.5 Gy (1750 rad) in 4 weeks – produced acute pneumonitis in two patients. One child had had actinomycin D and the other vincristine. The pneumonitis presented as an acute respiratory illness with dyspnoea and often pyrexia. Chest X-rays, showed pneumonic changes in both lung fields. The response to steroids and antibiotics is usually very prompt with symptoms and chest X-ray clearing rapidly. Pneumonitis recurred in one child after a further course of actinomycin D. Both children died later of their malignancy, but if they had survived, a long-term risk of lung fibrosis and a reduction in respiratory capacity could be expected.

Kidneys

Radiation tolerance of the whole of both or one kidney was described by Kunkler et al.[5] in adults. Children who received doses in excess of the 23 Gy (2300 rad) using kilovoltage showed both acute and chronic nephritis. This would be equivalent to a megavoltage dose of 27 Gy (2700 rad) in 5½ weeks or 24 Gy (2400 rad) in 4 weeks. In the first MRC trial[1] with actinomycin D and vincristine in two patients, acute radiation nephritis occurred 6–8 weeks after irradiation at respective kidney doses of 20 Gy (2000 rad) and 15 Gy (1500 rad). As both were achieved by shielding the kidney after this dose when the central axis dose was 30 Gy (3000 rad) in 4 weeks, these doses were given over a shorter time and were effectively higher, being equivalent to 23 Gy (2300 rad) and 20 Gy (2000 rad) in 4 weeks, which whilst below previous tolerance, proved too high in combination with chemotherapy. The children presented with an acute nephritis but later recovered. They would both be candidates for chronic renal damage and hypertension as described by Kunkler et al.[5] in adults. This complication of radiation should now be avoided. If the other kidney in nephroblastomas has to be included in the field it is safer to shield it from the posterior field for the whole of the treatment thus reducing the dose to less than 15 Gy (1500 rad) in 4 weeks when the midline dose is 30 Gy (3000 rad) in 4 weeks.

Sequelae of treatment 39

Late radiation effects

Children have been successfully treated with radiotherapy since the early 1940s, and there are now a considerable number who have gone through development and are well into the adult age range. In the author's institution it was decided that any patient treated with radiotherapy as a child should never be dismissed from follow-up. This has enabled the study of the different effects which have resulted from the radiation they received as children. A complete survey of all such patients has not yet been achieved but the effects can be described. They can be divided into three main physical effects: skin and soft tissue; skeletal; and endocrine. To this should be added the possible psychological effects which may follow the physical problems, and also the development of any second malignant disease.

Skin and soft tissue effects

The main changes were in patients treated in the early days with kilovoltage radiation, when the maximum dose on each field was received on the skin. For some techniques this produced considerable scarring, telangiectasia and atrophy, as shown in *Figure 3.3*.

As well as skin atrophy there was a thinning of the subcutaneous tissue with loss of fat deposits, leading to thin necks in those who had mantle treatments with kilovoltage and megavoltage dosages (*Figure 3.4*). In those having abdominal

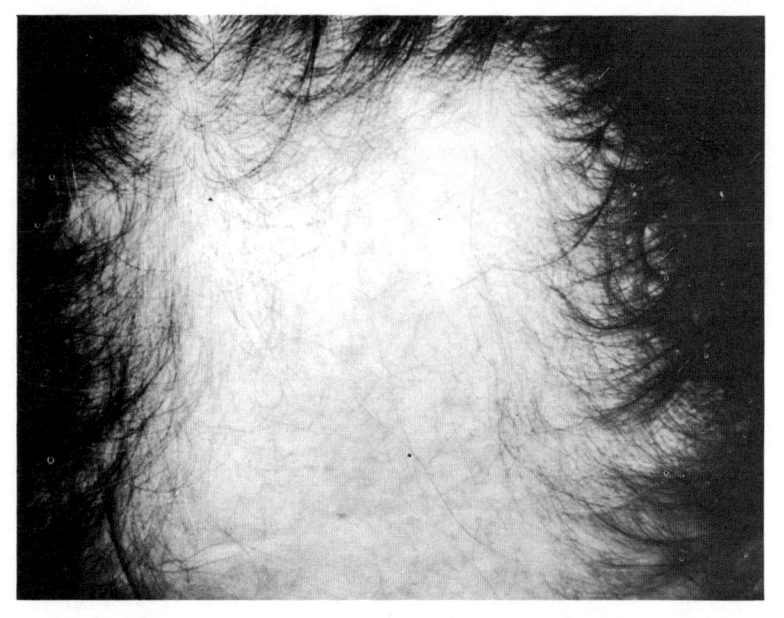

Figure 3.3 Scarring and permanent epilation of the scalp after radiotherapy

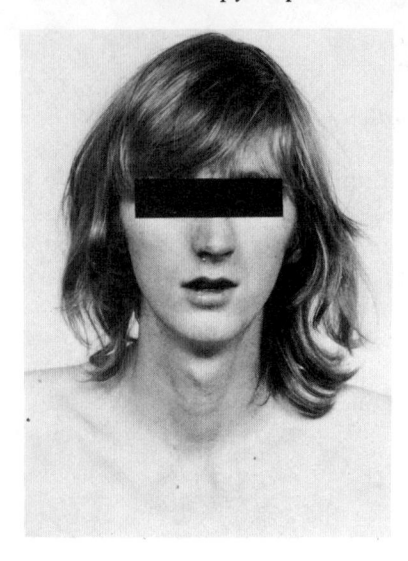

Figure 3.4 The thin neck after whole-neck irradiation

treatment, a lack of subcutaneous fat over the abdomen led to a thin waist. Some loss also occurs in muscle bulk, and was accentuated by lack of bone growth in all patients.

Skeletal effects

As mentioned earlier, radiation has an adverse effect on actively growing bone and therefore skeletal abnormalities are certain to occur. The younger the child, the greater is the final abnormality likely to be. Obviously, to treat part of a limb in a child under 5 years old will result in a greater degree of shortening than a child treated over the age of 12 years when there is less potential growth remaining. This effect on growing bone leads to the following variety of deformities.

(1) Shortened limbs.
(2) Shortening of the spine, now usually symmetrical, but before the bone effect was understood, radiation was given to half the spine resulting in scoliosis. It is now accepted that if part of the spine has to be included then the whole width of the vertebra must be irradiated, so that scoliosis is avoided.
(3) Lack of development of pelvis and clavicles if these are in the field.
(4) Asymmetry of face and jaws when part of the face is irradiated unilaterally.

Other effects on bone have been noted during follow-up. An important recent discovery has been the development of slipped femoral epiphyses in children receiving whole abdomen radiation[3]. These occur before puberty and may be bilateral. The authors has seen six such patients, usually presenting with pain and a limp. It is essential that this condition should be detected quickly as prompt orthopaedic attention and pinning of the epiphysis results in a normal functioning hip. Prevention is also important – it was previously thought that the whole femoral head was protected by the shielding shown in *Figure 3.5a*, but a radiograph (*Figure 3.6a*) reveals that this is not the case. Satisfactory shielding is shown in *Figure 3.5b* and confirmed by X-ray in *Figure 3.6b*.

Another skeletal change observed is the development of exostoses on bones within the radiation field. These may be multiple and grow only slowly or scarcely at all, but if any marked growth occurs they should be removed because of the possibility of later malignant change. *Figure 3.7* and shows an example which has not changed during many years follow-up.

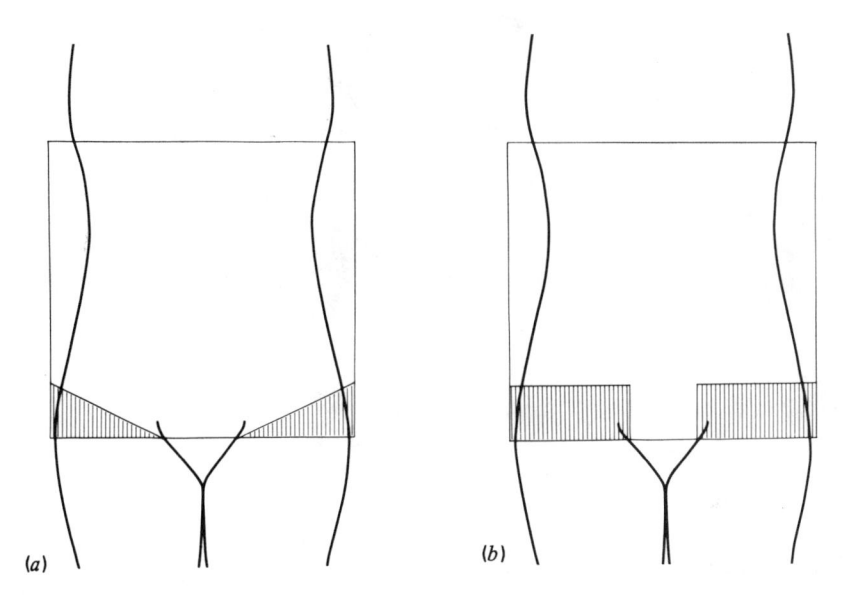

Figure 3.5 (*a*) The shielding previously used, which was thought to shield femoral heads. (*b*) Shielding now used to cover femoral heads

Endocrine effects

PITUITARY-HYPOTHALAMIC REGION
A study of long-term surviving patients who had been irradiated for brain tumours of various types[2] showed that many of them were shorter than normal, even when their spines had not been irradiated. Further investigation revealed that they were growth hormone deficient[9]. Growth hormone assays were therefore performed on children treated more recently, both for brain tumours and the cranial prophylaxis used in acute lymphoblastic leukaemia. These tests were performed where possible before radiation and several times after treatment, and a reduction in growth hormone levels after radiation has been detected. The radiation dosages received by the pituitary-hypothalamic region using the different techniques was calculated

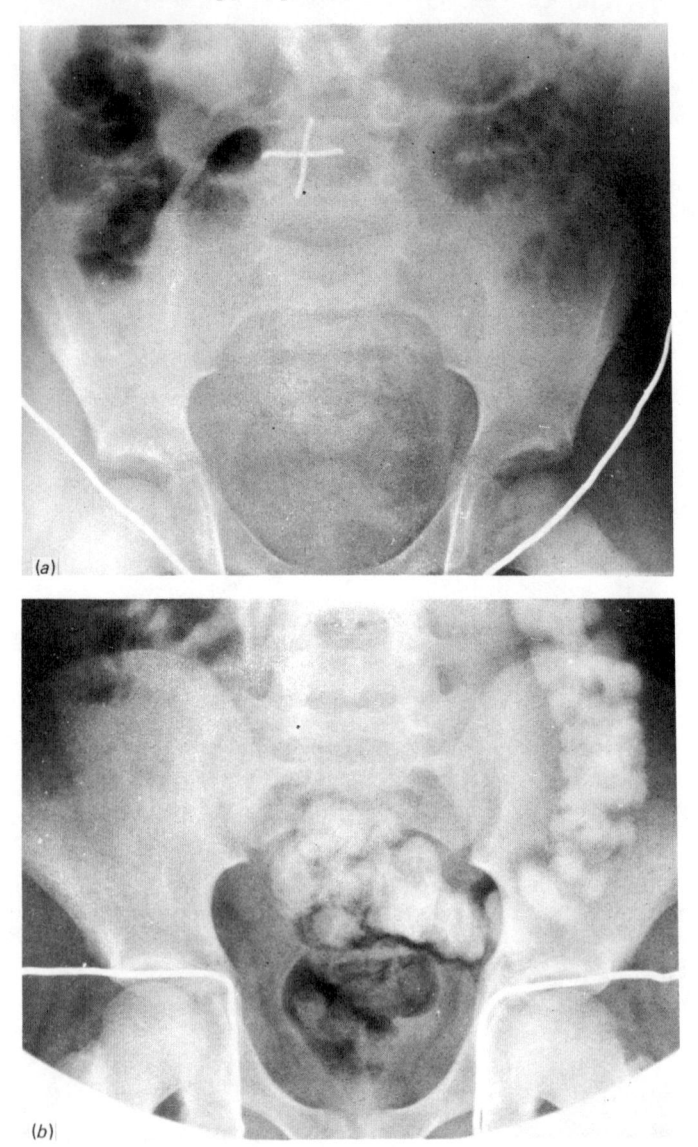

Figure 3.6 (*a*) Radiograph which shows that the shielding in *Figure 3.5a* did not protect the whole femoral head. (*b*) Radiograph confirming protection of femoral heads by the shielding in *Figure 3.5b*

for each patient, and it was shown that at dosages of 29 Gy (2900 rad) and over in four weeks, growth hormone deficiency developed. It is now the author's practice to investigate growth and growth hormone function in all children who have had cranial radiation. It is found that whilst some children have a degree of growth hormone deficiency their growth, at least for a time, may be reasonable. However, if they are surviving some time after their treatment and growth has slowed considerably or even ceased, then they should be treated with growth hormone.

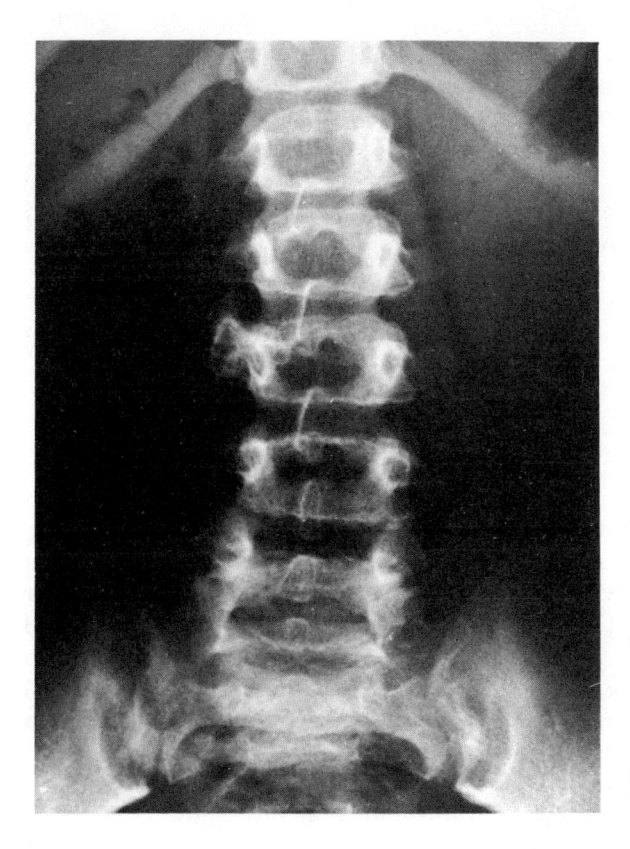

Figure 3.7 Radiograph showing exostosis on lumbar vertebra after radiation

THYROID

Radiation to the neck may affect function of the thyroid gland in both adults and children, particularly in patients having mantle X-ray therapy for Hodgkin's disease. There has been some evidence that recovery may occur in adults, but this does not seem to be the case in those children studied[8]. Biochemical tests of thyroid function, repeated annually, show a compensated dysfunction, characterized by raised thyroid-stimulating hormone and normal levels of tri-iodothyronine (T3) and thyroxine (T4). In those patients treated when children, they have never been observed to revert to normal and in one, T3 and T4 fell to hypothyroid levels 17 years after treatment. Three patients developed thyroid adenomas which had to be removed. A trial is at present being conducted to see whether early thyroxine replacement in these children will improve their growth particularly, and possibly prevent the development of the adenomas which could later become malignant.

GONADS

Ovaries

In the past it was considered necessary to treat many children's tumours with whole-abdomen irradiation. The changing pattern of management has meant that this is now only necessary in a few patients, so that it is largely possible to avoid irradiating the ovaries. Previous experience has shown that after whole-abdomen irradiation or pelvic irradiation, most girls will have ovarian failure and will fail to develop at puberty[10]. Results, however, are not always predictable, and some girls, despite pelvic radiation at quite high doses, developed normally had menses and in two cases have been pregnant, although in most cases where a dose of 30 Gy (3000 rad) in 4 weeks had been given, normal development did not take place. It is important that this should be recognized and that hormone replacement therapy should be instituted. Whilst for some children ovarian radiation can be avoided, there are still some ovarian tumours and pelvic rhabdomyosarcomas which do require radiation and in these, ovarian dysfunction is likely to occur.

Testis
Whole-abdomen irradiation in boys did not, except in the few cases of testicular tumours, include the scrotum in the direct field of therapy. It was considered that the doses of scattered radiation received were unlikely to be enough to produce testicular damage. This seemed to be borne out as normal development occurred at puberty in all these boys. However, some of these patients were not able to father children, and investigations of long-term survivors showed that many of them had either a complete absence of sperm or very low counts[11]. These changes occurred when the testis had received doses which were between 5 and 10 Gy (500–1000 rad) in 4 weeks. At higher doses of 30 Gy (3000 rad) in 4 weeks, hormone production and therefore pubertal development were also affected and these boys need hormone replacement therapy. As with the girls, these changes will be seen less often in boys with nephroblastoma since the radiation fields now used rarely include the whole abdomen and pelvis.

These conditions are the main late physical changes which occur after radiation therapy in childhood. For completeness, mention must be made of second malignancies in children who have had malignant disease in childhood, and psychological problems associated with their illness, sequelae and recovery.

Second malignancies

The author has seen patients who have developed second malignancies later in life – it seems likely that certain individuals who have had one form of malignant disease have a high chance of developing another, and this may or may not be related to the patient's treatment for the first cancer. In these patients, 50 per cent were not related to any previous radiation treatment, whereas the remainder occurred within the radiation field. One patient with the basal-naevoid syndrome is of interest in that following a medulloblastoma in childhood he later developed basal cell carcinomas both inside and outside the radiation field. These were thickest in relation to the spinal field at the edge, in the region of falling dose. The true incidence of second malignancies is not yet known, and will only be answered by registration of late effects on a national and international basis.

Psychological problems

These arise because, as a result of their disease and the sequelae of treatment, these children are different from their peers. It is important that all who handle them in follow-up should be aware of the problems they may have, and be prepared to listen to their worries and spend time explaining how we and they need to deal with their problems.

LIMITATIONS OF RADIOTHERAPY

Radiation is, at present, used as part of the local control of malignant disease, although in certain cases this may result in the irradiation of quite large portions of the body. It is still, however, a local treatment and cannot contribute to the control of micrometastases which, particularly in many children's tumours, can now be controlled by chemotherapy. Even local control by radiotherapy can be limited by certain tumour factors. The main biological factors which affect the radiosensitivity of a tumour are (1) its tissue of origin and type of neoplasm, which determines the sensitivity to radiation, and (2) the effect of anoxia.

As tumours increase in size they outgrow their blood supply and certainly, in the centre of any large tumour mass there are necrotic cells which have died because of lack of oxygen. Many cells in the tumour are anoxic and obviously, the larger the tumour, the greater the percentage of anoxic cells. It has been shown that cultured anoxic cells are more resistant to radiation than those which are normally oxygenated. This problem is to some extent diminished by using fractionated radiation, so that as oxygenated cells are destroyed and the tumour becomes smaller, previously anoxic cells become oxygenated and are then more sensitive to later fractions. Possible ways of resolving this problem are to increase oxgenation by treating patients in hyperbaric oxygen (which is not physically easy) or by using neutron radiation which is effective whatever the oxygenation of the cells. Neither of these possibilities has been shown to be so effective as to come into regular use in all centres, and the problems at the moment have not been solved. Other possibilities at the present time are that certain substances, notably misonidazole, may increase radiosensitivity and hence tumour destruction. These also are still in the experimental stage. It is not known whether the normal tissues will also show a greater sensitivity with no improvement in the Therapeutic Ratio.

These biological factors are the limitations of radiation therapy both in children and adults. Fortunately more tumours are radiosensitive in children, but there is always the problem of the increased sensitivity of normal tissue to be taken into account. However, with carefully planned and executed radiation techniques some of the sequelae seen in the past can be avoided.

THE FUTURE

It is difficult to predict the future of radiotherapy in children with malignant disease. In some instances, e.g. Stage I Wilms' tumour, it seems likely that we will be able to dispense with local radiation to the abdomen. In other cases it has become an essential part of the management, which was not originally envisaged, such as for cranial prophylaxis and the local treatment of testicular relapse in acute lymphoblastic leukaemia. At present it does not appear that it can be dispensed with for local control in other tumours, particularly those of the brain and rhabdomyosarcoma. The author predicts the greatest potential for the integration of chemotherapy and radiation therapy and in finding the right moment to deliver each. It would be of great benefit to be able to reduce the volume needing to be irradiated if tumour bulk could first be reduced using chemotherapy. This would also have a beneficial effect on radiosensitivity, as smaller tumours would have less anoxic cells and be more easily destroyed, possibly with lower doses. This needs continued investigation and assessment. If management timing were right, possible benefits would be more children cured, which is the first priority, and fewer radiation sequelae. However this still has to be achieved, and of course the sequelae of chemotherapy and combined therapy still have to be discovered, something which will only be seen as more children survive.

References

1 ARNEIL, G. C., HARRIS, F., EMANANUEL, I. G., YOUNG, D. G., FLATMAN, G. E. and ZADANY, R. B. Nephritis in two children after irradiation and chemotherapy for nephroblastoma. *Lancet*, **1,** 960–963 (1974)

2 BAMFORD, F. N., MORRIS JONES, P. H., BEARDWELL, C. G., PEARSON, D., RIBEIRO, G. G. and SHALET, S. M. Residual disabilities in children treated for intracranial space-occupying lesions. *Cancer*, **37,** 1149–1151 (1976)

3 CHAPMAN, J. A., DEAKIN, D. P. and GREEN, J. H. Slipped upper femoral epiphysis after radiotherapy. *Journal of Bone and Joint Surgery*, **62,** 337–339 (1980)

4 D'ANGIO, G. J., FARBER, S. and MADDOCK, C. L. Potentiation of X-ray effects by actinomycin D. *Radiology*, **73,** 175 (1959)

5 KUNKLER, P. B., FARR, R. F. and LUXTON, R. W. The limit of renal tolerance to X-rays. *British Journal of Radiology*, **25,** 190–201 (1952)

6 MOORE, J. V. Experimental combinations of cytotoxic drugs and radiation (in press)

7 PEARSON, D., DEAKIN, D. P., HENDRY, J. H. and MOORE, J. V. The interaction of actinomycin D and radiation. *International Journal of Radiation Oncology, Biology and Physicis*, **4,** 71–73 (1978)

8 ROSENSTOCK, J. D., SHALET, S. M., BEARDWELL, C. G., MORRIS JONES, P. H. and PEARSON, D. Thyroid disfunction following external irradiation to the neck for Hodgkin's disease in childhood. *Clinical Radiology*, **28,** 511–515 (1977)

9 SHALET, S. M., BEARDWELL, C. G., BAMFORD, F. N., MORRIS JONES, P. H., PEARSON, D. and RIBEIRO, G. G. Growth hormone deficiency in children with brain tumours. *Cancer*, **37,** 1144–1148 (1976)

10 SHALET, S. M., BEARDWELL, C. G., MORRIS JONES, P. H., ORRELL, D. H. and PEARSON, D. Ovarian failure following abdominal irradiation in children. *British Journal of Cancer*, **32,** 655–658 (1976)

11 SHALET, S. M., BEARDWELL, C. G., JACOBS, H. S. and PEARSON, D. Testicular function following irradiation of the human pre-pubertal testes. *Clinical Endocrinology*, **9,** 225 (1978)

4
Extramedullary leukaemia
Osborn B. Eden

INTRODUCTION

Over the last two decades the remarkable progress made in the management of childhood acute lymphoblastic leukaemia (ALL) now means that in most series 50 per cent of patients with ALL can be expected to be alive and disease-free 5 years from diagnosis. Long-term cure is now feasible. The other forms of childhood leukaemia, comprising less than 15 per cent of all cases, generally have poor prognoses but where survival has been prolonged similar incidence of overt extramedullary relapse as seen in ALL are evident. Consequently discussion will focus on ALL.

The improved survival has been attributed to many factors including improved accuracy and timing of diagnosis, support during infection, control of haemorrhage by platelet transfusions, and the careful combination of drugs rather than the use of sequential single agents[70, 87]. The use of 'prophylaxis' for the central nervous system (CNS) has been considered a prerequisite for long-term disease-free survival. Prior to its introduction at least 50 per cent of children developed CNS leukaemia whilst in systemic remission[30, 31, 52] and few of these eventually survived. The hypothesis is that cells present around the arachnoid vessels from an early stage of the disease can regain access to the systemic circulation if not destroyed and will be capable of reseeding the marrow[36, 87]. This theory has recently been challenged since the occurrence of meningeal relapse in at least one series has failed to influence total survival or duration of haematological remission for standard risk patients[77a]. With anxiety about the toxicity of CNS 'prophylaxis' radiation doses have been reduced or even omitted in some trials[42, 70]. Concurrent awareness of the heterogeneity of ALL necessitates caution before abandonment of the 'established' approach but review of the method, timing and results of different forms of 'prophylaxis' is appropriate.

The increasing incidence of testicular relapses within 2 years of cessation of maintenance therapy has led to discussion of new 'sanctuaries'. As for the CNS, the gonads have long been recognized as sites of disease [39, 80, 112] in those dying of leukaemia, but apparently isolated relapse (incidence 5–30 per cent of boys in remission)[21, 51, 60, 105] has been unmasked as survival times have lengthened. Again the possibility of reseeding and its contribution to the significantly inferior prognosis for boys compared to girls requires scrutiny.

The presence of multiple organ involvement has been well documented. Recent attempts to identify microfoci of disease have highlighted weaknesses in our diagnostic acumen[67]. CNS disease produces obvious symptoms and signs whilst testicular swelling is easily detected clinically but leukaemic infiltration elsewhere may lie undetected. Although this chapter reviews extramedullary disease, it must be emphasized that the majority of patients with such deposits will finally succumb to haematological relapse and it is the relationship between the two and their prevention which must be considered.

CENTRAL NERVOUS SYSTEM LEUKAEMIA

Incidence

CNS relapse became more frequent as combination drug therapy improved duration of haematological remission. Evans *et al.*[31] in 1970 reported a 50–70 per cent incidence with approximately half of these occurring in systemic remission. Median time from diagnosis to CNS relapse was 9 months prior to specific 'prophylaxis'[31]. Approximately 5 per cent of patients have CNS disease at diagnosis[121] with an increased risk in infants, adolescents, T-cell disease and those with a white cell count greater than 100×10^9/l (100 000/mm^3). It can occur in all forms of leukaemia[50] including acute myeloblastic (AML)[81], acute myelomonocytic, acute monocytic and chronic myeloid leukaemia[61], but with lower incidence probably as a result of inferior survival[31]. If duration at risk is considered, CNS relapse in AML is as frequent as in ALL. Without attempts at prevention the rate of CNS relapse has been estimated to be 4 per cent per month for 2 years and thereafter 1 per cent per month[11]. With 'prophylaxis' primary CNS relapse is reduced to a cumulative incidence of 1–10 per cent in different series.

Pathogenesis

It is now accepted that CNS involvement results from leukaemic cells lying in the walls of superficial arachnoid veins migrating into the surrounding adventitia[66, 73, 91, 127]. As cell numbers increase the arachnoid trabeculae are destroyed with subsequent penetration of cerebospinal fluid channels over the surface of the brain. With further growth there is extension into deeper arachnoid tissues impinging on grey and white matter. Finally there may be disruption of the pia–glial membrane resulting in direct infiltration of neural tissue. Leukaemic cells do not directly penetrate the capillaries of the parenchyma but reach it only after arachnoid disruption. Meningeal leukaemia has never been shown to result from lumbar punctures performed when there are circulating blasts[70]. In fact the use of early lumbar punctures, in conjunction with early intrathecal chemotherapy, has tended to decrease the incidence of CNS relapse. Meningeal and parenchymal disease rather than being separate entities should be viewed as differing degrees of the same process. Parenchymal disease is now usually seen following attempted eradication of overt meningeal disease with developing cellular resistance. Occasional isolated nodular infiltrates have been reported, for which no clear pathogenetic process has been defined[73]. Rarely isolated peripheral or cranial nerves, or the spinal cord and nerve roots can be involved. The patient can thus present with a wide variety of signs and symptoms. This constellation is reported more frequently in AML[116].

Signs and symptoms

Not surprisingly from the mode of development overt meningeal leukaemia presents with the features of raised intracranial pressure. Disturbance of the arachnoid tissues interferes with cerebospinal fluid (CSF) flow and absorption. Usually all ventricles are dilated and basal obstruction may be present. Headache, nausea, vomiting, lethargy and irritability are expected[8, 32, 46, 47, 52, 56, 82, 85, 110]. Subtle personality changes may be noted, with some patients developing anorexia and experiencing visual disturbance (especially diplopia), vertigo and ataxia. Less commonly, presentation with convulsions or coma can occur. Insatiable appetite is a suggestive symptom in the absence of steroids, but is more likely in advanced parenchymal infiltration. The most frequent signs are papilloedema (reports from 40–70 per cent)[47, 71], nuchal rigidity, cranial nerve palsies (most commonly III, IV, VI, then VII) weight gain and separation of cranial sutures.

The absence of papilloedema does not exclude the diagnosis. Any leukaemia patient presenting with headache and vomiting must be suspected of having meningeal disease unless an adequate alternative is defined. To complicate matters, abdominal pain (of unknown pathogenesis) can occur and resolves with intrathecal medication[56, 62]. Low-grade fever is most commonly due to infection but it has also been reported in meningeal relapse.

Cerebrospinal fluid analysis

In frank relapse there is pleocytosis in the CSF (median 0.5×10^9/l, 500/mm^3, ranging up to 65×10^9/l, 65 000/mm^3) but sometimes the numbers are low. Improved cytological preparations from sedimentation or centrifugation methods permits morphological identification of lymphoblasts[57] but they are frequently accompanied by small numbers of neutrophils, mature lymphocytes and monocytoid cells of marcrophage lineage. Cytochemistry, surface marker studies and chromosomal analysis are all possible on CSF and have confirmed identity with original marrow cells[66]. The cell count does not correlate with the immediate treatment response but with counts in excess of 1×10^9/l (1000/mm^3) early recurrence is likely[47]. The protein is elevated above 40 mg/100 ml in 20–50 per cent of cases[8, 52, 121] (up to 1060 mg/100 ml) and glucose decreased below 40 mg/100 ml in 55–70 per cent, but neither are consistent diagnostic features[52, 121]. The opening lumbar thecal pressure is elevated in 90 per cent of cases[52] (median in one series, 335 mm H$_2$O) but no correlation between cell numbers and pressure exists. Caution must be expressed regarding the state under which the pressure is recorded. Evans et al.[29] reported elevated pressures without identifiable CNS disease in leukaemic patients given general anaesthesia and the author has recorded a transient pressure of 100 mm Hg following ketamine induction of anaesthesia despite the patient walking into the treatment room and suffering no sequelae[18]. Any anaesthetic induction can elevate CSF pressure as indeed can crying. The absence of focal lesions in the majority of patients presumably explains the low risk of 'coning' following lumbar punctures even in those with raised thecal pressures[88]. Those rare cases of localized deposits or where there is a continued CSF dural leak increases the risk of uncal herniation[5].

Electroencephalographic changes are frequently present, including diffuse dysrhythmias, nonspecific θ- and δ-wave activity, but are nonspecific[52, 110]. For instance, the prolonged administration of prednisolone has been associated with an increase in 4–7 cycles/s activity especially over the posterior hemispheres[9]. It is rare nowadays to see any major degree of sutural diastasis, but this was formerly a useful diagnostic feature in preadolescent patients[52]. Erosion of the sellae turcica was also occasionally seen[110]. Serial head circumference measurements might have a place in the very young patient[114].

Lumbar puncture early in the course of ALL, at times of thrombocytopenia and circulating blast cells, carries a risk of bleeding into the CSF but has not increased the incidence of subsequent CNS leukaemia, perhaps because the schedule employing early lumbar puncture also includes repeated intrathecal injections of methotrexate started at the time of the first lumbar puncture. Extensive spinal subarachnoid haemorrhage and local haematoma has been reported following lumbar puncture (platelets less than $10 \times 10^9/l$)[122]. Spinal subdural haematoma has been reported[135]. Essential lumbar punctures can be covered by platelet transfusion with maintenance of levels above $50 \times 10^9/l$ (50 000/mm^3) for a minimum of 18–24 hours thereafter.

Factors predisposing to central nervous system relapse

Early CNS relapse occurs more frequently (1) in those under 2 or over 10 years at diagnosis, (2) where the initial white count is high ($50 \times 10^9/l$, 50 000/mm^3), (3) in the presence of marked organomegaly and lymphadenopathy[69, 89, 131] and (4) in T-cell ALL. In one study there was a higher incidence of CNS leukaemia in those with lowest initial platelet count[131]. If it is true that leukaemic cells are more likely to enter the CNS through the walls of the arachnoid veins, extravasation at lower platelet counts will occur more often, and with high white cell counts, greater cell spillage will occur. The increased proportion of cells in active replication cycles in T-cell ALL will lead to an earlier onset of signs and symptoms. The leucocyte count principally appears to affect the time of onset of CNS disease. No particular type of systemic chemotherapy has been shown to reduce the incidence of CNS relapse apart from the recent possible role of intermediate dose (500 mg/m^2) intravenous methotrexate infusions given early in remission. To be effective, especially in high risk groups, 'prophylaxis' must occur when cell numbers in the arachnoid veins are minimal[131]. Once cells have replicated and advanced into the adventitia, intrathecal medication is unlikely to be effective[91]. The seeding of the CNS is thought to occur usually early in the course of the disease with the blast cells subsequently protected from cytocidal concentrations of systemic chemotherapy by the blood –CSF barrier[94]. Indeed, the low concentrations of antileukaemic drugs in the CSF might predispose to the development of resistance in this population of cells.

Treatment of overt relapse

The optimum treatment of overt CNS relapse remains in doubt. Intrathecal methotrexate 0.25–0.5 mg/kg can produce a remission of 5 months duration[76], whilst cytarabine (cytosine arabinoside) 50–70 mg/m^2 has produced a shorter remission of only 1–2 months. If the methotrexate is given every 5–7 days in a dosage of 12 mg/m^2 until the CSF is clear of leukaemic cells and thereafter every 8 weeks, median remissions of only 8 months have been produced[118]. When no intrathecal maintenance was given after initial blast cell clearance of the CSF, remission duration was 3–4 months in the study. Primary cranial and craniospinal irradiation alone have proved equally ineffective in eradicating overt CNS leukaemia, achieving a remission of 7 months. Combining intrathecal methotrexate 15 mg/m^2 with intrathecal hydrocortisone 15 mg/m^2 every 4–5 days until normalization of the CSF is achieved, and then every 8 weeks, has lengthened remissions to 10 months. If cytarabine 30 mg/m^2 is added, the median remission duration has approached 16 months[58, 120]. Prolonged intrathecal medication has proved superior to combined cranial irradiation plus short intrathecal courses[115]. The UK Medical Research Council (MRC) trial showed an improved median remission of 19 months using intrathecal methotrexate 10 mg/m^2 to clear the CSF followed by craniospinal irradiation (25 Gy, 2500 rad cranial, 10 Gy, 1000 rad spinal) compared with cranial irradiation only[133]. CNS recurrence was found in only two out of nine who received craniospinal irradiation versus all eight who had only cranial therapy[75, 133]. In *Figure 4.1* the possibility of long term curability is seen with two patients off all therapy. On this protocol five children died of marrow relapse despite apparent total freedom from CNS recurrence.

It has been calculated that to remove all blasts from the meninges 10 intrathecal injections are required since each dose of 10 mg/m^2 on average reduces the CSF cell count by 1 log from an expected level of between 10^8 and 10^9 cells at relapse[107]. In practice this approach fails because of the inaccessibility of blasts in deep perivascular sites to intrathecal drugs alone, hence the value of combined modality therapy.

Higher concentrations of intrathecal methotrexate or increased frequency of injections, especially with irradiation, are associated with potentially severe toxicity including paralysis[104], encephalopathy[55], dementia and even death[1]. Increased risk from high drug concentration can result from delayed elimination or increased dosage and in meningeal leukaemia there is an observed alteration of transfer of

Extramedullary leukemia

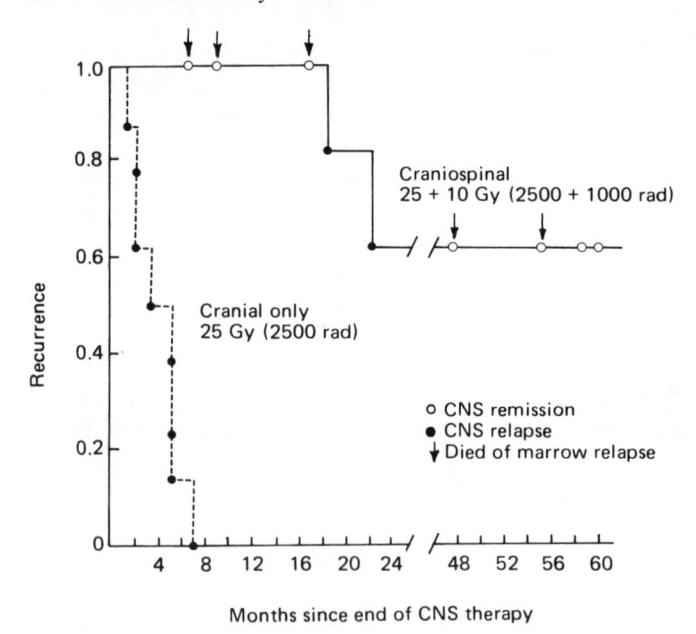

Figure 4.1 Long-term follow-up of incidence of meningeal recurrence in patients on MRC meningeal leukaemia trial. (From Willoughby[134], (Courtesy of the Publishers, *CNS Complications of Malignant Disease*. Copyright © 1979, Macmillan Press)

methotrexate from the CSF to the blood. Haghbin[43] used lower intrathecal or intraventricular dosages (6.25–7 mg/m^2) with as good results and no serious toxicity. The established method of calculating intrathecal dosage by surface area may lead to excessive dosage for older patients and an age-related schedule may more closely parallel actual CSF volume. The standard dosages of 10–12 mg/m^2 may have no greater therapeutic value compared to a lower dosage schedule. After intrathecal methotrexate 10 mg/m^2 in patients with active CNS disease, toxic levels greater than 10^{-6} M have been maintained in the CSF for several days[4]. Although there was no serious toxicity following radiotherapy in the previously unirradiated children in the MRC meningeal leukaemia trial[133], there is a small hazard when this therapy is given to previously irradiated patients[134]. Repeat CNS irradiation should not be given within 6 months of previous cranial irradiation because the risk of encephalopathy would then be unacceptably high. In such cases, maintenance intrathecal methotrexate at 6–8 week intervals would be an alternative, although also not entirely free from possible CNS toxicity.

Therefore, although intrathecal methotrexate will clear the CSF of free cells in over 90 per cent of cases[75], the majority of patients will relapse no matter how they are maintained. Hustu and Aur[51] reported three of eight patients remaining free of recurrence at 31, 35 and 74 months treated for meningeal relapse with intrathecal methotrexate and craniospinal irradiation.

Superior results have been obtained at the Memorial Sloan-Kettering Cancer Centre, New York, using initial intrathecal cytarabine plus methotrexate, followed by insertion of an Ommaya reservoir for intraventricular methotrexate every 8 weeks in addition to low dosage (6 Gy, 600 rad) neuraxis radiation. Prolonged disease-free survival for up to 5 years was obtained in 7 out of 10 patients treated[44]. There were fewer symptoms of meningeal irritation when the drugs were given directly into the ventricles.

The tendency of haematological relapse to follow CNS disease has led to the suggestion that second CNS relapses may have been reseeded from the intervening marrow relapse. The MRC group and others adopted reinduction and intensification of systemic treatment during and after CSF clearance of blast before craniospinal irradiation. Weekly intravenous vincristine with oral prednisolone (or prednisone) and, in the current MRC schedule, intravenous doxorubicin (adriamycin) have been used. Intramuscular asparaginase during this phase is a reasonable alternative to doxorubicin. Intermediate doses of methotrexate might carry a risk of inducing encephalopathy.

Even more experimental approaches to the treatment of overt CNS disease have been the use of ventriculolumbar perfusion of CSF with methotrexate to produce a more even drug distribution. Although successful in animals they are of dubious practical value for patients. The small proportion with long-term survival after CNS relapse emphasizes the importance of CNS preventive therapy in the initial treatment of childhood ALL.

Central nervous system prophylaxis

D'Angio et al.[14] used radiation for treatment of overt meningeal leukaemia as early as 1953 and following animal experimentation further evidence for its efficiency came from Sullivan's report[114] of five cases treated. Following the pioneering work of Pinkel[37, 38, 86] and his group at St. Jude, Memphis, from 1962 onwards using craniospinal and subsequently cranial irradiation with intrathecal methetrexate as prophylaxis, it has been possible to lower the incidence of CNS relapse from over 50 per cent of all patients in remission to less than 10 per cent in all forms of childhood ALL[89].

Craniospinal radiation, (24 Gy, 2400 rad) or cranial radiation only (24 Gy) plus 5–6 intrathecal injections of methotrexate 12 mg/m^2 have proved effective. However both the acute and chronic effects of these treatment schedules have raised doubts about their appropriateness for all patients. Spinal irradiation in a total dose of 24 Gy causes considerable bone marrow suppression making interruptions in systemic treatment necessary at an early stage of treatment when full tumouricidal therapy is essential. Long-lasting (1 year) lymphopenia especially of thymic-dependent type (T cells) has also been recorded. Reduction of dosage to 10 Gy (1000 rad) for the spinal field has reduced but not removed the liability to enforced interruption of treatment and even death from infection. Neutrophil numbers, phagocytosis and bacterial killing can also be affected by craniospinal treatment. Consequently spinal irradiation has been replaced in most treatment plans by intrathecal methotrexate. This is designed to erradicate leukaemic cells in the spinal extension of CSF and arachnoid but cannot be depended upon to reach all cranial foci. 'Optimum' prophylaxis currently consists of cranial irradiation for the arachnoid and 5–6 injections of methotrexate into the lumbar theca, but we do not know that this is needed for all patients. The US Children's Cancer Study Group are currently evaluating the need for irradiation in their selected 'low risk' group of patients (aged 3–7 years with white cell count less than $10 \times 10^9/l$ (10 000/mm^3) at presentation), there being a very low incidence of CNS relapse in this category of patients[10].

Three methods of CNS prophylaxis were compared in a previous trial[41] from the same group:

(1) intrathecal methotrexate 6 doses of 12 mg/m^2 only;
(2) 3 intermediate dose methotrexate infusion 5 mg/m^2 given as one-third bolus followed by two-thirds dose infused over 24 hours, plus a total of 6 doses intrathecal methotrexate 12 mg/m^2; and
(3) 24 Gy (2400 rad) cranial radiation in 12 fractions and intrathecal methotrexate 6 doses of 12 mg/m^2.

The incidence of primary CNS relapse was lower in all prognostic categories where cranial radiation was used. However, the disease-free survival of standard risk patients (aged more than 2 years and less than 10 years with a white cell count of less than $20 \times 10^9/l$ (20 000/mm^3) was significantly better for those who received intermediate dose methotrexate infusions. There was no significant difference in overall survival between the three treatment groups for standard risk patients. In high risk patients (more than 2 years or less than 10 years, white cell count greater than $20 \times 10^9/l$ (20 000/mm^3) the disease-free survival was best in those receiving cranial radiation. After intrathecal methotrexate alone the CNS relapse rate was unacceptably high and patients on this treatment arm were subsequently recalled for irradiation. It was concluded that 12 mg/m^2 twice a week for 3 weeks was not effective CNS prophylaxis for the patients on this study but did not exclude the efficacy of intrathecal methotrexate for prophylaxis given in other schedules and in certain subgroups of patients[41], hence their new study.

The postulate that CNS blasts could reseed the marrow if not eradicated should be proven if we can demonstrate a lowered marrow relapse rate where CNS prophylaxis is most effective. This has never been confirmed and indeed such recent analyses have shown no significant influence on total survival or haematological remission lengths for those receiving effective CNS prophylaxis[77a]. This finding is relevant to the question as to whether all categories of patients require cranial irradiation.

Although early trials and the US Children's Cancer Study Group report suggested an inadequate response when intrathecal medication was used alone for unselected patients, the more complex L2 and L10 protocols using no radiation but 3 doses of intrathecal methotrexate in induction; 1 in consolidation with intravenous carmustine (BCNU) (L2) or two doses of intrathecal or intraventricular methotrexate every 8 weeks in maintenance has been associated with a low incidence of CNS relapse[43].

Acute radiation damage during therapy is rare. The transient 'benign' somnolence syndrome lasting 7–30 days some 5–7 weeks following completion of cranial irradiation in dosages in excess of 20 Gy (2000 rad) is well known[36]. It is accompanied by transitory EEG changes and occasionally temporary increases in CSF protein[84]. Increase in procoagulant activity has also been reported[22, 40], due to a lipid-protein moiety (possibly a myelin degradation product). Elevation is thought to represent disturbed myelination. The activity has been seen to rise during CNS prophylaxis and then gradually fall. Some patients show persistence at high levels or a fall in activity and then late rises. The rise is thought to be greatest in the youngest children but for all, significant rises only occur when irradiation is combined with intrathecal methotrexate. Parker et al.[84] showed no increased risk of CNS relapse in those with somnolence but a possible decreased risk in boys. The numbers, however, were small.

Computerized axial tomography has been used to demonstrate intracerebral damage in ALL. Ramu et al.[95] identified ventricular dilation (8/32) increased subarachnoid space (9/32), areas of decreased attenuation coefficient (4/32) and calcification (1/32) on scans taken 19–67 months after 24 Gy (2400 rad) cranial radiation plus 5 doses of intrathecal methotrexate followed by monthly injections for 30 months. Other workers also using maintenance intrathecal methotrexate have produced similar results, but 28 patients who received 21 Gy (2100 rad) orthovoltage radiation to the cranium (10–15 fractions over 11–22 days) with limited intrathecal methotrexate, followed 20 months to 7 years after the prophylaxis, yielded 26 normal scans, one with marginal ventricular enlargement and one with moderate dilation[15]. The first had initial retinal haemorrhages and the second was born prematurely and had a low IQ identified prior to the diagnosis of leukaemia. The need for prospective studies and the influence of differences in radiation techniques could be important. It is likely that it is the combination of radiation (more than 20 Gy, 2000 rad) plus intrathecal or systemic methotrexate which may cause CNS toxicity[90]. The exact cumulative dose of intrathecal methotrexate which is 'safe' is not known but systemic cumulative dosages in excess of 500 mg/m^2 have been suggested to be potentially toxic. Leukoencephalopathy is rare but clinically less apparent changes might be more common[55]. Whether those without scan changes are also at long-term risk remains uncertain. There is controversy regarding verbal, performance and full IQ tests but general agreement is that children being treated for leukaemia show some defects of cognitive function, those treated at under 2 years of age being most affected[26, 27]. Only the results of long-term prospective studies will distinguish between temporary treatment-related factors (emotional effects, school deprivation and hospital attendance) and the true organic effects of therapy. Hypothalamic-pituitary axis function has also been studied extensively. Although reports of impaired growth hormone responses have been made[108], the vast majority of patients, after a decrease in growth rate during the first year of treatment, subsequently resume a normal growth pattern[109, 123]. Spinal irradiation has been associated with some truncal shortening.

New approaches to prevention

The above-mentioned anxieties have led to a reduction in recommended radiation dosages, e.g. 18 Gy (1800 rad) instead of 24 Gy (2400 rad) and the cessation of maintenance intrathecal methotrexate after cranial radiation.

A recent trial has shown no significant difference between those receiving 1800 or 2400 rad with respect to CNS relapse, haematological relapse or total survival, both for good and poor-risk patients[79]. The patients with high white cell counts, irrespective of their treatment, have a higher incidence of CNS relapse and may require alternative approaches to decrease this risk. Early (day 1) intrathecal methotrexate has been introduced as well as consolidation with systemic methotrexate as bolus injection or infusion following remission induction, but before radiotherapy. The systemic and intrathecal treatment have been combined to improve peak CSF levels. The advantage of such treatment is that it may reach multiple sanctuary sites enabling some delay in radiotherapy. With adequate precautions, methotrexate given in this way is relatively nontoxic to the marrow. Freeman et al[35]. reported CSF methotrexate levels of greater than 10^{-5} M at 2 hours falling to less than 10^{-6} M at 24 hours after an intrathecal injection of 12 mg/m^2, but when this was given concurrently with 500 mg/m^2 intravenously over 6 hours the levels were 5×10^{-5} at 2 hours and greater than 10^{-6} M at 24 hours (*Figure 4.2*).

The cytocidal concentration of methotrexate has been estimated as 10^{-6} M for human tumour cells. Peak values may be important but duration of exposure to such concentrations may be equally important. With the combined modes of

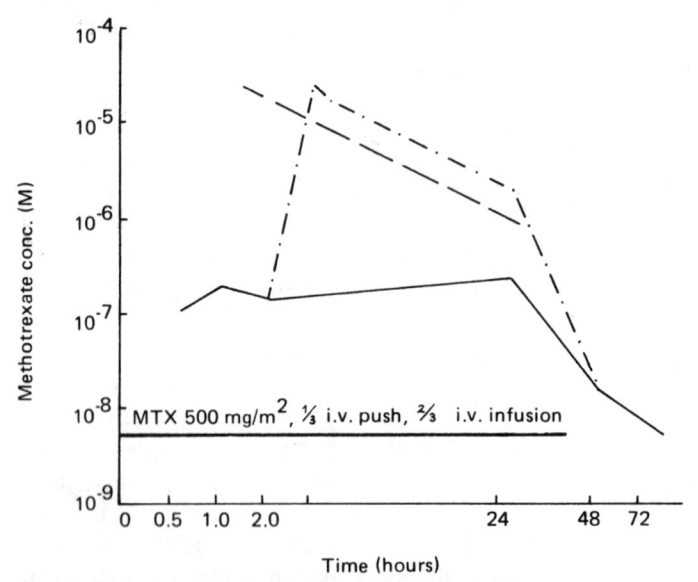

Figure 4.2 Methotrexate concentrations in lumbar CSF in 60 patients when administered intravenously at 500 mg/m^2 (—); in 5 patients following intrathecal administration at 12 mg/m^2 (---); and in 8 patients following both high-dose intravenous methotrexate 500 mg/m^2 plus intrathecal 12 mg/m^2 (-·-·-). (Intrathecal methotrexate given concurrently with one-third intravenous push.) Points on curves are geometric means of the value from the patients. (After Freeman, Wang and Sinks[35])

administration it was hoped to achieve more even CNS distribution of methotrexate. Ventricular CSF concentration is very variable after lumbar intrathecal injection. Analysis of patients developing leukoencephalopathy has shown that these dosages of systemic methotrexate 500 mg/m^2 should not be given after cranial irradiation although three doses given before radiotherapy have not been associated with increased toxicity[90].

In those at high risk or who have had CNS relapse, the use of an Ommaya reservoir[44] permits direct ventricular injection of methotrexate and more even CSF distribution of the drug. The risks of infection, misplacement of the cannula and maldistribution of the drug can, in some cases, outweigh the demonstrated improved remission duration[96]. Necrotizing encephalopathy and dementia have been reported, presumably when free drainage of CSF from the ventricles is impaired.

Zuelzer et al.[136] suspected that late meningeal relapse could not be due to cells lying dormant within the CNS for long periods, i.e. years, but that reseeding occurred from the marrow or other extramedullary sites and that a single initial course of prophylaxis might therefore fail to protect the CNS. They used a schedule of repeated low dose (1 Gy, 100 rad) craniospinal irradiation and intrathecal methotrexate 12 mg/m^2 every 10 weeks, starting at week 4 of induction and spread throughout 3 years of treatment (total cumulative dose 15 Gy, 1500 rad). The CNS relapse rate was 8 per cent after 36 months of the study, but longer follow-up will be needed to confirm the efficacy of this approach.

A number of systemically adminisered drugs are known to reach the CSF in the presence of overt disease. Asparaginase was reported to objectively improve the CSF findings when given intravenously or intramuscularly[124] in dogs, and in both dogs and monkeys[99] has been given intrathecally without undue toxicity. Both intrathecal and intraventricular asparaginase have been given in human patients with overt disease with inadequate response[125]. Riccardi et al.[99] using rhesus monkeys demonstrated that after 1000 units/m^2 of *Escherichia coli* and *Erwinia* asparaginase given intrathecally, although the enzyme activity rapidly declined, CSF asparagine was absent for 7 days. When 6000 units/m^2 were given intravenously daily for 3 days, negligible enzyme was found in CSF but asparagine was absent for 5 days. The use of systemic asparaginase may therefore have a place in enhancing CNS leukaemic cell kill but may also play a role in the toxic effects of treatment due to the hydrolysis of this essential amino acid derivative, asparagine. A recent description of cerebrovascular complications during or soon after induction therapy which included longer courses of asparaginase known to cause deficiencies of antithrombin, plasminogen, fibrinogen and factors IX and Xi, requires further scrutiny[92].

The nitrosoureas are a group of drugs with the ability to cross the blood–brain barrier. Carmustine (BCNU) which is relatively unionized and lipid-soluble was reported by Rall in 1963[93] to control meningeal leukaemia in five patients (dosage 15–150 mg/m^2) when given systemically. Toxicity was marked – in particular there was acute vomiting and protracted marrow depression. Both carmustine and the related oral agent lomustine (CCNU) have been incorporated into treatment protocols for leukaemia and lymphoma in the hope of enhancing the effects of systemic and intrathecal methotrexate in the prevention of CNS involvement, especially when radiotherapy has been omitted[45, 74]. In one critical trial of the efficacy of intravenous carmustine in the control of childhood CNS leukaemia the drug appeared inactive[115].

The discussion has focussed on ALL but there would appear to be an equal incidence in AML and in the acute transformation of chronic myeloid leukaemia if survival is extended. For AML, intrathecal cytarabine would appear to have an improved efficiency compared with its action in ALL, although intrathecal methotrexate and irradiation are also effective. Early trials showed an equal effect for the two drugs[130]. Cytarabine is a very active systemic agent against AML but is rapidly inactivated to arabinosyl uracil. Most schedules use 8–12 hourly intravenous injections or even continuous infusions. Given by the latter method, CSF levels can be maintained at 60 per cent of serum levels since cytidine deaminase is virtually absent within the brain or CSF. The half-life of a single intrathecal dose of 50 mg/m^2 is 2 hours and cytocidal levels can be maintained for 24-hour periods afterwards. However, intrathecal cytarabine has produced only short-term remissions for overt CNS disease, especially in ALL. Tetrahydrouridine can increase cytosine plasma levels by blocking its deamination[98]. In rhesus monkeys, tetrahydrouridine increased entry of cytarabine into the CSF after an intravenous injection of both. When both agents were given intrathecally (tetrahydrouridine 6 mg/kg and cytarabine 1 mg/kg into an Ommaya reservoir), the CSF concentration of cytarabine was considerably increased and its disappearance slowed. When given in this way, the concentration was 20 times greater than if cytarabine was given alone; and when tetrahydrouridine was injected intravenously a 12-fold increase occurred. No neurotoxicity was found in the monkeys, and therefore, the use of tetrahydrouridine to alter CSF cytosine pharmocokinetics may be applicable to patients. Caution should be expressed, however, for the use of cytarabine in young children less than 5 years, since seizures have been noted after intrathecal injections of this drug[19].

Conclusions

From our current understanding of acute leukaemia, highlighted by extensive searches for residual disease during remission, we know that leukaemic cells are present within the CNS from onset of the disease[67]. Improved methods of CSF analysis using cytocentrifugation or sedimentation with cytochemical and membrane marker analysis have made identification of the occasional leukaemic cell possible. Monitoring of the efficacy of initial cell kill is possible although we are still looking at free cells, not those around the arachnoid veins. We must continue our search for agents or modes of administration of current drugs which will enable all areas of the body to be penetrated without undue toxicity.

GONADAL RELAPSE

As with the CNS, the testes have long been recognised as sites of infiltration in those dying of leukaemia, with an incidence reported from 28 to 97 per cent[33, 39, 80,

[97, 117]. More controversial has been the concept of isolated testicular relapse, its prognosis and whether the testes are more prone to harbouring cells than the ovaries.

Givler[39] reported that 69 per cent of 70 cases of ALL at autopsy had testicular infiltration, but only five had been in apparent remission when the swelling was first noted. All five relapsed haematologically 3–17 months thereafter. Nies et al[80]. found that 3 out of 10 patients with testicular infiltration at autopsy also had renal involvement and one had parenchymatous brain disease. A recent autopsy review[97] identified gonadal infiltration in 25 of 39 boys and 6 of 12 girls. Where the testes were infiltrated the majority had other organ infiltration and in those without testicular involvement, multiple organ infiltration was the rule. The authors conclude that the involvement of the testis is simply an index of the presence of recurrent leukaemia. Certainly the previously reported poor prognosis of overt testicular relapse would support this concept. However, Till et al.[129] in a study of long-term survivors reported 10 patients with gonadal involvement, of whom two were in haematological remission. The boy was alive 7 years after testicular irradiation and the girl 11 years after bilateral oophorectomy. Mathe et al.[67] found one case of testicular infiltration amongst 14 biopsied during apparent remission. He found simultaneous hepatic and renal involvement. Two out of 13 boys in another series[65] investigated after 3 years or more of continuous complete

Table 4.1 Incidence of testicular infiltration (overt) in some ALL trials (for boys entered into treatment and achieving remission)

Trial	Ref.	Testis first (%)	Total incidence (%)	Male:female survival difference
UKALL	21			
I		4	10	+
II		12	24	++(25%)
II (Ord. + Mod.)		20	29	++(30%)
Intensive		7	13	+
South Western Oncology Group (1977)	117		33	++
Hosp. St Louis	105	6.4	15	+
(WBC > 100 × 10^9/l	106	–	48	
St Jude Series	51			
Total I–IVA		5	10.7	+ (10%)
V–VII		10.6	16.8	
Berlin 1970–76	100			
(n = 50)		6	8	±(6%)
Norwegian Study	72			
(n = 58)		0	0	0

UKALL = Medical Research Council Trials for ALL
0 = No sex difference; ± = less than 10 per cent; + = 10–20 per cent; ++ = 20–30 per cent.

remission, showed testicular infiltration without other evidence of disease, as shown by bone marrow aspirate, lumbar puncture, intravenous pyelography, skeletal surveys, electroencephalography, ophthalmologic examination, percutaneous liver and kidney biopsies, gallium scans, pelvic ultrasonography and cranial computerized tomography. No ovarian enlargement was seen in a group of girls studied. In the MRC series[21], 60 cases of testicular relapse were observed from August 1970 to December 1976 but only 29 occurred during first remission without other evidence of leukaemic recurrence. Only 5 of 29 remain free of disease 51–79 months post testicular relapse[24]. Thirteen early haematological, three meningeal and five testicular relapses have occurred. One patient had a combined testicular and CNS relapse, one a testicular and bone marrow relapse and one, widespread lymph node relapse.

None of this evidence answers the question of how isolated the testicular infiltration is. Even at presentation the possibility of reseeding already having occurred must be likely, either along lymphatic channels or via the bloodstream. In most series the increased incidence of testicular relapse paralleled the appearance of an inferior prognosis for boys compared with girls[3]. If girls have an equal incidence of gonadal infiltration why do they survive so much better[97] (*Table 4.1*)? The sex difference in 5-year disease-free survival varies from 10 to 30 per cent and is greatest where high testicular relapse rates are reported. This difference persists even if careful stratification is made for other unfavourable prognostic features, e.g. T-cell disease with male preponderance, but is not totally explicable on the basis of overt testicular relapse alone. Where testicular biopsy has been performed at the end of maintenance treatment, approximately 10 per cent showed identifiable leukaemic cells, and in the more favourable trial results to date the margin between boys and girls is of this order. These results have been achieved by intensification of induction and consolidation therapy, and indeed this may give a clue to the pathogenesis of testicular infiltration.

Pathogenesis

Because of its position the testis is easily available for assault by doctors. Some have even suggested that its high frequency of involvement is purely a reflection of this exposure but the sex differential has not been explained in any alternative way. The availability and ease of biopsy has led to early testicular biopsies being performed to ascertain whether leukaemic cells are present from diagnosis, as in the CNS. No clear evidence has accrued but the failure of histological methods alone to identify small foci of cells must be borne in mind (*see below*). Nevertheless it is assumed that cells are seeded into the testes at the time of circulating leukaemic cells. The site of accumulation is presumed to be around the vessels of the interstitium (*Figures 4.3., 4.4 and 4.5*).

Earlier reports[103] of the testis being an immunologically privileged site for survival of foreign grafts or even tumour cells, attributed to the lymph vessels having a long retroperitoneal pathway from the testis to kidney level before entering nodes, have been challenged by more recent work[132].

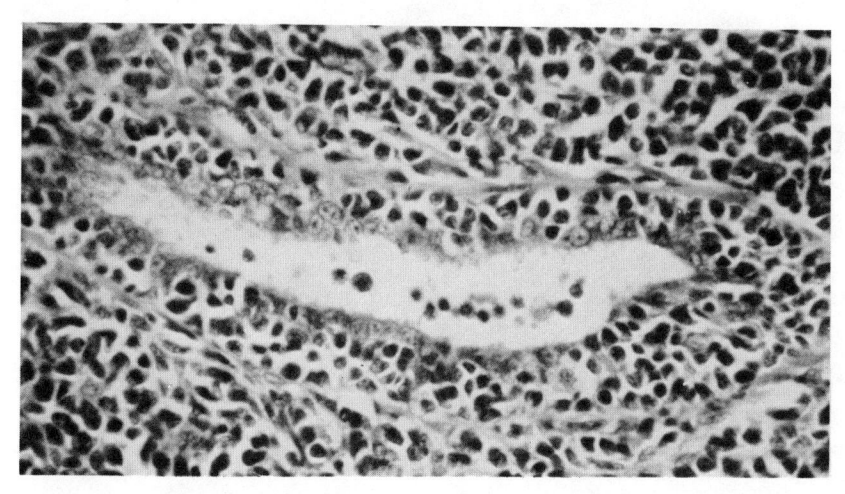

Figure 4.3 Heavy testicular infiltration by lymphoblasts showing distortion of but not penetration into tubule

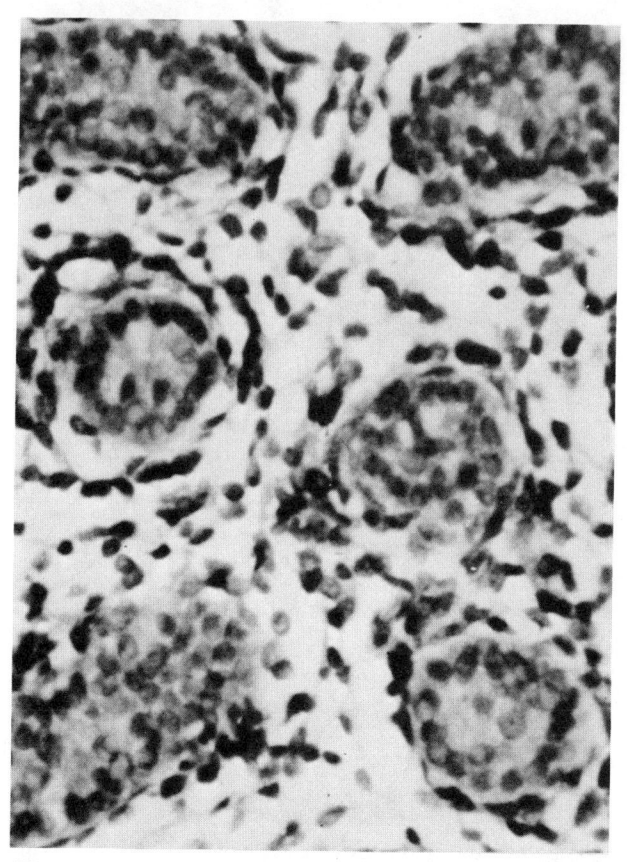

Figure 4.4 Minimal diffuse infiltration of the interstitium diagnosed by biospy

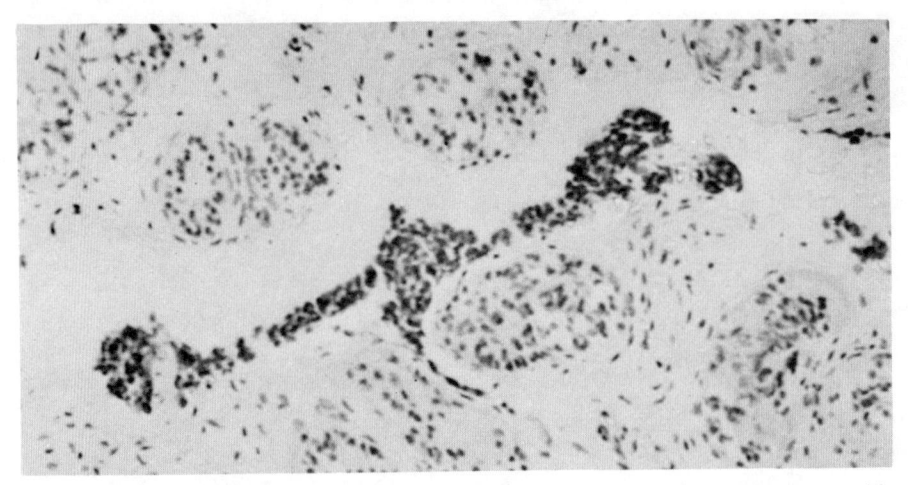

Figure 4.5 Single focal infiltrate rarely seen on biopsies? Reason for false-negative biopsies or is it diffuse 'missed' cells

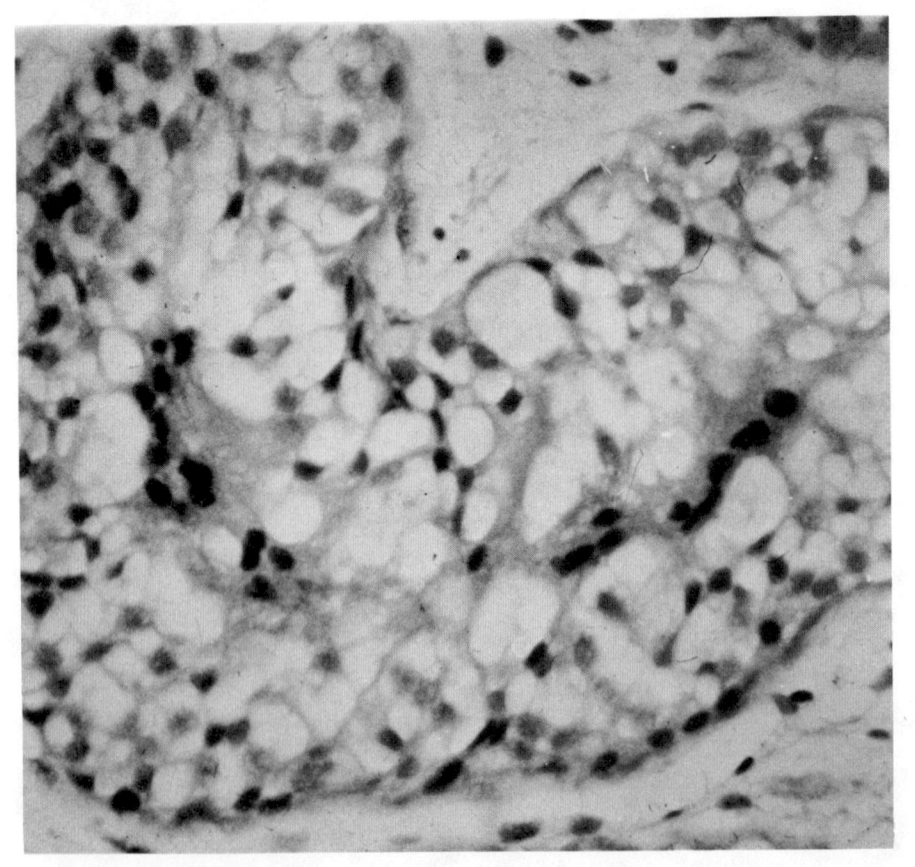

Figure 4.6 Tubular damage from chemotherapy – pyknotic cells, vacuolation, degeneration and reduced spermatogenesis (H & E stain)

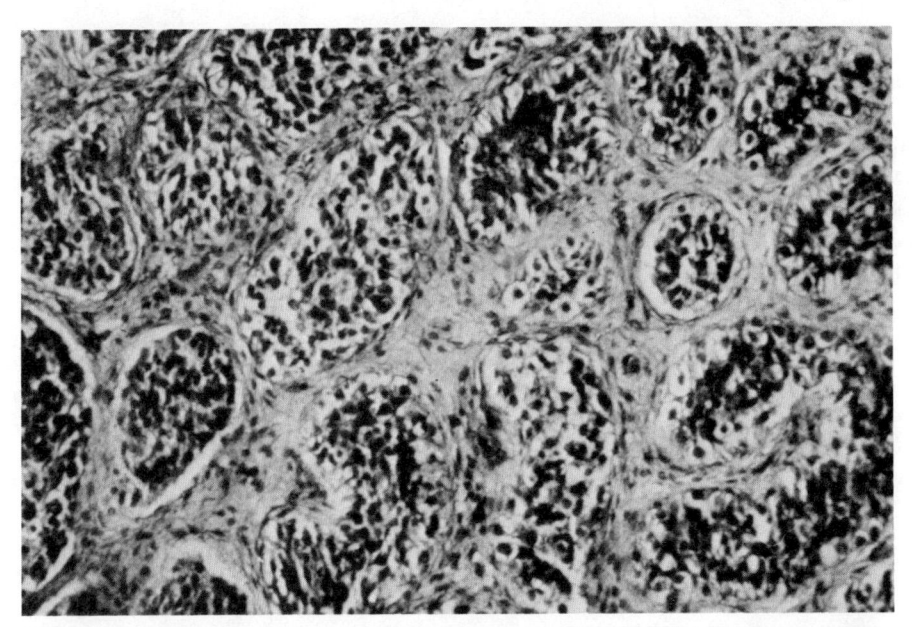

Figure 4.7 Interstitial fibrosis after 2 years treatment for ALL (picro-Mallory stain)

Speculation about a blood–testis barrier has ensued but only that surrounding the seminiferous tubules has been demonstrated[17]. Only one case from 170 testicular biopsies reviewed showed leukaemic cells crossing the basement membrane of the tubules[23] although Kuo et al.[60] observed invasion and accumulation beneath the Sertoli-cell layer. Cells may reach the interstitium but, as in the CNS, suspected decreased drug concentration at the site has been suggested. Certainly, toxic effects of chemotherapy are noted on biopsies[20,63] (*Figures 4.6 and 4.7*) with, in some instance, marked fibrosis. In such cases it is easy to envisage the survival of a few cells in a drug-protected fibrotic environment. Unfortunately for this argument, no clear evidence of a correlation between interstitial fibrosis and subsequent overt testicular relapse or haematological relapse has emerged from the biopsy studies. This would be necessary to confirm reseeding from small foci in a damaged testis.

Presentation of relapse

'Isolated' testicular relapse has been reported in 10–33 per cent of boys whose maintenance therapy has been stopped after 2–3 years[2,21]. Clinically overt testicular relapse presents with painless swelling of the scrotum noted by patient, parents or attending physician. The testes may merely feel firm but not be enlarged. Rarely 'soreness' or mild pain is reported[21]. The testicular relapse may be submerged in signs of generalized relapse[21]. Of the 60 MRC cases observed until December 1976 on UKALL Trials I–III[21], four groups could be defined. A small number (4) having testicular swelling at diagnosis of leukaemia, those with previous haematological relapse (14), those with no previous relapse but concurrent marrow or meningeal relapse (13) and finally the important[29] 'isolated' relapses (29). In this group the right testicle was swollen in 9 cases, the left in 11, with bilateral enlargement in 9. Histologically 11 out of 17 were bilaterally involved. It must generally be assumed that involvement is bilateral and treatment planned accordingly[21,112]. The majority of isolated relapses occur in the first 2 years after cessation of maintenance chemotherapy except in those with high white cell counts where sporadic cases occur whilst on chemotherapy (*Figure 4.8*). Beyond 2 years

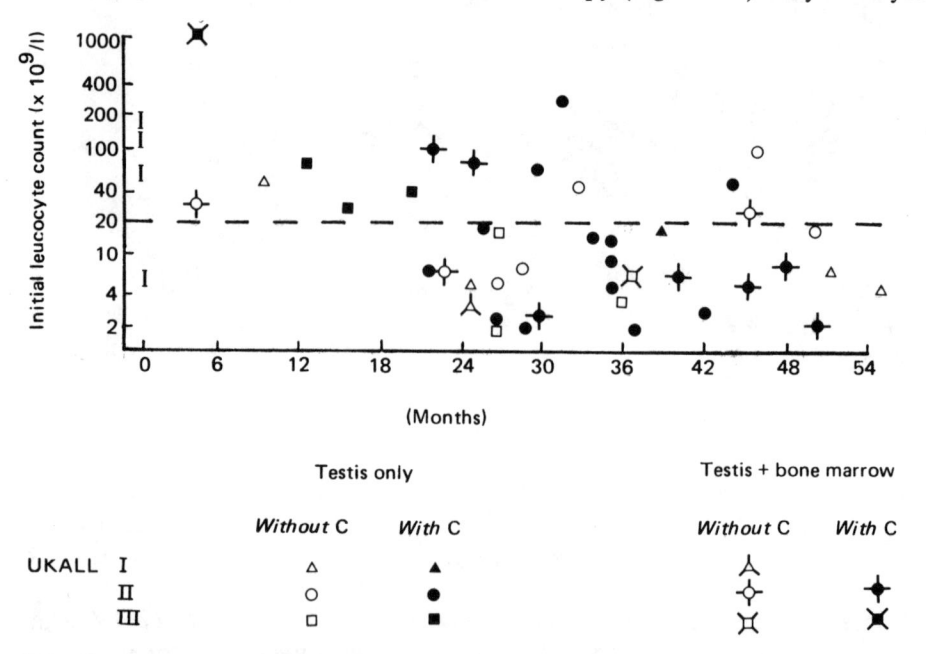

Figure 4.8 Testicular disease in ALL 1970–76 (MRC). Initial leucocyte count, time from diagnosis and treatment. Most testicular relapses occurring after cessation of maintenance for white cell count greater than 20×10^9 per litre. After 2 years from diagnosis initial white cell count has no influence on incidence. I = Infiltrate at diagnosis. C = cyclophosphamide. (From Eden et al.[21], courtesy of the Editor and Publishers, *British Medical Journal*)

initial white cell count has no influence on incidence of relapse. Testicular relapse on maintenance therapy carries a poor ultimate prognosis[21], as is the case for other forms of relapse on therapy.

Predisposing factors and prevention

The effect of initial white count is on timing of relapse and is probably a reflection of total body tumour load (*Figure 4.8*). Mediastinal mass is probably not an independent variable but reflects white cell count and cell type. Initial lymphadenopathy, haemoglobin levels greater than 7.5 g/dl and platelet counts less than

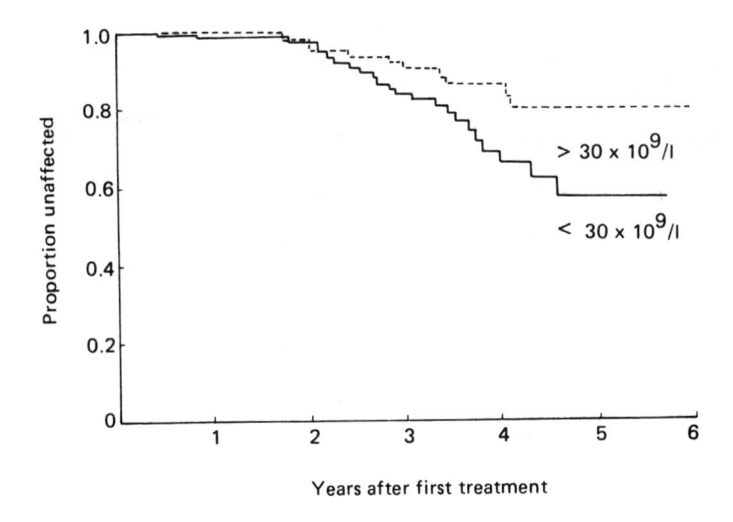

Figure 4.9 Incidence of testicular relapse by initial platelet count from the time of initial leukaemia treatment ($P < 0.05$). Data from MRC UKALL Trials I–III. (From Eden et al.[21], courtesy of the Editor and Publishers, *British Medical Journal*)

$30 \times 10^9/l$ ($30\,000/mm^3$) have been implicated as predisposing factors for those relapsing on treatment[78]. The lymphadenopathy and higher haemoglobin may be reflections of rapid cell proliferation and relative preservation of red cell numbers. In the MRC series[21] the risk of developing testicular leukaemia increased with platelet counts below $30 \times 10^9/l$ ($30\,000/mm^3$) but no correlation with actual haemorrhagic signs or symptoms at onset could be found (*Figure 4.9*). Pretreatment splenomegaly and lymphadenopathy may also be predisposing factors when the relapse occurs off treatment[78]. When the rate of testicular relapse after stopping systemic chemotherapy at 2 or 3 years is superimposed no difference is seen[21]. In series where maintenance was continued for 5 years there appears to be more than a delaying effect and at first analysis relapse rate is reduced[78]. The initial evidence suggesting that cyclophosphamide and cytarabine therapy increased the incidence of testicular relapse has not been borne out and the highest incidence of isolated relapse in MRC trials has occurred in the modified UKALL III regime (*Table 4.2*) where vincristine, prednisolone, asparaginase, mercaptopurine and methotrexate (oral and intrathecal) only were utilized[21]. From the MRC series the abandonment of craniospinal irradiation in 1973 paralleled the increase in testicular relapse whilst a contrasting influence (increased frequency for those given craniospinal irradiation) was noted by the US Children's Cancer Study Group[78]. In the St Jude[51] series 2 of 58 (3 per cent) boys receiving no cranial or craniospinal irradiation developed testicular relapse as against 12 of 111 (11 per cent) who received such CNS prophylaxis. Overall length of total disease-free survival have to be taken into consideration when analyzing these data but the 'necessary' interruption of early treatment to provide irradiation to the head (with or without spine) may be a crucial factor which will be discussed below.

Table 4.2 Testicular relapses (overt and occult) on MRC Trials I–VI inclusive showing the increasing diagnosis from 1970–1975. Follow-up time is still too short on UKALL V to predict ultimate incidence. IV and VI for high-risk patients have overall decreased time at risk since 2–3-year disease-free survival is significantly reduced. T = Testicular relapse; M = Meningeal relapse, H = Haematological relapse

Trial	'Isolated' (%)	Combined (T ± H ± M) (%)	Minimum follow-up from initial diagnosis (years)
I	4	6	9.0
II	12	12	7.0
III			
Ord. + Mod.	20	9	5.0
Intensive*	7	13	6.0
IV*	7	2	3.0
V	7	1	2.0
VI*	3	1	0.5

*For high risk patients.

It has also been shown that no age is either exempt nor particularly prone to testicular relapse. Incidence of overt testicular relapse has increased as overall survival has improved[14]. It is probable that an increasing awareness of the possibility has led to earlier biopsy and diagnosis. If the testicular swelling is slight it may be missed at times of marrow relapse. The trend observed by the author does not exclude other theories of causation of which the most likely is the failure to prescribe or take full dosages of chemotherapy early in treatment. Those series where incidence is highest have reduced chemotherapy dosage after the first month of treatment during CNS prophylaxis in an effort to disease previously noted major infection risks[64]. Where consolidation phases or sustained higher dose therapy have been utilized frequency of gonadal relapse has been considerably decreased.

Husta and Aur[51] reported a higher testicular relapse rate in patients not given an intensive consolidation phase consisting of high-dose intravenous mercaptopurine daily for 3 days intravenous methotrexate daily for 3 days, intravenous cyclophosphamide for 1 day following induction (10/82 as agaisnt 4/87) or periodic pulses of vincristine and predinsolone in maintenance (7/76) as against 6/93). However, these differences are minimal compared with the findings of Haghbin et al.[45] using the 3-year L2 protocol from 1969–73 (a multiple drug schedule with vincristine, prednisolone and daunorubicin induction; cytarabine, thioguanine, asparaginase and carmustine consolidation, an eight-drug maintenance regime and CNS treatment using introthecal methotrexate only, but with no interruption to systemic treatment). Forty-one boys treated on this regime suffered no testicular relapses.

Cranial irradiation has been omitted in some other trials and replaced by 3 intermediate doses of methotrexate (500 mg/m^2) at 3-weekly intervals with 8 doses of intrathecal methotrexate (first dose on day 1 of treatment). Of 95 patients[72] entered in one such trial, 81 per cent were in complete remission at a median time of 34 months (3–55 months) with no increase in CNS relapse (5 of 95) but even more interestingly, there are no cases yet of testicular relapse among 58 boys entered. It is too early to draw firm conclusions at this stage but such consolidation looks promising. Riehm et al.[100], by intensifying and prolonging the induction phase of treatment, particularly for patients with high initial white cell count, have eliminated the sex difference in prognosis and reduced gonadal relapse. In Riehm's Berlin–Frankfurt 1976 study[48] early results indicate that the probability of continued complete remission after 44 months for all boys is 0.74 ± 0.06 (89 entered) and for girls, 0.78 ± 0.06 (69 entered). These are remarkable results which if sustained point the way to a reappraisal of early therapy once remission is achieved.

An alternative approach has been the use of prophylactic sanctuary irradiation. Of 361 males[78] achieving remission, 76 were randomized to receive 24 Gy (2400 rad) to the whole neuraxis plus 12 Gy (1200 rad) to an extended field including liver, spleen, kidneys and gonads. Only one had testicular relapse after discontinuing maintenance at 3 years. Of 285 patients on the alternative three arms of treatment with no sanctuary radiation, 19 testicular relapses have occurred (eight after cessation of treatment). Twelve grays (1200 rad) to the gonads provided protection from testicular relapse whilst on maintenance and reduced the relapse rate thereafter. In two MRC trials, UKALL VI for high-risk patients (from January 1978 to March 1980) and UKALL VII (June 1979 to March 1980) a randomization to include 18 Gy (1800 rad) testicular irradiation was included. Analysis is premature but no testicular relapses have occurred in either trial for those receiving radiotherapy (none of 43 and none of 24 respectively), whilst on UKALL VI five have occurred among 77 patients not receiving the irradiation. There are no cases yet amongst 19 unirradiated boys in UKALL VII. There have been no sigificant differences in haematological or CNS relapses nor in infection risks between either groups. Testicular irradiation at this dosage will almost certainly sterilize the patient although hormonal status may be preserved. It has been suggested that prophylactic testicular irradiation might be restricted to those with high risk of extramedullary relapse rather than being used for all boys. Criteria might include those with initial high white cell counts $(20 \times 10^9/\text{l}, 20\,000/\text{mm}^3)$[78], T-cell disease, marked splenomegaly and lymphadenopathy, haemoglobin levels greater than 7.5 g/dl and platelet counts less than $30 \times 10^9/\text{l}$ ($30\,000/\text{mm}^3$). Prognostic markers of this type are not totally independent of the therapy given so each collaborative group needs to identify its own adverse criteria.

A further approach has been to biopsy the testes of all boys before discontinuation of their maintenance chemotherapy. Bilateral wedge biopsies are required for adequate histological examination using both haematoxylin/eosin (*Figures 4.3, 4.4 and 4.5*) and picro-Mallory stains for cellular and connective tissue assessment (*Figure 4.7*). Eighteen of 170 biopsies[23] were infiltrated by leukaemic cells prior to clinical evidence of testicular enlargement. Only six of these patients remain in complete continuous remission at a median of 32 months after the biopsy. These six received aggressive local and systemic treatment. Ten per cent of biopsies are difficult to interpret because of inadequate crushed material or the presence of inflammatory and large mesenchymal cells. False negative biopsies occurred in 7 per cent of boys in a survey among MRC childhood leukaemia centres, clinical relapse developing later in these patients at a median time of 12 months. Two false-positive biopsies also occurred. No local treatment was given, yet the patients never developed testicular leukaemia. These results demonstrate the difficulties of predicting occult infiltration by such methods. New approaches including staining or terminal DNA nucleotidyltransferase (TdT, a nuclear marker of lymphoblasts and thymocytes) in fixed paraffin sections have enhanced our ability to demonstrate individual cells where conventional histological methods have failed (*Figure 4.10*)[126].

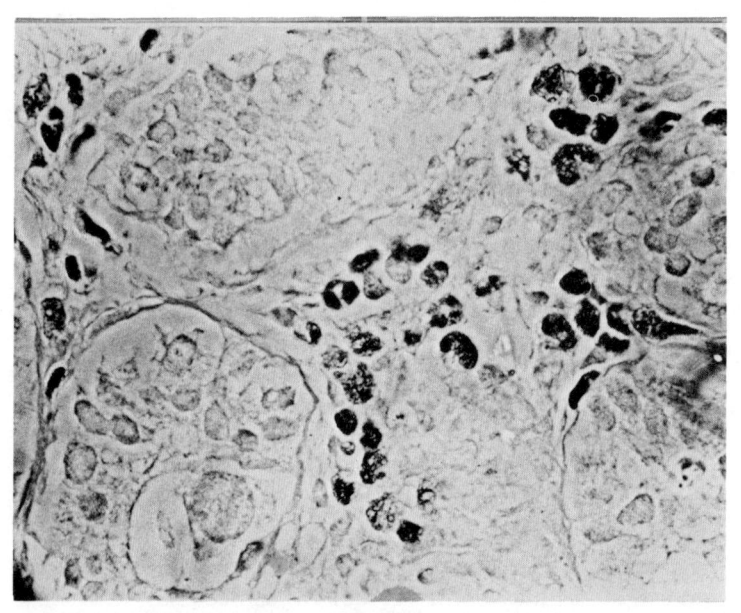

Figure 4.10 Formalin-fixed paraffin-embedded testicular tissue stained by an immunoperoxidase method for terminal DNA nucleotidyltransferase, showing individual lymphoblasts. (Courtesy of Thomas, A., and Janessy, G., Department of Immunology, Royal Free Hospital, London)

Fibrosis and reduced spermatogenesis have been noted in approximately 40 per cent of testes[23, 63] and altered morphology of the spermatogonia in 30–40 per cent of cases (*Figures 4.6 and 4.7*). A possible recovery of spermatogenesis with time has been suggested. Subsequent sperm counts as these patients pass beyond puberty should clarify this. No specific drugs can be implicated as causing the damage. Despite the changes it is thought that endocrine function will be preserved. These effects of chemotherapy may lessen the grounds for anxiety concerning irradiation of the gonads. It would nevertheless be preferable if a systemic chemotherapeutic approach could be developed to prevent persistence of leukaemic cells within the gonads and other sanctuary sites. Baum *et al.*[2] reported the results of five laparotomies in boys with apparently isolated testicular relapse (four overt, one occult). Three patients had positive nodes (iliac in three, para-aortic in two, mesenteric and inguinal in one), and one had liver and splenic involvement.

Although retrograde spread from the testis may possibly be the cause of this nodal involvement, therapy should also be systemic so as to include all areas of potential involvement. Testicular involvement may indeed be an index of widespread disease but this would not explain the inferior overall survival in males. If early intensive therapy eliminates this sex difference[48] this fact would favour the testis acting as a sanctuary site.

Treatment of overt relapse

Possible forms of local treatment include orchidectomy or radiotherapy. Of the 29 patients with isolated testicular relapses in the MRC series[21], six had unilateral orchidectomy only and four showed subsequent involvement of the other testis. Seventeen patients had radiotherapy in dosages ranging from 9 to 25 Gy (900–2500 rad) (mean 18.4 Gy, 1840 rad, median 17 Gy, 1700 rad) to the scrotum and inguinal regions with four relapsing after 9, 20, 25 and 10 Gy (900, 2000, 2500 and 1000 rad) respectively. Six had orchidectomy followed by irradiation in dosages from 14 to 20 Gy (1400–2000 rad) with no relapse. Either orchidectomy plus radiotherapy or radiotherapy alone in doses of over 20 Gy (2000 rad) appear necessary for local eradication of disease. Previous reports that lower doses (12 Gy, 1200 rad) were sufficient are not confirmed in this series[112].

The possibility of systemic 'reseeding' or that testicular involvement was a marker of systemic leukaemic recurrence during apparent remission has not always been considered. Systemic treatment following overt relapse in the testis has been variable. Only five of the 29 (*Figure 4.11*) in the MRC series are alive and free of disease 51–79 months (median 57 months) after testicular relapse and all five have received chemotherapy for a further 18–24 months. Three were continued on their

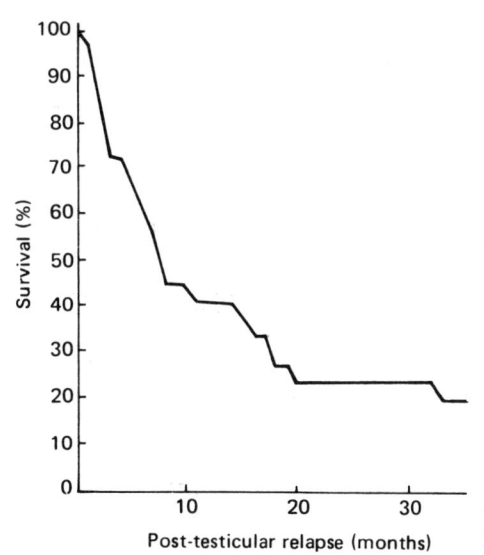

Figure 4.11 Disease-free survival from the time of 'isolated' testicular relapse in UKALL Trials I–III. Total group of 29 patients

original maintenance therapy, whilst two had multiple drug combination chemotherapy. No specific optimal regime has emerged and neither reinduction nor intensification have guaranteed continuing remission in all patients. Initial presentation with a low white cell count followed by adequate local treatment, plus 24 months further chemotherapy appear to be necessary requirements for long term survival after overt testicular relapse. From the whole series the next relapse was meningeal in three, at 11, 15 and 18 months. Only two out of the 29 had received any form of repeated preventive CNS therapy. Two of the meningeal relapses occurred in boys with otherwise favourable prognostic features and one has shown prolonged survival (46 months after testicular relapse). Further preventive treatment of the CNS seems necessary, perhaps in the form of 5–6 doses of intrathecal methotrexate[119]. The poor survival from this series where treatment was not standardized, contrasts with the results at the Hospital for Sick Children, Great Ormond Street, London[128]. The use of intensive reinduction, radiation in a dosage of 24 Gy (2400 rad) to the scrotum and lower third of the inguinal canals, and five intrathecal injections of methotrexate, has produced a mean second remission duration of 18.6 months in 10 boys with no deaths and three now off treatment. Even if there are later relapses when the 2 years of chemotherapy is stopped, these results are superior to those previously recorded (mean remission 35 weeks). Prevention must be the aim of initial treatment but if testicular relapse occurs it should be treated aggressively.

OTHER EXTRAMEDULLARY SITES

Before multiple drug regimes improved disease-free survival, autopsies at time of relapse identified infiltration of many organs[80, 111]. Thirty to seventy per cent of patients at all ages have been reported to have haemorrhages or leukaemic cell infiltrates of the heart (usually small interstitial foci) or pericardium[6, 101]. Indeed pericardial effusions can be the initial manifestation of ALL[53, 101] especially in T-cell disease, but usually responds rapidly to induction chemotherapy. At relapse there can be subclinical recurrence of pericardial effusion. Even if cardiac infiltration is present together with anaemia it rarely causes symptoms or signs with present-day management. Pulmonary infiltration either nodal or diffuse, producing an alveolar-capillary block syndrome, was reported in varying incidence in different series[77, 102]. Although rare, the latter can radiologically mimic infective interstitial pneumonitis (cytomegalovirus or *Pneumocystis carinii*, 'methotrexate pneumonitis' or even haemorrhage). Again symptoms are rarely present and autopsy-proven infiltration can be undetected in life. Hilar and/or mediastinal lymphadenopathy is more common, occurring in about 7–10 per cent of cases of ALL[68]. Enlargement can be rapid with life-threatening tracheal compression or superior vena caval obstruction. Raised plaque-like nodules have been reported in the ileal mucosa, stomach and colon with rarer diffuse infiltration with convoluted brain-like appearance of the mucosal folds and multiple leukaemic polyposis. Rarely, however, do any such lesions become obvious in life although pain, anorexia, nausea, vomiting, diarrhoea or constipation and bleeding are all quite common[13]. The lacrymal and salivary glands can be enlarged but painless in childhood ALL (Mikulicz syndrome)[49].

Enlargement of the kidneys is frequently reported at diagnosis but rarely causes problems[116]. However those with large tumour load during induction therapy may be precipitated into renal failure by a combination of cell lysis, haemorrhage, renal infiltration and hyperuricaemia. The one case in Mathe's series[67] of patients in apparent remission with testicular relapse when extensively investigated had hepatic and renal involvement, whilst one of five in Baum's series[2] had hepatic and splenic involvement. Of 28 patients in another series[65] undergoing investigation (intravenous pyelography, skeletal survey, electroencephalography, opthalmologic examination, liver and kidney biopsies testicular biopsies in 13 boys, gallium scan, pelvic ultrasonography, computed tomography scans of head, bone marrow and CSF cytology), the only organ involvement identified were two cases of testicular infiltration. Follow-up is too short yet to be certain of the accuracy of such multiple organ surveillance for residual disease whilst the patient is in remission.

A recent report of the rare occurrence of ocular deposits[83] emphasize the problems of initial seeding and failure of eradication in areas with protection by natural barriers or where decreased antileukaemic drug concentrations occur. The anterior portion of the eye is normally excluded from prophylactic cranial radiotherapy fields to protect the lens from later radiation-induced cateract. Aur and Hustu[51] reported five cases of leukaemic iritis. Two had received no CNS radiation, three had previous relapses (one CNS, two CNS + haematological). There were leukaemic cells in the CSF of the latter three at the time of ocular involvement. Four of five of these patients subsequently developed haematological relapse.

As in the testes, if the disease site is truly isolated, aggressive treatment may enable long term survival, but more often the focal site is an index of actual or potential full blown relapse.

Conclusions

The currently used criteria for systemic remission (less than 5 per cent blast cells in the bone marrow) are crude indices of disease status. With new enzyme markers in cells or fixed tissues (e.g. terminal DNA nucleotidyltransferase[12,54] or hexosaminidase[7,28]) concentration of CSF cells (centrifugation[57,113] or sedimentation[16]) and the application of immunological techniques to detect residual leukaemic cells[59], we can hope to identify more accurately residual blast cells and potential pharmacologic sanctuaries. However, this more retrospective approach must not interrupt the search for the optimum induction treatment which reaches the 'total body' before cell resistance or tissue damage affords protection for small numbers of residual leukaemic cells. Failure of initial disease eradication cannot, it appears, be salvaged by mere prolongation of maintenance therapy[25].

References

1 BACK, E. H. Death after intrathecal methotrexate. *Lancet*, **2,** 1005 (1969)
2 BAUM, E., NESBIT, M., TILFORD, D., HEYN, R. and KRIVIT, W. Extent of disease in pediatric patients with acute lymphocytic leukaemia experiencing an apparent isolated testicular relapse (abstract). *Proceedings of the American Association of Cancer Research*, **20,** 435 (1979)
3 BAUMER, J. H. and MOTT, M.G. Sex and prognosis in childhood acute lymphoblastic leukaemia. *Lancet*, **2,** 128–129 (1978)
4 BLEYER, W. A., DRAKE, J. C. and CHALMAR, B. A. Neurotoxicity and elevated cerebrospinal fluid methotrexate concentration in meningeal leukaemia. *New England Journal of Medicine*, **289,** 770 (1973)
5 BOGGS, D. R., WINTROBE, M. M. and CARTWRIGHT, G. E. The acute leukaemias. *Medicine*, **41,** 163 (1962)
6 BREGANI, P. and PERROTTA, P. Il cucre nelle leucemie (aspetti clinica ed elettrocardiografici), *Folia Cardiologica*, **19,** 193 (1960)
7 BROADHEAD, D. M., BESLEY, G. T. N., MOSS, S. E., BAIN, D., EDEN, O.B. and SAINSBURY, C. P. Q. Recognition of abnormal lysosomal enzyme patterns in childhood leukaemia by isoelectric focusing with special reference to some properties of abnormally expressed components. *Leukaemia Research*, **5,** 29–40 (1981)
8 BRODER, L. E. and CARTER, S. K. *Meningeal Leukaemia*, New York, Plenum Press (1972)
9 BUTCHER, D. M., HARDISTY, R. M., LANGE, L. and PAMPRIGLIONE, G. EEG studies in children with leukaemia. *Electroencephalography and Clinical Neurophysiology*, **28,** 209 (1970)
10 CHILDREN'S CANCER STUDY GROUP, Protocol 161 in progress (personal communication)
11 COCCIA, P., MILLER, D. R., KERSEY, J. *et al.* Relationship of blast cell surface markers and morphology (FAB) in childhood acute lymphocytic leukaemia (ALL) (abstract). *Blood*, **54** (Suppl. 1), 182a (1979)
12 COLEMAN, M. S., GREENWOOD, M. F., HUTTON, J. J., BOLLUM, F. J., LAMPKIN, B. and HOLLAND, P. Serial observations on terminal deoxynucleotidyl transferase and lymphoblast surface markers in acute lymphoblastic leukaemia. *Cancer Research*, **36,** 120–127 (1976)
13 CORNES, J. S. and JONES, T. G. Leukaemic lesions of the gastrointestinal tract. *Journal of Clinical Pathology*, **15,** 305 (1962)
14 D'ANGIO, G. J., EVANS, A. E. and MITUS, A. Roentgen therapy of certain complications of acute leukaemia in childhood. *American Journal of Roentgenology*, **82,** 54 (1959)
15 DAY, R. E., KINGSTON, J., THOMSON, J. L. G., BULLAMORE, J. and MOTT, M. G. CT brain scans after CNS prophylaxis for acute lymphoblastic leukaemia. *CNS Complication of Malignant Disease*, edited by J. M. A. Whitehouse and H. E. M. Kay, 197–201. London, Macmillan (1979)
16 DYKEN, P. R. Cerebospinal fluid cytology. Practical clinical usefulness. *Neurology*, **25,** 210–217 (1975)

17 DYM, M. and FAWCETT, D. W. The blood–testis barrier in the rat and the physiological compartmentation of the seminiferous epithelium. *Biology of Reproduction*, **3,** 308–326 (1970)
18 EDEN, O. B. (personal communication)
19 EDEN, O. B., GOLDIE, W., WOOD, T. and ETCUBANAS, E. Seizures following intrathecal cytosine arabinoside in young children with acute lymphoblastic leukaemia. *Cancer*, **42,** 53–58 (1978)
20 EDEN, O. B., GOWING, N. and KAY, H. E.M. On behalf of the MRC Working Party on Leukaemia in Childhood. Structural changes within the testes consequent upon treatment of acute lymphoblastic leukaemia of childhood. *Proceedings of the Tenth Meeting of the International Society of Paediatric Oncology* (Sept 1978, Brussels)
21 EDEN, O. B., HARDISTY, R. M., INNES, E. M., KAY, H. E. M. and PETO, J. Testicular disease in acute lymphoblastic leukaemia in childhood – report on behalf of the Medical Research Council's Working Party on Leukaemia in Childhood. *British Medical Journal*, **1,** 334–338 (1978)
22 EDEN, O. B., MILLAR, J. B., BELTON, N., GILES, M. and UTTLEY, W. S. Detection of evidence for demyelination in childhood leukaemia. Proceedings of Paediatric Research Society. *Archives of Disease in Childhood*, **54,** 801 (1979)
23 EDEN, O. B. and RANKIN, A. On behalf of Medical Research Council Working Party on Leukaemia in childhood. Testicular biopsies in childhood lymphoblastic leukaemia. *Proceedings of the Twelfth Meeting of the International Society of Paediatric Oncology* (Budapest, 1980)
24 EDEN, O. B., RANKIN, A. and KAY, H. E. M. (unpublished observations)
25 EDITORIAL. Second remissions in childhood acute lymphoblastic leukaemia. *British Medical Journal*, **282,** 760–761 (1981)
26 EISER, C. Intellectual abilities among survivors of childhood leukaemia as a function of CNS irradiation. *Archives of Disease in Childhood*, **53,** 391–395 (1978)
27 EISER, C. and LANSDOWN, R. A retrospective study of intellectual development in children treated for acute lymphoblastic leukaemia. *Archives of Disease in Childhood*, **52,** 525–529 (1977)
28 ELLIS, R. B., RAPSON, N. T., PATRICK, A. D. and GREAVES, M. F. Expression of hexosaminidase isoenzymes in childhood leukaemia. *New England Journal of Medicine*, **298,** 476 (1978)
29 EVANS, A. The cerebospinal fluid of leukaemic children without CNS manifestation. *Pediatrics*, **31,** 1024 (1963)
30 EVANS, A. E. Central nervous system involvement in children with acute leukaemia. A study of 921 patients. *Cancer*, **17,** 256–258 (1964)
31 EVANS, A., GILBERT, E. S. and ZANDSTRA, R. The increasing incidence of central nervous system leukaemia in children. *Cancer*, **26,** 404 (1970)
32 FALKSON, G., VAN EDEN, E. B. and FALKSON, H. C. Meningeal leukaemia. *Medical Proceedings of Johannesburg*, **15,** 13 (1968)
33 FINKLESTEIN, J. Z., DYMENT, P. G. and HAMMOND, G. D. Leukaemic infiltration of the testes during bone marrow remission. *Pediatrics*, **43,** 1042–1045 (1969)

34 FREEMAN, A. I., WANG, J. J. and SINKS, L. F. High dose methotrexate in acute lymphocytic leukaemia. *Cancer Treatment Reports*, **61,** 727–731 (1977)

35 FREEMAN, J. E., JOHNSTONE, P. G. B. and VOKE, J. M. Somnolence after prophylactic cranial irradiation in children with acute lymphoblastic leukaemia. *British Medical Journal*, **4,** 523 (1973)

36 FREI, E. for Acute Leukaemia, Group B. The effectiveness of combinations of antileukaemic agents in inducing and maintaining remissions in children with acute leukaemia. *Blood*, **26,** 642 (1965)

37 GEORGE, P., HERNANDEZ, K., HUSTU, H. O., BERELLA, L., HOLTON, C. and PINKEL, D. A study of 'total therapy' of acute lymphocytic leukaemia in children. *Journal of Pediatrics*, **72,** 399–408 (1968)

38 GEORGE, P. and PINKEL, D. CNS radiation in children with acute lymphocytic leukaemia in remission. *Proceedings of the American Association for Cancer Research*, **6,** 22 (1965)

39 GIVLER, R. L. Testicular involvement in leukaemia and lymphoma. *Cancer*, **23,** 1290–1295 (1969)

40 GRAEBNER, J. E. and STUART, M. J. Spinal-fluid procoagulant activity. A sensitive indicator of central-nervous-system damage. *Lancet*, **11,** 285–288 (1978)

41 GREEN, D. M., FREEMAN, A. I., SATHER, H. N., SALLAN, S. E., NESBIT, M. E., CASSADY, J. R., SINKS, L. F., HAMMOND, D. and FREI, E., III. Comparison of 3 methods of CNS prophylaxis in childhood ALL *Lancet*, **1,** 1398–1401 (1980)

42 HAGHBIN, M. Chemotherapy of acute lymphoblastic leukaemia in children. *American Journal of Haematology*, **1,** 201–209 (1976)

43 HAGHBIN, M. Antimetabolites in the prophylaxis and treatment of central nervous system leukaemia. *Cancer Treatment Reports*, **61,** 661–666 (1977)

44 HAGHBIN, M. and GALICICH, J. H. Use of the Ommaga reservoir in the prevention and treatment of CNS leukaemia. *American Journal of Pediatric Hematology and Oncology*, **1,** 111 (1979)

45 HAGHBIN, M., TAN, T. C., CLARKSON, B. D., MIKÉ, V., BURCHENAL, J. H. and MURPHY, M. L. Treatment of acute lymphoblastic leukaemia in children with 'prophylactic' intrathecal methotrexate and intensive systemic chemotherapy. *Cancer Research*, **35,** 807–811 (1975)

46 HAGHBIN, M. and ZEULZER, W. W. A long-term study of cerebospinal leukaemia. *Journal of Pediatrics*, **67,** 23 (1965)

47 HARDISTY, R. M. and NORMAN, P. M. Meningeal leukaemia. *Archives of Disease in Childhood*, **42,** 411 (1967)

48 HENZE, G., LANGERMANN, H. J., SCHELLONG, G. and RIEHM, H. Therapy results of the BFM studies in childhood acute lymphoblastic leukaemia. *Proceedings of the Twelfth Meeting of the International Society of Pediatric Oncology* (Budapest, 1980)

49 HIRD, A. J. Mikulicz's syndrome *British Medical Journal*, **2,** 416 (1949)

50 HUNT, W. E., BOURONCLE, B. A. and MEAGHER, J. N. Neurologic complications of leukaemias and lymphomas. *Journal of Neurosurgery*, **16,** 135 (1959)

51 HUSTU, H. O. and AUR, R. J. A. Extramedullary Leukaemia Clinics in *Haematolgy*, **7,** 313–337 (1978)

52 HYMAN, C. B., BOGLE, J. M., BRUBAKER, C. A., WILLIAMS, K. and HAMMOND, D. CNS

involvement by leukaemia in children. 1. Relationship to systemic leukaemia and description of clinical and laboratory manifestations. *Blood*, **25,** 1 (1965)

53 JAFFE, N., TRAGGIS, D. G. and TEFFT, M. Acute leukaemia presenting with pericardial tamponade. *Paediatrics*, **45,** 461 (1970)

54 JANOSSY, G., HOFFBRAND, A. V., GREAVES, M. F., GANESHAGURU, K., PAIN, C., BRADSTOCK, K. F., PRENTICE, H. G., KAY, H. E. M., LISTER, A. Terminal transferase enzyme assay and immunological membrane markers in the diagnosis of leukaemia: a multiparameter analysis of 300 cases. *British Journal of Haematology*, **44,** 221–234 (1980)

55 KAY, H. E. M., KNAPTON, P. J. and O'SULLIVAN, J. P. Encephalopathy in acute leukaemia associated with methotrexate therapy. *Archives of Disease in Childhood*, **47,** 344–354 (1972)

56 KOCH, K., REIQUAM, C. W. and BEATTY, E. C. JR. Acute Childhood leukaemia. Unusual complications. *Rocky Mountain Medical Journal*, **63,** 50 (1966)

57 KOMP, D. M. Cytocentrifugation in the management of central nervous system leukaemia. *Journal of Pediatrics*, **81,** 992 (1972)

58 KOMP, D., FALLETTA, J., RAGAB, A. and HUMPHREY, G. B. Is cranial radiation necessary for CNS prophylaxis in ALL of childhood? *Proceedings of the American Society for Clinical Oncology*, **16,** 1046 (1975)

59 KUMAR, S., CARR, T. F., HANN, I. M., MORRIS JONES, P. and EVANS, D. I. K. Immunological detection of residual leukaemic disease in the bone marrow of children with acute lymphoblastic leukaemia. *British Medical Journal*, **1,** 544 (1978)

60 KUO, T. T., TSCHANG, T. P. and CHU, J. Y. Testicular relapse in childhood acute lymphocytic leukaemia during bone marrow remission. *Cancer*, **38,** 2604–2612 (1976)

61 KWAAN, H. C., PIERRE, R. V. and LONG, D. L. Meningeal involvement as first manifestation of acute myeloblastic transformation in CGL. *Blood*, **33,** 348 (1969)

62 LASCARI, A. D. Personal experience. In *Leukaemia in Childhood*. Springfield, Illinois, C. C. Thomas (1973)

63 LENDON, M., HANN, I. M., PALMER, M. K. SHALET, S. M. and MORRIS JONES, P. H. Testicular histology after combination chemotherapy in childhood for acute lymphoblastic leukaemia. *Lancet*, **11,** 439–441 (1978)

64 MACLENNAN, I. C. M. and KAY, H. E. M. Analysis of treatment in childhood leukaemia. IV. *Cancer*, **41,** 108–111 (1978)

65 MAHONEY, D. H., GONZALES, E. T., FERRY, G. D., WILSON, C. J., VON NOORDEN, G. K. and FERNBACH, D. F. Occult disease in children with acute leukaemia prior to discontinuation of therapy. *Blood*, **54,** Suppl. 1, 197A (1979)

66 MASTRANGELO, R., ZUELZER, W. W., ECKLUND, P. S. and THOMPSON, R. I. Chromosomes in the spinal fluid. Evidence for metastatic origin of meningeal leukaemia. *Blood*, **35,** 227 (1970)

67 MATHE, G., SCHWARZENBERG, L., MERZ, A. M., COTTON, A., SCHNEIDER, M., ARNIEL, J. L., SCHLUMBERGER, J. R., POISSON, J. and WAJCNER, G. Extensive histological and cytological survey of patients with acute leukaemia in 'complete remission'. *British Medical Journal*, **1,** 640–642 (1966)

68 MATHEW, P. M., PRANGNELL, D. R., COLE, A. J. L., HILL, F. G. H., SHAH, K. J., MORRIS-JONES, P. H., MARTIN, J., PALMER, M. K., THOMPSON, E. N., EDEN, O. B., MOTT, M. G. and MANN, J. R. Clinical haematological and radiological features of children presenting with

lymphoblastic mediastinal masses. *Medical and Paediatric Oncology*, **8,** 193–204 (1980)

69 MELHORN, D. K., GROSS, S., FISHER, B. J. and NEWMAN, A. J. Studies on the use of 'prophylactic' I/T amethopterin in childhood leukaemia. *Blood*, **36,** 55 (1970)

70 MILLER, D. R. Acute lymphoblastic leukaemia. *Paediatric Clinics of North America*, **27,** 269–291 (1980)

71 MITUS, A., Dexamethasome – its effectiveness in the treatment of the acute symptoms of meningeal leukaemia. *American Journal of Diseases in Childhood*, **117,** 307 (1969)

72 MOE, P. J.*et al.* High dose methotrexate in ALL in childhood: report on a national program. *Pediatric Research*, **13,** 951 (1979)

73 MOORE, E. W., THOMAS, L. B., SHAW, R. K. and FREIREICH, E. J. The CNS in acute leukaemia. A post mortem study of 117 consecutive cases with particular reference to haemorrhages, leukaemic infiltration and the syndrome of meningeal leukaemia. *Archives of Internal Medicine*, **105,** 451 (1960)

74 MOTT, M. G. (on behalf of United Kingdom Children's Cancer Study Group). Combination chemotherapy ± low dose irradiation for non-Hodgkins lymphoma. In *Non-Hodgkins Lymphoma in Children*, edited by J. Graham. New York, Masson (1980)

75 MRC FIRST MENINGEAL TRIAL reported by Willoughby, M. L. N., *Paediatric Haematology*, Edinburgh, Churchill, Livingstone, 1977.

76 MURPHY, M. L. Leukaemia and lymphoma in children. *Pediatric Clinics of North America*, **6,** 611–638 (1959)

77 NATHAN, D. J. and SANDERS, M. Manifestation of acute leukaemia in the parenchyma of the lung. *New England Journal of Medicine*, **252,** 797 (1955)

77a NESBIT, M. E., D'ANGIO, G. J., SATHER, H. N.*et al.* Effect of isolated CNS leukaemia on bone marrow remission and survival in childhood ALL. *Lancet*, **1,** 1386–1388 (1981)

78 NESBIT, M. E., ROBINSON, L., ORTEGA, J. A., SUTHER, H., DONALDSON, M. and HAMMOND, D. Testicular relapse in childhood acute lymphoblastic leukaemia. Association with pretreatment patient characteristics and treatment. *Cancer*, **45,** 20009–2016 (1980)

79 NESBIT, M. E., SATHER, H. N., ROBISON, L. L., ORTOGA, J., LITTMAN, P. S., D'ANGIO, G. J. and HAMMOND, G. D. Presymptomatic CNS therapy in previously untreated childhood ALL. Comparison of 1800 rad and 240 rad. *Lancet*, **1,** 461–466 (1981)

80 NIES, B. A., BODEY, G. P., THOMAS, L. B., BRECKER, G. and FREIREICH, E. J. The persistence of extra meduallary leukaemia infiltrates during bone marrow remission of acute leukaemia. *Blood*, **26,** 133–141 (1965)

81 NIES, B. A., MALONGREN, R. A., CHU, E. W., DELVECCHIO, P. R., THOMAS, L. B. and FREIREICH, E. J. Cerebospinal fluids cytology in patients with acute leukaemia. *Cancer*, **18,** 1385 (1965)

82 NIES, B. A., THOMAS, L. B. and FREIREICH, E. J. Meningeal leukaemia, a follow up study. *Cancer*, **18,** 546 (1965)

83 NINANE, J. The eye as a sanctuary in acute lymphoblastic leukaemia. *Lancet*, **1,** 452–453 (1980)

84 PARKER, D., MALPAS, J. S., SANDLAND, R., SHEAFF, P. C., FREEMAN, J. E. and PAXTON, A.

Outlook following 'somnolence syndrome' after prophylactic cranial irradiation. *British Medical Journal*, **1,** 554 (1978)
85 PIERCE, M. Leukaemia in children: treatment of 22 cases with 6–mercaptopurine. *Annals of the New York Accademy of Sciences*, **60,** 415 (1954)
86 PINKEL, D. Five year following up of total therapy of childhood lymphocytic leukaemia. *Journal of American Medical Association*, **216,** 648–652 (1971)
87 PINKEL, D. Treatment of acute leukaemia. *Pediatric Clinics of North America*, **23,** 117–129 (1976)
88 POCHEDLY, C. *The Child with Leukaemia.* Springfield, Illinosis, C. C. Thomas (1973)
89 POCHEDLY, C. Prophylactic CNS therapy in childhood acute leukaemia. *American Journal of Pediatric Hematology and Oncology*, **1,** 119 (1979)
90 PRICE, R. A. and JAMIESON, P. A. The central nervous system in childhood leukaemia, II. Subacute leukoencephalopathy. *Cancer*, **35,** 306–318 (1975)
91 PRICE, R. A. and JOHNSON, W. W. The central nervous system in childhood lymphocytic leukaemia. The arachnoid. *Cancer*, **31,** 520 (1973)
92 PRIETS, J. R., RAMSAY, N. K. C., LATCHAW, R. E., LOCKMAN, L. A., HASEGAWA, D. K., COATES, T. D., COCCIA, P. F., EDSON, J. R., NESBIT, M. E. and KRIVIT, W. Thrombotic and haemorrhagic strokes complicating early therapy for childhood acute lymphoblastic leukaemia. *Cancer*, **46,** 1548–1555 (1980)
93 RALL, D. P., BEN, M. and MCCARTHY, D. M. BCNU toxicity and initial clinical trial. *Proceeding of the American Association for Cancer Research*, **4,** 55(1963)
94 RALL, D. P. and ZUBROD, C. G. Mechanisms of drug absorption and excretion. *Annual Reviews in Pharmacology and Toxicology*, **2,** 109 (1962)
95 RAMU, N., POPLACK, D. G., PIZZO, P. A., ADORHATO, B. J. and DI CHISO, G. *New England Journal of Medicine*, **298,** 815–818 (1978)
96 RATCHESEN, R. A. and OMMAYA, A. K. Experience with subutaneous cerebrospinal fluid reservoir. Preliminary report of 60 cases. *New England Journal of Medicine*, **279,** 1025 (1968)
97 REID, H. and MARSDEN, H. B. Gonadal infiltration in children with leukaemia and lymphoma. *Journal of Clinical Pathology*, **33,** 722–729 (1980)
98 RICCARDI, R., CHABNER, B., GLAUBIGER, D., MASTRANGELO, R. and POPLACK, D. Alteration of cerebrospinal fluid pharmacokinetics of cytosine arabinoside by tetrahydrouridine. *Proceedings of the American Association for Cancer Research*, **21,** 641 (1980)
99 RICCARDI, R., HOLCENBERG, J., GLAUBIGER, D. and POPLACK, D. L-asparaginase pharmacokinetics and L-asparaginase in the cerebrospinal fluid (abstract) *Proceedings of the American Society of Clinical Oncology*, **21,** 69 (1980)
100 RIEHM, H., GADNER, H. and WELTE, K. Die West-Berliner Studie zur Behandlung der akuten lymphoblastischen Leukaemie des kindes Erfahrungsbericht nach 6 Jahren. *Klinische Padiatrie*, **189,** 89–102 (1977)
101 ROBERTS, W. C., BODEY, G. P. and WESTLAKE, P. T. The heart in acute leukaemia: a study of 420 autopsy cases. *American Journal of Cardiology*, **21,** 388 (1968)
102 ROSS, J. S. and ELLMAN, L. Leukaemia infiltration of the lungs in the chemotherapeutic era. *American Journal of Clinical Pathology*, **61,** 325–341 (1974)
103 RUSSEL, P. S. and MANCUO, A. P. The biology of tissue transplantation. *New England*

Journal of Medicine Medical Progress Series, **15,** Boston, Little, Brown and Co. (1965)

104 SARKI, J. H., THOMPSON, S. and SMITH, F. Paraplegia following intrathecal chemotherapy. *Cancer*, **29,** 370–374 (1972)

105 SCHAISIN, G., JACQUILLAT, C., WEIL, M. AUCLERC, M. F, DESPREZ CURELY, J. P. and BERNARD, J. Rechute a localisation gonadique au cours des leucemies aigues. 113 cas. *Nouvell Presse Medicale*, **6,** 1029–1032 (1977)

106 SCHAISON, G. Personal communication.

107 SELAWRY, O. S. and ODOM, S. On eradication of leukaemic meningopathy. *Proceedings of the American Association for Cancer Research*, **9,** 62 (1968)

108 SHALET, S. M., BEARDWELL, C. G., MORRIS-JONES, P. H. and PEARSON, D. Growth hormone deficiency after treatment of acute leukaemia in children. *Archives of Disease in Childhood*, **51,** 489 (1976)

109 SHALET, S. M., PRICE, D. A., BEARDWELL, C. G., MORRIS-JONES, P. H. and PEARSON, D. Normal growth despite abnormalities of growth hormone secretion in children treated for acute leukaemia. *CNS Complications of Malignant Disease*, edited by J. Whitehouse and H. E. M. Kay, 202–217. London, Macmillan (1979)

110 SHAW, R. K., MOORE, E. W., FREIREICH, E. J. and THOMAS, L. B. Meningeal leukaemia. A syndrome resulting from increased intracranial pressure in patients with acute leukaemia. *Neurology*, **10,** 823 (1960)

111 SIMONE, J. V., HOLLAND, E. and JOHNSON, W. Fatalities during remission of childhood leukaemia. *Blood*, **39,** 759 (1972)

112 STOFFEL, T. J., NESBIT, M. E. and LEVITT, S. H. Extramedullary involvement of the testes in childhood leukaemia. *Cancer*, **35,** 1203–1211 (1975)

113 STOKES, H. B., O'HARA, C. M., BUCHANAN, R. D. and OLSON, W. H. An improved method for examination of cerebrospinal fluid cells. *Neurology*, **25,** 901–906 (1975)

114 SULLIVAN, M. P. Intracranial complications of leukaemia in children. *Pediatrics*, **20,** 757 (1957)

115 SULLIVAN, M. P., HAGGARD, M. E., DONALDSON, H. H. and KRALL, J. Comparison of the prolongation of remission in meningeal leukaemia with maintenance intrathecal methotrexate and i.v. BCNU. *Proceedings of the American Association for Cancer Research*, **11,** 77 (1970)

116 SULLIVAN, M. P. and HRGOVCIC, M. *Extramedullary Leukemia in Clinical Pediatric Oncology*, edited by W. W. Sutow, T. J. Vietti and D. J. Fernbach, 227–251. St. Louis, Mosby (1973)

117 SULLIVAN, M. P. and HRGOVIC, M. *Extramedullary Leukemia in Clinical Pediatric Oncology*, edited by W. W. Sutow, T. J. Vietti, and D. J. Fernbach, St. Louis, Mosby (1977)

118 SULLIVAN, M. P., HUMPHREY, G. B., VIETTI, T. J., HAGGARD, M. G. and LEE, E. Superiority of conventional intrathecal methotrexate therapy with maintenance over intensive intrathecal methotrexate therapy maintained or radiotherapy (2000–2500 rad tumour dosage) in treatment of meningeal leukaemia. *Cancer*, **35,** 1066 –1073 (1975)

119 SULLIVAN, M. P., PEREZ, C. A., HERRON, J., SILVA-SUISA, M., LAND, V., DYMENT, P. G., CHAN, R. and AYALA, A. G. Radiotherapy (2500 rad) for testicular leukaemia. *Cancer*, **46,** 508–515 (1980)

120 SULLIVAN, M. P., SUTOW, W. W., TAYLOR, H. G. and WILBUR, J. R. Intrathecal (I.T) comination chemotherapy for meningeal leukaemia using methotrexate (MTX) cystosine arabinoside (CA), and hydrocortisone (HDC). *Proceedings of the American Association for Cancer Research*, **12,** 45 (1971)

121 SULLIVAN, M. P., VIETTI, T. J., FERNBACH, D. J., GRIFFITH, K. M., HADDY, T. B. and WATKINS, W. L. Clinical investigations in the treatment of meningeal leukaemia: Radiation therapy regimens vs. conventional intrathecal methotrexate. *Blood*, **34,** 301–319 (1969)

122 SULLIVAN, M. P. and WINDMILLER, J. Side effects of amethopterin (methotrexate) administered intrathecally in the treatment of meningeal leukaemia. *Medical Record and Annals*, **50,** 92 (1966)

123 SWIFT, P. G. F., KEARNEY, P. J., DALTON, R. G., BULLIMORE, J. A., MOTT, M. G. and SAVAGE, D. C. L. Growth and hormonal status of children treated for acute lymphoblastic leukaemia. *Archives of Disease in Children*, **53,** 890 (1978)

124 TALLAL, L., TAN, C., OETTGEN, H., WOLLNER, N., MCCARTHY, M., HELSON, L., BURCHENAL, J., KARNOFSKY, D. and MURPHY, M. L. *E. coli* L-asparaginase in the treatment of leukaemia and solid tumours in 131 children. *Cancer*, **25,** 306 (1970)

125 TAN, C. and OETTGEN, H. Clinical experience with L-asparaginase administered intrathecally. *Proceedings of the American Society for Cancer Research*, **10,** 92 (1964)

126 THOMAS, J. A., JANOSSY, G. and BOLLUM, F. J. (personal commnication)

127 THOMAS, L. B. Pathology of leukaemia in the brain and meninges. P.M. studies of patients with acute leukaemia and of mice given inoculations of L1210 leukaemia. *Cancer Research*, **25,** 1555 (1965)

128 TIEDEMANN, K., CHESSELLS, J. M. and SANDLAND, M. R. Management of testicular relapse in childhood ALL *Proceedings of the Twelfth Meeting of the International Society of Pediatric Oncology* (Budapest, 1980)

129 TILL, M. M., HARDISTY, R. M. and PIKE, M. C. Long survivals in acute leukaemia. *Lancet*, **1,** 534–538 (1973)

130 WANG, J. J. and PRATT, C. B. Intrathecal arabinosyl cytosine in meningeal leukaemia. *Cancer*, **25,** 531–534 (1970)

131 WEST, R. J., GRAHAM-POLE, J., HARDISTY, R. M. and PIKE, M. C. Factors in pathogenesis of central nervous system leukaemia. *British Medical Journal*, **3,** 311–314 (1972)

132 WHITMORE, W. F. and GITTES, R. F. Studies on the prostate and testes as immunologic privileged sites. *Cancer Treatment Reports*, **61,** 217–222 (1977)

133 WILLOUGHBY, M. L. N. Treatment of overt meningeal leukaemia. Results of second MRC meningeal leukaemia trial. *British Medical Journal*, **1,** 864 (1976)

134 WILLOUGHBY, M. L. N. The management of childhood CNS leukaemia. *CNS Complications of Malignant Disease*, edited by J. M. A. Whitehouse, and H. E. M. Kay, 70–79. London, Macmillan (1979)

135 WOLCOTT, G. J., GRUNNET, M. L., LAHEY, M. E. Spinal subdural haematoma in a leukaemia child. *Journal of Pediatrics*, **77,** 1060 (1970)

136 ZUELZER, W. W., RAVINDRANATH Y., LUSHER, J. M., SARNAIK, S. and CONSIDINE, B. IMFRA (intermittent intrathecal methotrexate and fractional radiation) plus chemotherapy in childhood leukaemia. *American Journal of Haematology*, **1,** 191–199 (1976)

5
Significance of immunological cell surface markers in childhood acute lymphoblastic leukemia

James H. Garvin, Jr. and Stephen E. Sallan

INTRODUCTION

Childhood acute lymphoblastic leukemia (ALL) is a heterogeneous group of diseases with differing clinical and laboratory findings. Although the outlook for children with ALL has improved in recent years, resulting in prolonged remission and probable cure for 40–50 percent of patients[28, 43, 64], the remainder relapse on or after cessation of conventional treatment. Analysis of patients who relapse suggests that these children may have biologically distinct forms of the disease. This chapter will discuss the immunological subtypes of ALL and their clinical significance.

LYMPHOBLAST IMMUNOLOGY

Normal lymphocytes and lymphoblasts

Normal lymphocytes are derived from bone marrow stem cell progeny which undergo maturation in the thymus (T cells) or bursal equivalent (B cells). T cells are generally associated with cell-mediated immunity and B cells with antibody production, although important interactions occur between these classes. T cells predominate in the peripheral circulation[33]. Normally, 20 percent of T cells are cytotoxic effector/suppressor cells responsible for cell-mediated lympholysis[21, 59], while the other 80 percent lack this function and serve primarily as helper cells for antibody elaboration, macrophage activation and hematopoietic differentiation[16]. Unaccounted for in this simple definition are the infinite differentiation stages between stem cell and mature lymphocyte. The transforming event from normal progenitor to leukemic cell can occur at any stage.

The recent availability of specific antisera to leukemic blasts has made it possible to classify patients with ALL on an immunological basis.

Diagnostic methods

Table 5.1 lists the cell surface markers on lymphocytes and lymphoblasts. Although morphologically indistinguishable, T cells can be identified by spontaneous rosette formation with sheep erythrocytes[33], and B cells by the presence of surface membrane immunoglobulin[50]. Receptors for complement and the F_c portion of the immunoglobulin molecule are characteristic of B cells but do occur in some T cells[6].

Table 5.1 Cell surface markers on lymphocytes and lymphoblasts

Marker	Cell identified	Other positive cells
Sheep erythrocyte receptor	Thymocytes, T cells, T lymphoblasts	–
Surface membrane immunoglobulin	B cells, B lymphoblasts	Monocytes
F_c receptors	B cells, monocytes	Some T cells
Complement receptors	B cells, monocytes	Some T cells
T cell antigens	Thymocytes, T cells, T lymphoblasts	–
Ia-like antigens	B cells, monocytes, non-T lymphoblasts	Some T cells
Common ALL antigen	Non-T, non-B lymphoblasts	AUL blasts CML blasts

AUL = acute undifferentiated leukemia.
CML = chronic myelogenous leukemia.

T cells specific heteroantisera have been prepared in rabbits against an E-rosette positive variant of ALL[8, 36, 65, 66, 73]. These antisera react only with normal thymocytes, circulating T cells and T lymphoblasts, defining T cell ALL.

An antiserum to the glycoprotein complex p23,30, isolated from a human B cell lymphoblastoid line, is highly specific for B cells and recognizes a human counterpart of the murine Ia (immune response-associated) antigen[8, 13, 65, 66, 73]. The presence of Ia-like antigen on lymphoblasts in patients with non-T, non-B cell ALL suggests that the disease is of pre-B cell origin[11].

Finally, antisera prepared against non-T lymphoblasts can detect a leukemia-associated antigen, the common ALL antigen (cALL or CALLA) in the majority of children with non-T, non-B cell ALL[5, 12, 13, 25, 39, 41, 51, 63]. The common ALL antigen is not expressed on normal adult or fetal lymphocytes and does not appear to be an altered normal antigen or virally induced. The antisera are reactive in certain individuals with acute undifferentiated leukemia (AUL), an entity not otherwise classifiable[4], and also some patients with Philadelphia chromosome positive chronic myelogenous leukemia (CML) in lymphoid blast crisis.

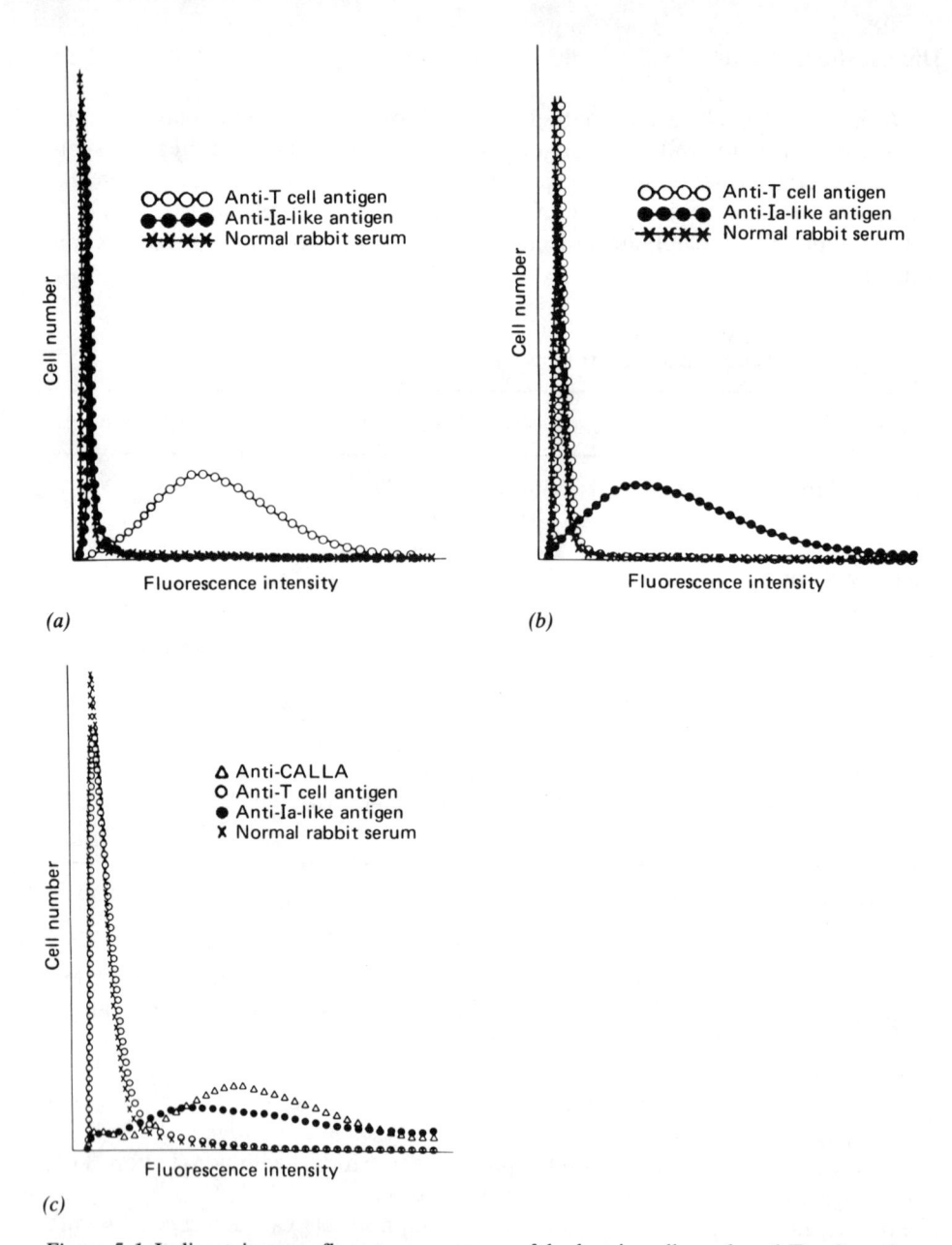

Figure 5.1 Indirect immunofluorescence assay of leukemic cells and anti-T cell antigen, anti-Ia-like antigen, and anti-CALLA using the fluorescence-activated cell sorter for analysis. In each sample, 40 000 cells were counted and presented as a histogram of number of cells versus intensity of fluorescence for each antigen. Normal rabbit serum is used as a negative control in each analysis. (*a*) Leukemic cells are anti-T cell antigen positive, anti-Ia-like antigen negative. (*b*) Leukemic cells are anti-T cell antigen negative, anti-Ia-like antigen positive. (*c*) Leukemic cells are anti-T cell antigen negative, anti-Ia-like antigen positive, anti-CALLA positive

Detection of lymphoblast surface antigens is based on immunofluorescence assay of leukemic cells with the corresponding antisera, using the fluorescence-activated cell sorter[7]. With this technique it is possible to detect leukemic cells of most patients with non-T cell ALL, some with CML lymphoid blast crisis and a few with AUL, while discriminating T cell ALL and acute myelogenous leukemia (AML) (*Figure 5.1*).

The common ALL antigen described by Brown *et al*. (cALL)[12] is variably and weakly expressed by certain non-leukemic cells, including normal bone marrow, fetal hematopoietic tissue, and marrow from children with various severe anemias and non-hematological malignancies. It is also detectable in neonatal leukemoid reactions, post-chemotherapy lymphocytosis and regenerating marrow of transplant recipients, as well as reacting with some T cell leukemic lines and in about 10 percent of T cell ALL patients. The CALLA antiserum[51], extensively absorbed with renewable cells lines, was unreactive with T cells (serologically defined) and did not react with any normal cells tested, including monocytes, stimulated T and B cells, normal and regenerating marrow cells, fetal thymocytes and lymphocytes, or T and B cell or myeloid leukemic cell lines. Monoclonal anti-CALLA antibodies have now been prepared from 'hybridomas'[38] generated *in vitro* by fusion of murine myeloma cells with spleen cells from mice immunized with CALLA positive lymphoblasts. The specificity of these antisera has been confirmed by indirect immunofluorescence assay with panels of leukemic and normal cells[61].

The cALL antigen has been isolated and partially characterized, and shown to be a single glycosylated polypeptide of a molecular weight of 100 000 daltons[70]. The fact that it is expressed in blasts from unrelated patients with at least two distinct types of leukemia (Philadelphia chromosome negative ALL and Philadelphia chromosome positive CML blast crisis) restricts its possible genetic origins and tends to exclude random mutation. The antigen appears to be released by ALL blasts[34], and it may be possible to devise a radioimmunoassay for its detection in serum.

CLINICAL SUBTYPES OF CHILDHOOD ACUTE LYMPHOBLASTIC LEUKEMIA

T cell acute lymphoblastic leukemia

T lymphoblasts, defined by E-rosette formation or reactivity with T cell specific antisera, characterize 15–20 percent of childhood ALL. They also occur in Sezary syndrome[10] and lymphoblastic lymphoma[35]. Numerous studies have confirmed the relatively short duration of remission and survival in T cell ALL compared to non-T cell ALL[13, 20, 64, 73]. The interpretation of results is complex because T cell positivity occurs most often in the clinically unfavorable setting of an older child, most often a boy, with organomegaly, thymic enlargement and an elevated white blood count. Where E-rosette negative but T cell antigen positive blasts have been encountered, the serological definition of T cell ALL has been the better predictor of clinical outcome[2].

Discrete stages of T cell differentiation in thymic 'compartments' can be defined on the basis of reactivity with monoclonal antibodies to T cell subsets[55, 56]. The tumor cells in most cases of T cell ALL are found to arise from the prothymocyte or early thymocyte compartment, and only rarely from the common or mature thymocyte compartment[58, 60]. As anticipated from their early thymic derivation, these leukemic blasts lack demonstrable T cell function compared to the abnormal cells of mature T cell compartment disease, i.e. Sezary syndrome, T cell chronic lymphatic leukemia (CLL) and mycosis fungoides, which may show typical helper or suppressor functions of peripheral T cells[10]. In a separate study, T cell leukemic blasts with higher proportions of F_c receptors appeared to represent more differentiated disease, possibly with a better prognosis[3]; these receptors are lacking in non-leukemic thymocytes[27] but are present on normal mature peripheral T lymphocytes[47].

B cell acute lymphoblastic leukemia

Lymphoblasts with characteristics of B cells, bearing surface membrane immunoglobulin (Sm Ig) detectable by immunofluorescence assay[50], occur in less than 5 percent of children with ALL. There is a clinical, morphological and cytogenetic relationship with Burkitt's lymphoma, and the prognosis is correspondingly very poor[22]. Other well characterized B cell lymphoproliferative disorders, such as CLL, Waldenström's macroglobulinemia and multiple myeloma[1, 52, 54], are exceedingly rare in childhood. However, recognition of a pre-B cell group in which the lymphoblasts have intracytoplasmic immunoglobulin (Cyt Ig) in a perinuclear distribution[11, 74] suggests that pre-B cell ALL is common and that these patients may have a relatively favorable prognosis[18].

The Ia-like antigen is expressed on normal and leukemic B lymphocytes, non-T, non-B cells, certain activated T cells, and also myeloid and erythroid progenitors[15, 29, 32, 37, 57, 76]. These antigens are not necessarily identical or even products of the same genes. Lymphocyte precursors migrating to the thymus to mature along the T cell pathway apparently lose the Ia-like antigen while acquiring T cell antigens. Since the HLA-related Ia-like antigens are critical in the initiation of a mixed lymphocyte response and the generation of cytotoxic T lymphocytes, the absence of these antigens on T cells may provide one of the explanations for the poor prognosis of T cell ALL patients.

Non-T, non-B cell acute lymphoblastic leukemia

About 80 percent of children with ALL have lymphoblasts which do not form E-rosettes, react with T cell specific antisera or bear surface immunoglobulin[13]. Clinical features include younger age, lack of thymic enlargement and organomegaly, and lower median initial white blood counts[45]. The prognosis for this group is relatively favorable compared to T cell patients, but not all patients do well. Elevated white blood count *per se* has been found to be an adverse factor in most

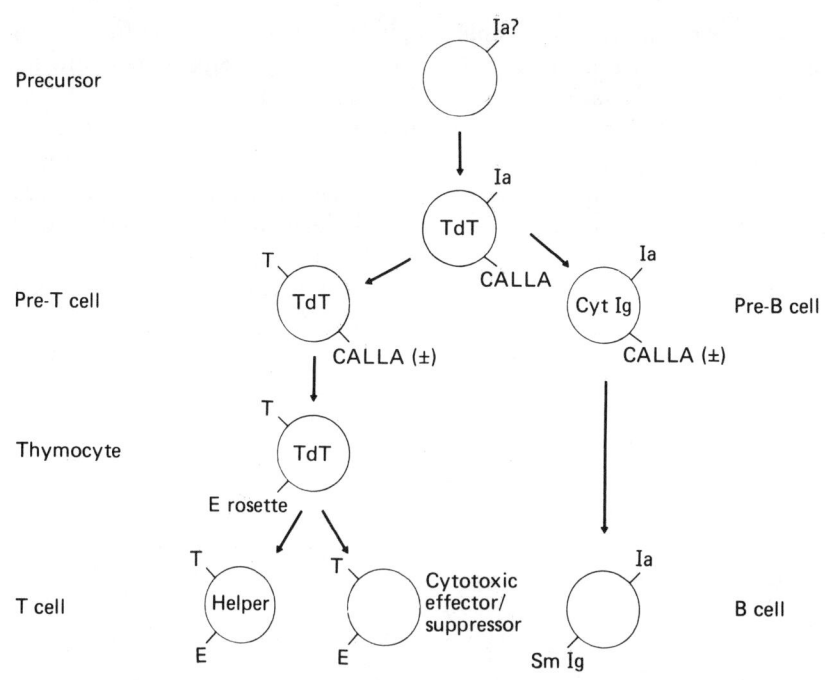

Figure 5.2 Appearance of cell surface markers in lymphocyte differentiation. Ia=Ia-like antigen; TdT = terminal deoxynucleotidyl transferase; CALLA = common ALL antigen; cyt Ig = cytoplasmic immunoglobulin; E = receptor for E-rosette formation with sheep red blood cells; Sm Ig = surface membrane immunoglobulin

studies[13]. Levels of terminal deoxynucleotidyl transferase (Td)[44], an enzyme distinguishing ALL from AML, are highest in non-T, non-B cell ALL[17], but prognostic subgroups have not emerged.

Non-T, non-B cell ALL blasts exhibit the antigenic variability of normal marrow cells[31], and express characteristics of normal prothymocytes (TdT activity[67]) and pre-B cells (Ia-like antigen, cytoplasmic IgM[74]). The common ALL antigen is associated with both T cell and B cell lineages, as seen from analysis of established leukemic cell lines[46], but is expressed at the precursor level and not in more mature T or B cells (*Figure 5.2*).

RESULTS OF TREATMENT

Between 1973 and 1977 cell marker studies were carried out in 93 children with ALL treated at the Children's Hospital Medical Center (CHMC) and the Sidney Farber Cancer Institute (SFCI) and followed from 2 to 6½ years (median 4 years)[64]. Three subsets of patients were defined serologically:

```
T cell+   Ia−   CALLA−
T cell−   Ia+   CALLA+
T cell−   Ia+   CALLA−
```

The T cell positive group were older children, predominantly males, usually with elevated white blood counts and mediastinal masses. Their prognosis was distinctly poorer than that of T cell negative patients. Moreover, the majority of relapses in the T cell positive patients occurred at extramedually sites, whereas extramedullary relapses were unusual in the T cell negative group. The latter were younger children without sex predilection or mediastinal masses. The median disease-free survival is presently undefined, and approximately 50 percent of these children remain in continuous complete remission 4 to 8 years from diagnosis, compared to a median disease-free survival of only 12 months in the T cell positive group ($P=0.001$) (*Figure 5.3*). Multivariate analysis confirmed the prognostic significance of T cell positivity when factors of age and white cell count were controlled.

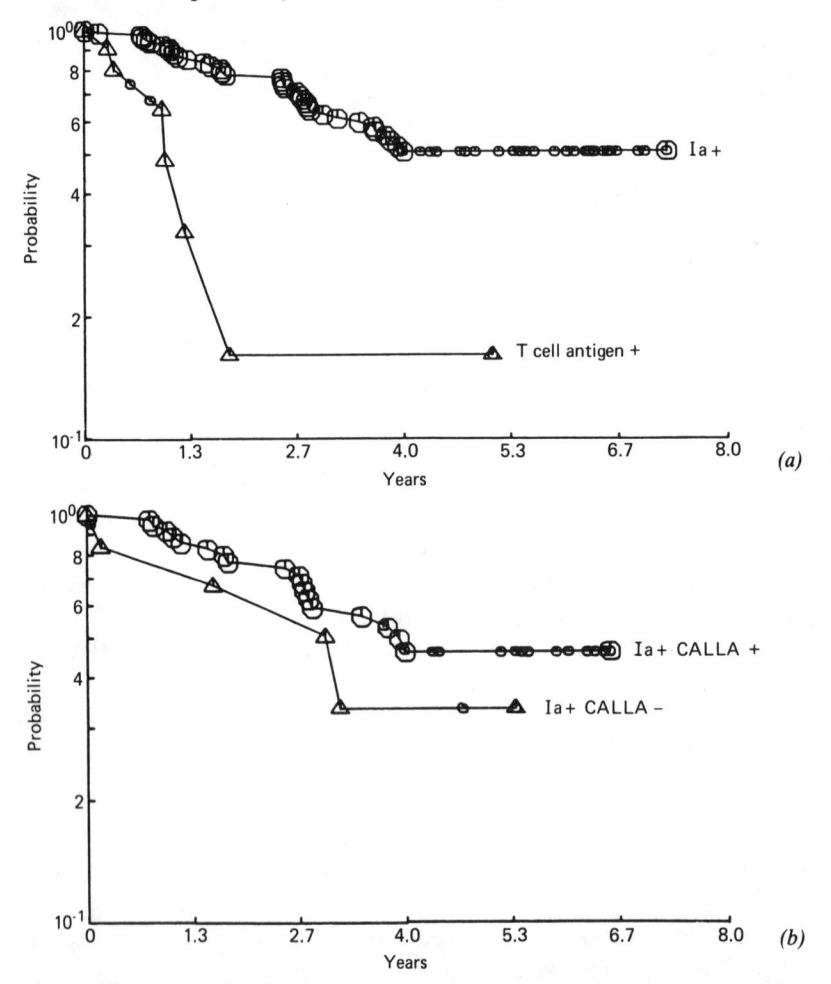

Figure 5.3 Disease-free survival for ALL patients on SFCI protocol 73-001 (64). (*a*) Disease-free survival for 73 Ia+ and 10 T cell antigen + patients. The difference is statistically significant ($P = 0.001$). (*b*) Disease-free survival for 41 Ia+ patients who were also tested for CALLA. Within the Ia+ group, the difference between CALLA+ and CALLA− patients is not statistically significant

Among Ia positive patients tested for CALLA, those who were CALLA positive had somewhat longer median disease-free survival than those who were Ia positive but CALLA negative. Thus, among the non-T cell ALL patients, CALLA negativity suggested a less favorable prognosis compared to the CALLA positive majority. In a subsequent program, 75 children with non-T cell ALL were treated between 1977 and 1979. After a median period of follow-up of 29 months, 46 of 73 evaluable patients are in continuous complete remission and the median time to relapse remains undefined.

With recognition of their poor prognosis, children with T cell ALL now receive more intensive chemotherapy. These patients also undergo thymectomy, and boys receive testicular irradiation. Between 1977 and 1980, 13 patients were entered, but only 3 remained in continuous complete remission for more than 15, 35 and 36 months after diagnosis, and median disease-free survival was only 11 months. Cell sorter analysis of blasts from T cell ALL patients revealed abnormal subset distributions, either exclusively cytotoxic effector/suppressor or exclusively helper cells, and the first group had notably longer survival than the second despite higher white counts[58].

Analysis of cell markers in 94 patients treated at the Hospital for Sick Children in London between 1974 and 1977 revealed 11 with T cell ALL, 2 with B cell ALL, 71 with cALL positive non-T, non-B cell ALL, and 10 with cALL negative non-T, non-B cell ALL[13]. Patients with T cell ALL had a median duration of remission of only 30 weeks, despite more intensive treatment and often prompt initial remission. Those with B cell ALL also fared poorly. Non-T, non-B cell ALL patients who were cALL positive had the best outcome, even in the presence of an elevated white blood count. The cALL negative group had an intermediate prognosis, and children who presented with a mediastinal mass tended to relapse early whereas those without mediastinal enlargement responded like the cALL positive group.

Studies from other large centers[9,48] are confirming that common ALL antigen negativity identifies a subgroup of non-T cell ALL patients with an adverse prognosis. Conversely, the more favorable outcome of common ALL antigen positive patients, even those with elevated white blood counts, confirms the importance of this marker. A related finding emerged from a large study in Germany; half of common ALL antigen positive patients also had T cell antigen detectable by heteroantisera, yet fared as well as or better than cALL positive/T cell negative patients and had significantly longer disease-free survival than cALL negative/T cell positive patients[71].

IMPLICATIONS FOR PATIENT MANAGEMENT

Diagnosis and monitoring of disease

With the identification of an ALL-associated antigen it should be possible to monitor the selective disappearance of leukemic blasts during induction therapy and to confirm continued remission or anticipated relapse. The comparison of lymphoblast markers at diagnosis and relapse generally shows a consistent pattern[26], and lymphoid cell lines *in vitro* usually remain stable in long-term culture. However, more detailed attempts at monitoring disease activity have not yet been entirely successful.

Among a series of patients with cALL positive ALL, AUL or CML blast crisis, followed up to 4 years with bi-monthly bone marrow aspirates, the number of cALL positive cells fell dramatically during induction chemotherapy in all but one[26]. Reappearance of more than 0.5 percent cALL positive blasts heralded relapse in some patients. Others had rapid emergence of blasts without prior increase in marker positivity. Some extramedullary relapses were associated with transient increases in cALL positive marrow cells. Certain patients relapsed with cALL negative blasts, and about 15 percent had 'phenotypic' shifts from cALL positive to negative, or the reverse. In theory, loss of the common ALL antigen in relapse could occur because of selection of an antigen negative mutant or minor pre-existing clone, or because of antibody-induced removal of cell surface antigen[40].

The availability of monoclonal antibodies produced by the hybridoma technique[38] may improve the accuracy of disease monitoring[42]. In addition, multiparameter assessment may allow earlier recognition of impending clinical relapse. For example, reversion to common ALL antigen positivity may be accompanied by increased TdT levels. Similarly, demonstration of premature chromosome condensation in bone marrow cells appears to have predictive value in anticipating relapse[30].

Therapy

Refinement of diagnosis and prognosis has led to new chemotherapy programs directed at specific types of ALL. Conventional therapy has been unsuccessful in maintaining remission in T cell ALL, perhaps due to differences in drug responsiveness of T and B lymphoblasts. For example, methotrexate and 6-mercaptopurine are relatively inactive against thymus-derived AKR murine leukemia in spite of being highly active in non-T cell disease, while cytosine arabinoside and cyclophosphamide show selective activity against the T cell variant[23] and have been incorporated into treatment regimens.

More recently, 2'-deoxycofomycin (DCF), an adenosine deaminase (ADA) inhibitor, has been used to treat patients with relapse T cell ALL[53]. T lymphoblasts have markedly elevated levels of ADA, and inhibition of the enzyme with subsequent accumulation of cytotoxic 2'-deoxyadenosine triphosphate is thought to be a mechanism of action of DCF[24, 68, 69]. In the future, DCF may be used during initial remission induction in T cell patients, with ADA levels measured to assess disease activity, and ultimately patients may be offered transplantation of autologous bone marrow[19] depleted of T lymphoblasts by prior exposure to DCF.

Children with non-T cell ALL who relapse on standard therapy have a poor prognosis with the chemotherapeutic agents available for subsequent treatment[62]. An alternative approach to management is syngeneic or allogeneic bone marrow transplantation. However, this therapy is available only to patients with histocompatible siblings and affords only a 30 percent likelihood of survival[72].

The recent availability of antisera directed against lymphoblasts offers a novel approach to transplantation, namely *in vitro* elimination of leukemic blasts with antileukemic antibodies (such as anti-CALLA antibody) in bone marrow harvested for autologous transplantation. Lack of reactivity with normal marrow cells is an obvious prerequisite. Initial experience showed uniform engraftment of treated marrow, although there was no prolonged survival[75]. Improved results may be anticipated with the development of monoclonal anti-CALLA antibodies and anti-T cell antibodies, assuring specific elimination of leukemic cells. Antibody treatment of bone marrow and peripheral blood from normal volunteers does not diminish expression of myeloid or erythroid progenitors in terms of colony forming units in cell culture[14] and appears not to compromise early lymphoid cells that are possibly important for hematopoietic and immune reconstitution following transplantation[49]. Preliminary observations in the authors' patients show that anti-CALLA antibody treated marrow infused in remission has the capacity to reconstitute patients prepared for transplantation by intensive chemotherapy and total body irradiation.

CONCLUSIONS

Analysis of lymphocyte cell surface markers has refined the diagnosis of childhood ALL and afforded new insights into the cellular origin, clinical heterogeneity and prognosis of this disorder. With the development of monoclonal antibodies to cell surface antigens, future prospects include standardized diagnosis, improved monitoring of disease activity and entirely new approaches to leukemia specific therapy.

References

1 AISENBERG, A. C., BLOCH, K. J. and LONG, J. C. Cell-surface immunoglobulins in chronic lymphocytic leukemia and allied disorders. *American Journal of Medicine*, 55, 184–191 (1973)

2 ANDERSON, J. K., MOORE, J. O., FALLETTA, J. M., TERRY, W. F. and METZGAR, R. S. Acute lymphoblastic leukemia: classification and characterization with antisera to human T-cell and Ia antigens. *Journal of the National Cancer Institute*, 62, 293–298 (1979)

3 BECK, J. D., HAGHBIN, M., WOLLNER, N., MERTELSMANN, R., GARRETT, T., KOZINER, B., CLARKSON, B., MILLER, D., GOOD, R. A. and GUPTA, S. Subpopulations of human T lymphocytes. VI. Analysis of cell markers in acute lymphoblastic leukemia with special reference to Fc receptor expression on E-rosette-forming blasts. *Cancer*, 46, 45–49 (1980)

4 BESSIS, M. Pathology of the leukemic cell, or reasons why some leukemias are unclassifiable. In *Unclassifiable Leukemias*, edited by Bessis, M., Brecher, G. 183–188. Berlin, Springer, (1975)

5 BILLING, R., MINOWADA, J., CLINE, J., CLARK, B. and LEE, K. Acute lymphocytic leukemia-associated cell membrane antigen. *Journal of the National Cancer Institute*, 61, 423–429 (1978)

6 BLOOM, B. R. and DAVID, J. R. (Editors) *In Vitro Methods in Cell-Mediated and Tumor Immunity*, 113–122, 137–142. New York, Academic Press (1976)

7 BONNER, W. A., HULETT, H. R., SWEET, R. G. and HERZENBERG, L. A. Fluorescence activate cell sorting. *Review of Scientific Instruments*, **43**, 404–409 (1972)

8 BORELLA, L., SEN, L. and CASPER, J. T. Acute lymphoblastic leukemia (ALL) antigens detected with antisera to E rosette-forming and non-E rosette-forming ALL blasts. *Journal of Immunology*, **118**, 309–315 (1977)

9 BOWMAN, W. P., MELVIN, S. L., AUR, R. J. A., MAUER, A. M. and NICKSON, J. Patterns of cell membrane markers and clinical prognostic features in acute lymphocytic leukemia (ALL) of childhood. *Proceedings of the American Association for Cancer Research and American Society for Clinical Oncology*, **20**, 156 (1979)

10 BROOME, J. D., ZUCKER-FRANKLIN, D., WEINER, M. S., BIANCO, C. and NUSSENZWEIG, V. Leukemic cells with membrane properties of thymus derived (T) lymphocytes in a case of Sezary's syndrome: morphologic and immunologic studies. *Clinical Immunology and Immunopathology*, **1**, 319–329 (1973)

11 BROUET, J. C., PREUD'HOMME, J. L., PENIT, C., VALENSI, F., ROUGET, P. and SELIGMANN, M. Acute lymphoblastic leukemia with pre-B-cell characteristics. *Blood*, **54**, 269–273 (1979)

12 BROWN, G., HOGG, N. and GREAVES, M. Candidate leukaemia-specific antigen in man. *Nature*, **258**, 454–456 (1975)

13 CHESSELLS, J. M., HARDISTY, R. M., RAPSON, N. T. and GREAVES, M. F. Acute lymphoblastic leukaemia in children: classification and prognosis. *Lancet*, **2**, 1307–1309 (1977)

14 CLAVELL, L. A., LIPTON, J. M. BAST, R. C., Jr., KUDISCH, M., PESANDO, J., SCHLOSSMAN, S. F. and RITZ, J. Absence of common ALL antigen on normal bipotent myeloid, erythroid, and granulocyte progenitors. *Blood*, **58**, 333–336 (1981)

15 CLINE, M. J. and BILLING, R. Antigens expressed by human B lymphocytes and myeloid stem cells. *Journal of Experimental Medicine*, **146**, 1143–1145 (1977)

16 CLINE, M. J. and GOLDE, D. W. Cellular interactions in haematopoiesis. *Nature*, **277**, 177–181 (1979)

17 COLEMAN, M. S., GREENWOOD, M. F., HUTTON, J. J., HOLLAND, P., LAMPKIN, B., KRILL, C. and KASTELIC, J. E. Adenosine deaminase, terminal deoxynucleotidyl transferase (TdT), and cell surface markers in childhood acute leukemia. *Blood*, **52**, 1125–1131 (1978)

18 CRIST, W., VOGLER, L., SARRIF, A., PULLEN, J., BARTOLUCCI, A., FALLETTA, J., HUMPHREY, G. B., VAN EYS, J. and COOPER, M. Clinical and laboratory characterization of pre-B-cell leukemia in children (abstract). *Blood*, **54**, (Suppl. 1), 183a (1979)

19 DICKE, K. A., McCREDIE, K. B., SPITZER, G., ZANDER, A., PETERS, L., VERMA, D. S., STEWART, D., KEATING, M. and STEVENS, E. E. Autologous bone marrow transplantation in patients with adult acute leukemia in relapse. *Transplantation*, **26**, 169–173 (1978)

20 DOW, L. W., BORELLA, L., SEN, L., AUR, R. J., GEORGE, S. L., MAUER, A. M. and SIMONE, J. V. Initial prognostic factors and lymphoblast erythrocyte rosette formation in 109 children with acute lymphoblastic leukemia. *Blood*, **50**, 671–682 (1977)

21 EVANS, R. L., LAZARUS, H., PENTA, A. C. and SCHLOSSMAN, S. F. Two functionally distinct subpopulations of human T cells that collaborate in the generation of cytotoxic cells responsible for cell-mediated lympholysis. *Journal of Immunology*, **120**, 1423–1428 (1978)

22 FLANDRIN, G., BROUET, J. C., DANIEL, M. T. and PREUD'HOMME, J. L. Acute leukemia with Burkitt's tumor cells: a study of six cases with special reference to lymphocyte surface markers. *Blood*, **45**, 183–188 (1975)

23 FREI, E., III, SCHABEL, F. M., Jr and GOLDIN, A. Comparative chemotherapy of AKR lymphoma and human hematological neoplasia. *Cancer Research*, **34**, 184–193 (1974)

24 GIBLETT, E. R., ANDERSON, J. E., COHEN, F., POLLARA, B. and MENWISSEN, H. J. Adenosine deaminase deficiency in two patients with severely impaired cellular immunity. *Lancet*, **2**, 1067–1069 (1972)

25 GREAVES, M. F., BROWN, G., RAPSON, N. T. and LISTER, T. A. Antisera to acute lymphoblastic leukemia cells. *Clinical Immunology and Immunopathology*, **4**, 67–84 (1975)

26 GREAVES, M. PAXTON, A., JANOSSY, G., PAIN, C., JOHNSON, S. and LISTER, T. A. Acute lymphoblastic leukaemia associated antigen. III. Alterations in expression during treatment and in relapse. *Leukaemia Research*, **4**, 1–14 (1980)

27 GUPTA, S. and GOOD, R. A. Subpopulations of human T lymphocytes. III. Distribution and quantitation in peripheral blood, cord blood, tonsils, bone marrow, thymus, lymph nodes, and spleen. *Cellular Immunology*, **36**, 263–270 (1978)

28 HAGHBIN, M., MURPHY, M. L., TAN, C. C., CLARKSON, B. D., THALER, H. T., PASSE, S. and BURCHENAL, J. A long-term clinical follow-up of children with acute lymphoblastic leukemia treated with intensive chemotherapy regimens. *Cancer*, **46**, 241–252 (1980)

29 HALPER, J., FU, S. M., WANG, C. Y., WINCHESTER, R. and KUNKEL, H. G. Patterns of expression of human 'Ia-like' antigens during the terminal stages of B cell development. *Journal of Immunology*, **120**, 1480–1484 (1978)

30 HITTELMAN, W. N., BROUSSARD, L. C., DOSIK, G. and McCREDIE, K. B. Predicting relapse of human leukemia by means of premature chromosome condensation. *New England Journal of Medicine,*, **303**, 479–484 (1980)

31 JANOSSY, G., BOLLUM, F. J., BRADSTOCK, K. F., McMICHAEL, A., RAPSON, N. and GREAVES, M. F. Terminal transferase-positive human bone marrow exhibits the antigenic phenotype of common acute lymphoblastic leukaemia. *Journal of Immunology*, **123**, 1525–1529 (1979)

32 JANOSSY, G., GOLDSTONE, A. H., CAPELLARO, D., GREAVES, M. F., KULENKAMPFF, J., PIPPARD, M. and WELSH, K. Differentiation linked expression of p28, 33 (Ia-like) structures on human leukaemic cells. *British Journal of Haematology*, **37**, 391–402 (1977)

33 JONDAL, M., HOLM, G. and WIGZELL, H. Surface markers on human T and B lymphocytes. I. A large population of lymphocytes forming nonimmune rosettes with sheep red blood cells. *Journal of Experimental Medicine*, **136**, 207–215 (1972)

34 KABISCH, H., ARNDT, R., BECKER, W. M., THIELE, H. G. and LANDBECK, G. Serological detection and partial characterization of the common-ALL-cell associated antigen in the serum of c-ALL patients. *Leukaemia Research*, **3**, 83–91 (1979)

35 KAPLAN, J., MASTRANGELO, R. and PETERSON, W. D., Jr. Childhood lymphoblastic lymphoma, a cancer of thymus-derived lymphocytes. *Cancer Research*, **34**, 521–525 (1974)

36 KERSEY, J. H., SABAD, A., GAJL-PECZALSKA, K., HALLGREN, H. M., YUNIS, E. J. and NESBIT, M. E. Acute lymphoblastic leukemic cells with T (thymus-derived) lymphocyte markers. *Science*, **182**, 1355–1356 (1973)

37 KOEFFLER, H. P., BILLING, R., LEVINE, A. M. and GOLDE, D. W. Ia antigen is a differentiation marker on human eosinophils. *Blood*, **56**, 11–14 (1980)

38 KÖHLER, G. and MILSTEIN, C. Continuous cultures of fused cells secreting antibody of predefined specificity. *Nature*, **256**, 495–497 (1975)

39 KOSHIBA, H., MINOWADA, J., PRESSMAN, D. Rabbit antiserum against a non-T, non-B leukemia cell line that carries the Ph1 chromosome (NALM-1): antibody specific to a non-T, non-B acute lymphoblastic leukemia antigen. *Journal of the National Cancer Institute*, **61**, 987–991 (1978)

40 LAMM, M. E., BOYSE, E. A., OLD, L. J., LISOWSKA-BERNSTEIN, B. and STOCKERT, E. Modulation of TL (thymus-leukemia) antigens by F ab fragments of TL antibody. *Journal of Immunology*, **101**, 99–103 (1968)

41 LEBIEN, T., HURWITZ, R., KERSEY, J. H. Characterization of a xenoantiserum produced against three molar KCL-solubilzed antigens obtained from a non-T, non-B (pre-B) acute lymphoblastic leukemia cell line. *Journal of Immunology*, **122**, 82–88 (1979)

42 LEVY, R., DILLEY, J., FOX, R. I., WARNKE, R. A human thymus-leukemia antigen defined by hybridoma monoclonal antibodies. *Proceedings of the National Academy of Sciences, USA*, **76**, 6552–6556 (1979)

43 MAUER, A. M. Therapy of acute lymphoblastic leukemia in childhood. *Blood*, **56**, 1–10 (1980)

44 McCAFFREY, R., HARRISON, T. A., PARKMAN, R., BALTIMORE, D. Terminal deoxynucleotidyl transferase activity in human leukemic cells and in normal thymocytes. *New England Journal of Medicine*, **292**, 775–780 (1975)

45 MILLER, D. R., PEARSON, H. A., BAEHNER, R. L. and McMILLAN, C. W. (Editors) *Smith's Blood Diseases of Infancy and Childhood*, 593–595. St. Louis, C. V. Mosby, (1978)

46 MINOWADA, J. Markers of human leukemia-lymphoma cell lines reflect hematopoietic cell differentiation. In *International Symposium on Human Lymphocyte Differentiation: Its Application to Cancer*, 337–344. Amsterdam, North-Holland Publishing Co. (1978)

47 MORETTA, L., FERRARINI, M., MINGARI, M. C., MORETTA, A. and WEBB, S. R. Subpopulations of human T cells identified by receptors for immunoglobulins and mitogen responsiveness. *Journal of Immunology*, **117**, 2171–2174 (1976)

48 MORGAN, E. and HSU, C. C. S. Prognostic significance of the acute lymphoblastic leukemia (ALL) cell-associated antigen in children with null-cell ALL. *American Journal of Pediatric Hematology-Oncology*, **2**, 99–102 (1980)

49 NETZEL, B., RODT, H., LAU, B., THIEL, E., HAAS, R. J., DÖRMER, P. and THIERFELDER, S. Transplantation of syngeneic bone marrow incubated with leukocyte antibodies. II. Cytotoxic activity of anti-cALL globulin on leukemic cells and normal hemopoietic precursor cells in man. *Transplantation*, **26**, 157–161 (1978)

50 PAPAMICHAIL, M., BROWN, J. C. and HOLBOROW, E. J. Immunoglobulins on the surface of human lymphocytes. *Lancet*, **2**, 850–852 (1971)

51 PESANDO, J., RITZ, J., LAZARUS, H., COSTELLO, S. B., SALLAN, S. and SCHLOSSMAN, S. F. Leukemia-associated antigens in ALL. *Blood*, **54**, 1240–1248 (1979)

52 PIESSENS, W. F., SCHUR, P. H., MOLONEY, W. C. and CHURCHILL, W. H. Lymphocyte surface immunoglobulins. Distribution and frequency in lymphoproliferative diseases. *New England Journal of Medicine*, **288**, 176–180 (1973)

53 PRENTICE, H. G., SMYTH, J. F., GANESHAGURU, K., WONKE, B., BRADSTOCK, K. F., JANOSSY, G., GOLDSTONE, A. H. and HOFFBRAND, A. V. Remission induction with adenosine-deaminase inhibitor 2′-deoxycofomycin in Thy-lymphoblastic leukaemia. *Lancet*, **2**, 170–172 (1980)

54 PREUD'HOMME, J. L. and SELIGMANN, M. Surface bound immunoglobulins as a cell marker in human lymphoproliferative diseases. *Blood*, **40**, 777–794 (1972)

55 REINHERZ, E. L., KUNG, P. C., GOLDSTEIN, G. and SCHLOSSMAN, S. F. A monoclonal antibody with selective reactivity with functionally mature human thymocytes and all peripheral human T cells. *Journal of Immunology*, **123**, 1312–1317 (1979)

56 REINHERZ, E. L., KUNG, P. C., GOLDSTEIN, G., LEVEY, R. H. and SCHLOSSMAN, S. F. Discrete stages of intrathymic differentiation: analysis of normal thymocytes and leukemic lymphoblasts of T-cell lineage. *Proceedings of the National Academy of Sciences, USA*, **77**, 1588–1592 (1980)

57 REINHERZ, E. L., NADLER, L. M., ROSENTHAL, D. S., MOLONEY, W. C. and SCHLOSSMAN, S. F. T-cell subset characterization of human T-CLL. *Blood*, **53**, 1066–1075 (1979)

58 REINHERZ, E. L., NADLER, L. M., SALLAN, S. E. and SCHLOSSMAN, S. F. Subset derivation of T-cell acute lymphoblastic leukemia in man. *Journal of Clinical Investigation*, **64**, 392–397 (1979)

59 REINHERZ, E. L. and SCHLOSSMAN, S. F. Con A-inducible suppression of MLC: evidence for mediation by the TH_2 + T cell subset in man. *Journal of Immunology*, **122**, 1335–1341 (1979)

60 REINHERZ, E. L. and SCHLOSSMAN, S. F. Regulation of the immune response: inducer and suppressor T-lymphocyte subsets in human beings. *New England Journal of Medicine*, **303**, 370–373 (1980)

61 RITZ, J., PESANDO, J. M., NOTIS-McCONARTY, J., LAZARUS, H. and SCHLOSSMAN, S. F. A monoclonal antibody to human acute lymphoblastic leukaemia antigen. *Nature*, **283**, 583–585 (1980)

62 RIVERA, G., MURPHY, S. B., AUR, R. J., VERZOSA, M. S., DAHL, G. V. and MAUER, A. M. Recurrent childhood lymphocytic leukemia: clinical and cytokinetic studies of cytosine arabinoside and methotrexate for maintenance of second hematologic remission. *Cancer*, **42**, 2521–2528 (1978)

63 RODT, H., NETZEL, B., THIEL, E., JAGER, G., HUHN, D., HAAS, R., GOTZE, D. and THIERFELDER, S. Classification of leukemic cells with T and O-ALL specific antisera. *Haematology and Blood Transfusion*, **20**, 87–96 (1977)

64 SALLAN, S. E., RITZ, J., PESANDO, J., GELBER, R., O'BRIEN, C., HITCHCOCK, S., CORAL, F. and SCHLOSSMAN, S. F. Cell surface antigens: prognostic implications in childhood acute lymphoblastic leukemia. *Blood*, **55**, 395–402 (1980)

65 SCHLOSSMAN, S. F., CHESS, L., HUMPHREYS, R. E. and STROMINGER, J. L. Distribution of Ia-like molecules on the surface of normal and leukemic human cells. *Proceedings of the National Academy of Sciences, USA*, **73**, 1288–1292 (1976)

66 SEN, L. and BORELLA, L. Clinical importance of lymphoblasts with T markers in childhood acute leukemia. *New England Journal of Medicine*, **292**, 828–832 (1975)

67 SILVERSTONE, A. E., CANTOR, H., GOLDSTEIN, G. and BALTIMORE, D. Terminal deoxynucleotidyl transferase is found in prothymocytes. *Journal of Experimental Medicine*, **144**, 543–548 (1976)

68 SMYTH, J. F. and HARRAP, K. R. Adenosine deaminase activity in leukaemia. *British Journal of Cancer*, **31**, 544–549 (1975)

69 SMYTH, J. F., POPLACK, D. G., HOLIMAN, B. J., LEVENTHAL, B. G. and YARBRO, G. Correlation of adenosine deaminase activity with cell surface markers in acute lymphoblastic leukemia. *Journal of Clinical Investigation*, **62**, 710–712 (1978)

70 SUTHERLAND, R., SMART, J., NIAUDET, P. and GREAVES, M. Acute lymphoblastic leukaemia associated antigen. II. Isolation and partial characterisation. *Leukemia Research*, **2**, 115–126 (1978)

71 THIEL, E., RODT, H., HUHN, D., NETZEL, B., GROSS-WILDE, H., GANESHAGURU, K. and THIERFELDER, S. Multimarker classification of acute lymphoblastic leukemia: evidence for further T subgoups and evaluation of their clinical significance. *Blood*, **56**, 759–772 (1980)

72 THOMAS, E. D., SANDERS, J. E., FLOURNOY, N., JOHNSON, F. L., BUCKNER, C. D., CLIFT, R. A., FEFER, A., GOODELL, B. W., STORB, R. and WEIDEN, P. L. Marrow transplantation for patients with acute lymphoblastic leukemia in remission. *Blood*, **54**, 468–476 (1979)

73 TSUKIMOTO, I., WONG, K. Y. and LAMPKIN, B. C. Surface markers and prognostic factors in acute lymphoblastic leukemia. *New England Journal of Medicine*, **294**, 245–248 (1976)

74 VOGLER, L. B., CRIST, W. M., BOCKMAN, D. E., PEARL, E. R., LAWTON, A. R. and COOPER, M. D. Pre-B-cell leukemia. A new phenotype of childhood lymphoblastic leukemia. *New England Journal of Medicine*, **298**, 872–878 (1978)

75 WELLS, J. R., BILLING, R., HERZOG, P., FEIG, S. A., GALE, R. P., TERASAKI, P. and CLINE, M. J. Autotransplantation after in vitro immunotherapy of lymphoblastic leukemia. *Experimental Hematology*, **7**, (Suppl. 5), 164–169 (1979)

76 WINCHESTER, R. J., MEYERS, P. A., BROXMEYER, H. E., WANG, C. Y., MOORE, M. A. and KUNKEL, H. G. Inhibition of human erythropoietic colony formation in culture by treatment with Ia antisera. *Journal of Experimental Medicine*, **148**, 613–618 (1978)

6
Histiocytosis
Stephan Ladisch

INTRODUCTION

The childhood histiocytic syndromes comprise a group of frequently severe diseases which remain poorly understood, especially with respect to their etiologies and pathogenesis. Consequently, therapy has been generally empirical and frequently unsuccessful. It is probably not an understatement to say that this group of diseases represents a major challenge for future study in the area of pediatric oncology.

Perhaps because of the difficulties which the childhood histiocytoses present to the pediatrician, there is an extensive literature on these diseases. This chapter will therefore not attempt to present a detailed summary of clinical, laboratory and pathological observations in childhood histiocytosis, but will emphasize areas of study in which progress has been made in recent years and which appear to be of most importance for future study. Selected references will be given to guide further reading on these topics.

Common to all of the childhood histiocytoses is an infiltration and accumulation of monocytes/macrophages at sites of disease activity. The origin of normal cells of this series is the bone marrow. Following maturation in the marrow, peripheral blood monocytes circulate (with a circulatory half-life of approximately 3 days) and ultimately are found in their final state of maturation, the tissue macrophage, in almost every organ of the body. These 'resident' macrophages are known by various names, the Kupffer cell in the liver, the Langerhans cell in the skin. Since a number of environmental stimuli (notably infection) are recognized as resulting in macrophage accumulation in involved organs, the origin of these infiltrating cells is of critical importance in understanding the pathogenesis of the childhood histiocytoses. To date, no firm direct evidence exists to support the concept that the well differentiated cells of this series (i.e. macrophages) proliferate in the end organs in which they may accumulate. Rather, such accumulations might be more appropriately viewed as the result of homing of effector cells to a site of need, as exemplified by the granulomas in tuberculosis or granulocytic infiltrates in bacterial abcesses. Thus, the only histological criterion which presently can be safely used to characterize an accumulation of macrophages as indicative of a malignant process is identification of the cells themselves as malignant by morphological criteria.

With respect to the role of monocytes/macrophages in host defense mechanisms, two important groups of functions are recognized. One group is 'non-specific'; it includes among others the phagocytic and microbicidal activities, which are well known. The second group includes specific immune functions. These functions, which are becoming increasingly appreciated and understood, include the production of immunoregulatory molecules, collaboration with lymphocytes in the cellular immune response, and engaging in cytotoxic function directed against foreign, tumor and virus-infected cells. For a detailed discussion of monocyte/macrophage properties and functions, the reader is directed to the excellent recent review by Poplack and Blaese[36].

While the most common and perhaps best recognized form of histiocytosis in children is histiocytosis X, there are a number of other syndromes which present diagnostic difficulties in their distinction from histiocytosis X. A review of progress and controversies regarding these syndromes will be a subject of this chapter. Disease processes in which histiocytic infiltrates are observed but accepted as being secondary to a clearly defined primary diagnosis will not be included (e.g. severe combined immunodeficiency disease and the graft-versus-host reaction). Instead, the discussion will focus on the following four disorders: (1) histiocytosis X, (2) familial erythrophagocytic lymphohistiocytosis, (3) maligant histiocytosis and (4) the virus-associated hemophagocytic syndrome.

HISTIOCYTOSIS X

Histiocytosis X is a term generally used to encompass three forms of childhood histiocytosis. The most common of these is eosinophilic granuloma, characterized by single or multiple lytic lesions of the bone. Pathological examination reveals a histiocytic infiltrate mixed with varying proportions of eosinophils and other mononuclear cells. The Hand-Schuller-Christian triad has classically been defined as consisting of the same lesions, diabetes insipidus and proptosis, although the expression of the complete syndrome in an individual patient is rare. Finally, Letterer-Siwe disease is a severe disseminated form of histiocytosis frequently involving multiple internal organs with organ dysfunction. Whether these three syndromes reflect a clinical spectrum of the same pathogenetic process or represent different disease processes is still debated. For this reason controversy exists even over what should be included under the designation histiocytosis X. However, in his original suggestion of the term in 1953, Lichtenstein noted that this was to be only a working term, the letter X serving to underline the lack of understanding of the etiology and pathogenesis of these apparently related disease processes[24]. He felt that the important future direction of study in histiocytosis X should be the delineation of the etiology of this diseases(s). His recommendation remains valuable almost 30 years later.

What is histiocytosis X? Although frequently grouped with neoplastic processes in reviews of pediatric oncology, there is in fact morphological or other evidence of malignancy in the histiocytes characterizing the lesions of histiocytosis X. Presumably, these cells represent a reaction to an unknown etiological agent or process. Given the lack of agreement as to whether the different clinical forms grouped together as histiocytosis X represent related or unrelated disease processes, the various classification systems applied to histiocytosis X represent stratification essentially by clinicopathologic criteria. While this may not invalidate their usefulness in predicting outcome in histiocytosis X, prognostication on this basis remains empirical and difficult. Only with a more basic understanding of histiocytosis X can one expect prognostic classification to be of more certain value.

An attempt at pathological subclassification of histiocytosis X was made by Newton and Hamoudi[30]. They described two types of lesions. The type II (favorable) lesion, almost uniformly observed in the lytic bone lesions of eosinophilic granuloma, revealed histiocytes in a syncytial pattern. Associated with these cells were giant cells and varying proportions of eosinophils. The lesions were focal and necrosis was sometimes observed. In contrast, the type I (unfavorable) lesion consisted of individual histiocytes, and no giant cells, eosinophils or necrosis were visible. The lesions were diffuse. Originally, it was proposed that the type I lesion was associated with Letterer-Siwe disease, while the type II lesion was associated with eosinophilic granuloma, with Hand-Schuller-Christian disease variably expressing type I or type II pathology. Subsequent investigators, however, have failed to confirm the segregation of the clinically severe (Letterer-Siwe) from the clinically mild (eosinophilic granuloma) forms of histiocytosis X on the basis of this pathological subclassification[32], finding the type I lesion generally associated with childhood histiocytic syndromes other than histiocytosis X. Most pathologists now agree that the type I lesion describes true malignant histiocytosis and not severe histiocytosis X[46].

The frequency of infection as the cause of death of children with histiocytosis X has led to histopathological studies of the thymus, searching for a possible thymic basis for immunodeficiency in these patients. In an autopsy study of 29 patients, Hamoudi et al.[11] delineated three patterns of thymic involvement. Four patients each demonstrated thymic involution and thymic dysplasia, the latter similar to that seen in congenital thymic dysplasia. The remaining 21 patients had dysmorphic changes with prominent histiocytic-fibrohistiocytic infiltration. Though this was an autopsy study of patients who had received therapy, Osband et al.[35] have recently confirmed the presence of thymic abnormalities by biopsy in five of seven newly diagnosed untreated children with histiocytosis X. Whether the patterns of thymic involvement will prove to be of prognostic value and to what extent these findings are linked to the immunological findings in histiocytosis X remain to be elucidated.

Another recent approach to pathological classification of histiocytosis X has been the estimation of the degree of infiltration of the lesions by eosinophils. Fredericksen and Thommesen[9] examined bone biopsies of affected areas of 27 patients diagnosed as having histiocytosis X with osseous lesions. The lesions of 10 patients had what the authors considered *marked* eosinophilic infiltration. None of the 10 were found to have extraosseous disease, and all 10 survived. In contrast, 11 of the 17 patients with only *mild* eosinophilic infiltration of the biopsied lesions also were found to have extraosseous disease. Nine of the 17 patients died. Neither extent of disease nor survival were clearly correlated to the degree of either lymphocytic or histiocytic infiltration of the lesions. Therefore, the conclusion of the study, which warrants confirmation by others, was that the degree of eosinophilic infiltration of bone lesions may constitute a criterion for the staging of histiocytosis X with respect to prognosis and extent of disease. The findings also provide indirect evidence supporting the hypothesis of an importance of the immune response in the pathogenesis and outcome of this disease.

It is becoming increasingly recognized that the one histopathological feature commonly and possibly uniformly present in histiocytosis X lesions is the electronmicroscopic finding of Langerhans granules[4] in the infiltrating histiocytic cells. These granules, also seen in normal Langerhans cells of the epidermis, but only rarely in other histiocytes, are straight or curved rods found almost exclusively in the cytoplasm of the affected cells[3]. To place the potential significance of these granules in perspective, both the nature of the granules and the functions of the normal cell (Langerhans cell) in which they are prominent have been studied. Although the ultrastructural detail has been well described, the nature of the granule remains a mystery. However, extensive evidence, recently comprehensively reviewed[44], indicates that the epidermal Langerhans cell is a terminally differentiated cell of the monocyte/macrophage series capable of performing immunological functions normally associated with other cells of this series. These include, for example, antigen binding, antigen presentation of lymphocytes and ability to induce the mixed lymphocyte reaction. Since electronmicroscopic evidence suggests a plasma membrane origin of Langerhans granules, it has been postulated that the granules represent structural membrane alterations caused by antigenic challenge and that such a challenge may underlie the development of histiocytosis X[25].

The true histiocytic origin of the cells seen in the lesions of histiocytosis X is no longer disputed. Surface membrane markers and functional properties, including both non-specific and F_c-receptor mediated phagocytosis, are shared by both normal monocytes/macrophages and the Langerhans granule-positive histiocytosis X cells isolated from patients with eosinophilic granuloma[31] and Letterer-Siwe disease[7]. Detailed morphological, histochemical and functional studies of the histiocytosis X cell are discussed in a recent review of this subject by Nezelof[33]. He concludes with the hypothesis that presence of the Langerhans granule defines a certain state of differentiation and functional maturity of a subset of cells of the monocyte/macrophage series, and that histiocytosis X represents an unusual accumulation of these cells, the stimulus for which is not yet known. It would appear that a better understanding of the Langerhans granule might be a key to the understanding of the pathogenesis of histiocytosis X.

The prominence in lesions of histiocytosis X of the macrophage, with its important immunological functions, has led some authors to propose that histiocytosis X is associated with disordered immunological function and/or immunoregulation. Leikin et al.[23] assessed the immunocompetence of 13 children with histiocytosis X, including 6 infants with Letterer-Siwe disease. Delayed hypersensitivity, lymphocyte blastogenic responses to mitogens and allogeneic cells, bacterial killing and leukocyte nitroblue tetrazolium dye reduction were normal. Isolated mild defects in the above parameters noted in several patients generally improved following chemotherapy. The authors therefore concluded that there is no evidence of a combined immunodeficiency disorder being associated with histiocytosis X. A larger study by the Children's Cancer Study Group confirmed these initial findings. The only frequent abnormality was the finding of increased serum IgM levels (in 67 percent of 49 patients studied)[22]. Finally, Thommeson et al.[42] have documented normal lymphocyte proliferative responses to mitogens in eight patients with eosinophilic granuloma and Hand-Schuller-Christian disease.

Recent findings of marked immunological abnormalities in familial erythrophagocytic histiocytosis (FEL)[14] and the prominent involvement of the macrophage in the pathological lesions of histiocytosis X have led to study of macrophage-dependent immune responses in histiocytosis X[15]. These studies of a small number of patients suggest that children with acute disseminated (Letterer-Siwe) disease have impaired lymphocyte proliferative responses to soluble specific antigens as well as plasma-mediated suppression of normal lymphocyte proliferative responses. In contrast, patients with solitary or multiple eosinophilic granulomas or the Hand-Schuller-Christian syndrome appear to have neither of these abnormalities. Increasing evidence of an immunoregulatory function of lipids and the consistent finding of hyperlipidemia in FEL (to be discussed later) led to quantitation of the circulating lipid level in these patients with histiocytosis X as well. These studies revealed moderate hypertriglyceridemia (plasma triglycerides of 150–300 mg%), apparently confined to those patients diagnosed as having Letterer-Siwe disease[16]. Whether the findings of depressed specific cellular immune function, hyperlipidemia and a plasma suppressor factor will reliably segregate the forms of histiocytosis X is the subject of a larger study being carried out at the present time.

Most recently, Osband et al. have evaluated patients with histiocytosis X for the presence of defective immunoregulation, as indicated by autocytotoxicity[35]. They obtained evidence of immunological autoreactivity in 12 of 17 patients tested; seven expressed lymphocyte cytotoxicity against autologous fibroblasts and seven had a circulating antibody to autologous erythrocytes. These *in vitro* findings were associated with a relative deficiency of circulating suppressor T lymphocytes *in vivo*. *In vitro* incubation of patient peripheral blood mononuclear cells with a crude thymic extract caused resolution of the autocytotoxicity, a result confirmed *in vivo* by administration of thymic extract. Clinical response is more difficult to evaluate, but a striking difference between the overall response of patients treated with thymic extract and historical controls (treated by chemotherapy and untreated) was not reported. However, as suggested by the authors, further studies should be undertaken since a clinical response in association with correction of the immunoregulatory imbalance they described would add further evidence for an immunological pathogenesis of histiocytosis X.

The definition of appropriate therapy is justifiably the major issue confronting physicians who care for children with histiocytosis X. Since Lahey[19] demonstrated in 1962 that the prognosis was not as hopeless as generally appreciated and suggested that therapy did in fact influence overall outcome, numerous investigators have attempted to improve the outcome by varied therapeutic approaches.

Histiocytosis

It is well recognized that unifocal and possibly multifocal eosinophilic granuloma (without extraosseous sites of involvement) is a self-limiting process with essentially no mortality and little morbidity. A recent review of the literature regarding the outcome of 686 patients with eosinophilic granuloma documents this point[41]. However, while the consensus appears to be that rather aggressive cytotoxic chemotherapy may be of benefit in the severe forms of histiocytosis X, there is little agreement about the details of the approach to treatment. Furthermore, no clear documentation of an effect of chemotherapy is available. The small size of most studies and the lack of agreement over a staging system complicate the evaluation of therapy.

To present an overview of the current status of outcome in histiocytosis X, the survival data of patients reported in nine arbitrarily selected articles have been compiled. These nine studies included 433 patients of whom 317 (72 percent) survived. Excluding patients identified by the authors of the original reports or determined from the clinical data presented as having monostotic eosinophilic granuloma, there were 391 patients with 'generalized' histiocytosis of whom 278 (71 percent) survived (*Table 6.1*, column A).

In order to estimate differences in survival among certain subgroups of patients with histiocytosis X, and to compare the survival statistics of different reports, an effort was made to classify patients into three groups (B, C and D in *Table 6.1*).

Table 6.1 Survival in histiocytosis X

Period	Reference	%Survival A	B	C	D
			(number of surviving patients/total number of patients)		
Prior to 1957	34	61 (23/38)	95 (16/17)	44 (7/16)*	33 (2/6)
Prior to 1957	2	81 (25/31)	100 (9/9)	86 (25/29)	0 (0/2)
1949–1969	6	82 (36/44)		100 (44/44)	0 (0/12)
1952–1978	32	52 (26/50)†		59 (20/34)	38 (6/16)
Prior to 1971	13	78 (52/67)†	100 (8/8)	91 (39/43)	54 (13/24)**
1966–1975	20	71 (59/83)	§	98 (48/50)	33 (11/33)
1969–1978	43	80 (20/25)	100 (5/5)	90 (18/20)	40 (2/5)
1970s	21	68 (19/28)	100 (7/7)	68 (19/28)	§
1970s	12	72 (18/25)	100 (1/1)	91 (10/11)	54 (7/13)
Total		71 (278/391)	98 (46/47)	76 (138/181)	37 (41/111)

A = All histiocytosis X, excluding monostotic eosinophilic granuloma.
B = 'Mild' – polyostotic eosinophilic granuloma, and monostotic eosinophilic granuloma not separated from polyostotic disease in the original report.
C = 'Moderate' – soft tissue involvement without organ dysfunction (includes Hand-Schuller-Christian disease).
D = 'Severe' – organ dysfunction, Letterer-Siwe disease.
* Oberman placed patients with clinical Letterer-Siwe syndrome but *with* bone lesions into the intermediate group II (C in this table); the 44% survival in group C is thus lower than expected in comparison with other studies where such patients are placed in group D on the basis of organ dysfunction.
† Polyostotic eosinophilic granuloma also excluded.
§ Excluded from study.
** Defines any patient with soft-tissue involvement only as 'severe'. A patient with diabetes insipidus and skin lesions only would fall in group D rather than group C, as in most other studies. The 54% figure may therefore overestimate survival in the 'severe' group.

Categorization of patients into one of these groups was based upon stated diagnosis and/or clinical information included in the original reports. While the stratification used is arbitrary and not universally accepted, it does allow certain general observations.

As previously reported[41] and generally well known, 'mild' histiocytosis, i.e. single or multiple eosinophilic granuloma without initial extraosseous involvement (column B) is characterized by essentially no mortality (98 percent survival). With soft tissue involvement but no organ dysfunction at diagnosis (this group generally includes Hand-Schuller-Christian disease), there was an overall mortality of 24 percent in 181 patients (column C). In contrast, 'severe' histiocytosis X (defined by the presence of organ dysfunction, or by the names acute disseminated histiocytosis X or Letterer-Siwe disease) shows a much higher mortality of 63 percent (column D).

Combining survival data of patients with the relatively mild forms (columns B and C) yields a survival figure of 86 percent (276/322). Since these 322 patients comprise almost three quarters of all the patients with generalized histiocytosis X in this table, the need to separate the small group with much lower survival (D) for purposes of analysis of treatment results should be clear. Restated, to report survival rates in histiocytosis X as a single figure is meaningless since such a figure will reflect primarily the relative numbers of patients included in a given study with disease of varying degrees of severity, and reflect only secondarily the efficacy of the therapy being tested. Numerous recent treatment reports, including some in *Table 6.1*, have delineated staging systems and given clinical data which allow the stratification of patients according to degree of disease activity. However, only rarely have these been used in the analysis of treatment results of the same study. The most likely explanation for this irony appears to be that the number of patients in each group was too small to allow confident conclusions regarding the effectiveness of therapy.

Another observation can be made concerning the effect of therapy in these studies, spanning a 60-year period. In spite of the variety of treatments used in these studies, there appear to be no striking differences in survival, and no clear trend of increased survival over the last half century emerges. Admittedly, the numbers are small, and perhaps a comprehensive review of all reported results would be a useful undertaking. Also, while survival (an absolute criterion of response) was chosen for preparing the table, clinical response as judged by specific, standardized criteria could be used for such an analysis. Despite these qualifications of the analysis, it would seem that not all that much progress has been made in effectively treating histiocytosis X.

Therefore, without improved understanding of the agent or process resulting in the development of histiocytosis X, it might be prudent to limit the amount of cytotoxic therapy used as much as possible, as has been suggested by others. Review of the literature, as exemplified by *Table 6.1*, does not indicate clear superiority of one cytotoxic chemotherapeutic regimen over another. Conclusions drawn in individual reports regarding improvements in therapy should be reviewed very critically since only results of adequately stratified treatment studies should be compared with each other.

Finally, lack of stratification may impart a direct risk to patients. Overall results may be biased by 'good response' of patients who really have mild disease which might have resolved spontaneously. Thus, children with relatively good prognosis could be exposed to an unwarranted risk of either acute or chronic drug effects of aggressive therapeutic regimens. To summarize, definition of the etiology and pathogenesis, careful diagnosis, pretreatment stratification, and the development and application of realistic response criteria are all necessary elements in attempts to improve the outcome in histiocytosis X.

FAMILIAL ERYTHROPHAGOCYTIC LYMPHOHISTIOCYTOSIS

Although rare, familial erythrophagocytic lymphohistiocytosis (FEL), first described by Farquhar and Claireaux[8], is almost always rapidly fatal. FEL demonstrates an autosomal recessive pattern of inheritance although no genetic marker has yet been identified. The pathogenesis of FEL is not understood. Clinically the disease is characterized by generalized symptoms and laboratory findings remarkably similar to those found in the Letterer-Siwe form of histiocytosis X and in malignant histiocytosis. A unique coagulation abnormality frequently results in fatal bleeding diatheses[28]. Pathological features distinguish FEL from these other syndromes. Mixed lymphohistiocytic infiltration of almost every organ, including the central nervous system, may be seen. The histiocytes in these infiltrates are morphologically normal, without malignant features. Marked phagocytosis by these cells of all peripheral blood elements, but especially erythrocytes, is the striking feature.

Two additional features of FEL, hyperlipidemia and defective immune function, are now recognized to be constant findings in FEL. First noted in FEL in 1965[29], hyperlipidemia was recently documented in all of four patients with active FEL[14]. The uniformity of this lipid abnormality, characterized by plasma triglyceride levels frequently above 500 mg%, has now been further confirmed[1, 18, 40]. Resolution of the hyperlipidemia in patients experiencing temporary clinical remission[1, 17] suggests that the hyperlipidemia is a secondary phenomenon, but its mechanism is not known. Nevertheless, the association of immunological dysfunction and hyperlipidemia in FEL[14], coupled with a now well appreciated role of lipids in regulation of the immune response, indicates that further studies of the hyperlipidemia of FEL might increase understanding of the pathogenesis of the disease.

The clinical resemblance of FEL to some immunodeficiency states has prompted investigation of immune function in FEL. Until recently, only isolated immunological defects had been reported. However, a comprehensive immunological study of four children with FEL has documented a previously unrecognized immunodeficiency syndrome which includes defects in both humoral and cellular immunity, and a plasma inhibitor of *in vitro* lymphocyte blastogenesis[14]. The cellular defects included skin test anergy and significant depression of lymphocyte proliferative responses, particularly in response to specific antigens. T cell cytotoxic effector function and antibody-dependent cellular cytotoxic effector function (by both K cells and monocytes) were impaired. Defects in humoral immunity included low resting antibody titers from previous immunizations (diptheria and tetanus) as well as poor ability to respond to primary immunization, particularly with pneumococcal polysaccharide. Natural antibody titers were also depressed. The plasma of patients with FEL caused suppression of normal lymphocyte proliferative responses to specific antigens *in vitro*, in relation to the degree of hypertriglyceridemia previously discussed. Unpublished studies of additional patients[18] and a recently published report[1] have confirmed the association of immunodeficiency with FEL. The possible role of immunodeficiency in the actual pathogenesis of the disease remains to be defined.

Treatment results in FEL have been dismal[37]. Most therapeutic regimens have employed cytotoxic/immunosuppressive chemotherapy without success. In individual cases, such therapy has resulted in partial or complete but temporary remissions[1, 26, 48]. However, the disease relapses in almost all cases, with lymphohistiocytic infiltrates present at autopsy. The very poor prognosis for children with FEL has resulted in a search for alternative approaches to therapy.

One such approach was based on the associated findings of immunodeficiency, plasma-mediated immunosuppression, and hyperlipidemia in FEL. These findings led to the hypothesis that a circulating factor with immunosuppressive activity could have a central role in the pathogenesis of the immunodeficiency in FEL. The resultant therapeutic approach has been to attempt to decrease plasma immunosuppressive activity and hyperlipidemia by multiple blood exchanges. Three patients with positive family histories and biopsy-proven FEL have been treated in this way[17, 18]. Complete clinical remission, associated with correction of the hyperlipidemia and complete recovery of immunological function, occurred in two of the three patients, including one who had never received steroids or cytotoxic chemotherapy. Subsequently however, both patients relapsed and died. While exchange therapy as used in these three cases is therefore not completely effective, the observations made during treatment allow several tentative conclusions to be drawn regarding the pathogenesis of FEL. First, the immunodeficiency is not a primary phenomenon but associated with the disease process. This was demonstrated by the complete recovery of immunological function during remission in two of the children, an observation which has recently found some support. Secondly, since one of the children never received cytotoxic chemotherapy, radiation therapy or steroids, it appears that the repeated removal of plasma (containing an as yet unidentified factor) is associated with complete remission of the disease process. The results provide evidence favoring the hypothesis suggested above, i.e. that a circulating factor is an important element in the pathogenetic evolution of FEL. Furthermore, they support the concept that the histiocytic proliferation in FEL is reactive and not autonomous, since clinical remission was confirmed by biopsy in one patient.

In conclusion, the occurrence of remission without the use of cytotoxic or immunosuppressive therapy allows the hope that in FEL, as in histiocytosis X, a better understanding of pathogenesis may ultimately lead to effective therapy for this disease.

MALIGNANT HISTIOCYTOSIS

Among the childhood histiocytoses, malignant histiocytosis (also known as histiocytic medullary reticulosis) is the only syndrome in which a large proportion of the histiocytes seen on pathological examination are neoplastic by morphological criteria. It should be emphasized that this disease is the only childhood histiocytosis in which the use of the term malignant (in its pathological meaning) is justified. Some confusion exists in the literature because severe histiocytosis X (Letterer-Siwe disease) has also variably been called malignant histiocytosis or malignant histiocytosis X. This use of the term 'malignant' in defining histiocytosis X should be abandoned.

Malignant histiocytosis is usually seen in older children or young adults[45]. However, the disease has been described in very young children. In the latter group, the clinical features, including fever, wasting, lymphadenopathy and organomegaly, as well as skin lesions and peripheral blood cytopenia, make the clinical distinction between this disease and both FEL and severe histiocytosis X difficult at times. However, the tumor cells should be readily distinguished pathologically from cells seen in the lesions of histiocytosis X and FEL[10].

Malignant histiocytosis is the only childhood histiocytic syndrome in which cytotoxic chemotherapy can be considered the proven treatment of choice. Although earlier results indicated a very poor prognosis for this disease, a recent study reported that 12 of 13 children receiving combination chemotherapy with vincristine, prednisone, cyclophosphamide and doxorubicin (Adriamycin) entered complete remission, and 9 of 13 have remained in complete remission for a period of 21 to more than 46 months[38]. Eight of these nine children were no longer receiving therapy. A probable central importance of doxorubicin (Adriamycin) in treatment regimens for malignant histiocytosis was suggested. This was confirmed by a second study, in which 75 percent disease-free survival was achieved among patients whose treatment included Adriamycin[49]. Overall, it appears that with appropriate therapy, significant long-term disease-free survival may be achieved in malignant histiocytosis, which is therefore the one childhood histiocytosis in which a beneficial effect of cytotoxic chemotherapy has been clearly documented.

VIRUS-ASSOCIATED HEMOPHAGOCYTIC SYNDROME

The final form of childhood histiocytosis to be discussed in this chapter is the virus-associated hemophagocytic syndrome (VAHS), recently defined in 19 patients by Risdall et al.[39]. Clinical features and laboratory findings include fever, constitutional symptoms, liver function and coagulation abnormalities, and peripheral blood cytopenias. In addition, patients had hepatosplenomegaly, lymphadenopathy, pulmonary involvement and frequently a skin rash. The syndrome was associated with proven active viral infection. Viral culture revealed herpes group viral infection in 14 patients and adenovirus infection in one. Biopsies showed histiocytic hyperplasia with hemophagocytosis. However, the infiltrating histiocytic cells had no malignant or neoplastic features. Clinically, this syndrome occurring in a young child could be easily confused with FEL, malignant histiocytosis or Letterer-Siwe disease. However, its pathological features should easily distinguish it from these other three syndromes.

As stressed by Risdall et al.[39], making the correct diagnosis is absolutely essential. Misdiagnosis as one of the other forms of childhood histiocytosis, which are still frequently treated with chemotherapy, could result in death of the patient by allowing a viral infection to overwhelm the host. In the original study[39], once the syndrome was recognized, no further immunosuppressive therapy was given to the patients, who were now classified as having a primary diagnosis of viral infection. Complete recovery occurred in 13 of the originally reported 19 patients.

Since the original report, VAHS has been diagnosed in additional patients. These include patients with chronic lymphocytic leukemia[27], a child with mucocutaneous lymph node syndrome[5], an infant[18] and a young adult[47] with serological evidence of Epstein-Barr viral infection and a newborn with disseminated herpes virus infection[18].

Many of the above cases occurred in patients who might have been expected to be immunosuppressed prior to the onset of the syndrome. Thus, recognition of this syndrome, most frequently occurring in immunosuppressed hosts, is critical to making the decision *not* to treat this histiocytic proliferation with cytotoxic chemotherapy.

SUMMARY AND CONCLUSIONS

Our understanding and treatment of the childhood histiocytoses is in need of great improvement. One problem lies in the need for more exacting criteria for differential diagnosis, or alternatively for more exacting and consistent application of the criteria that already exist. Discrimination between the various syndromes should be possible, however, by careful pretreatment evaluation, including determination of the morphological characteristics of the infiltrating histiocytes. Some features distinguishing the severe forms of childhood histiocytosis from each other are summarized in *Table 6.2*.

It seems extremely important that in studies of histiocytosis X, patients be stratified (prior to treatment) according to the severity of the disease. Probably even more important than a particular system of stratification would be the universal acceptance of such a scheme, thus allowing comparisons between different treatments. A rigid set of universally accepted criteria for the evaluation of response in histiocytosis X is also needed. Finally, despite the rarity of these diseases, randomization of patients between a new treatment and previously accepted treatments, and possibly no treatment at all, would seem to be essential. The recent treatment of histiocytosis X with thymic extract exemplifies this point[35]. When the authors compared their results with the outcome of treated or untreated historical matched controls, they found only a slight improvement, not amenable to statistical analysis, associated with the new treatment.

This chapter will close with a theoretical consideration of the approach to treatment of the childhood histiocytoses. Although a presumed proliferation and

Table 6.2 Characteristic features of severe childhood histiocytic syndromes

	Letterer-Siwe disease	FEL	Malignant histiocytosis	VAHS
Morphological findings				
Degree of histiocytic infiltration	+	+++	+++	+++
Degree of erythrophagocytosis	+	+++	+++	+++
Morphological evidence of malignancy	−	−	+	−
Langerhans granules in histiocytes	+	−	−	−
Immunological Studies				
Cellular immunity	↓	↓		
Plasma suppressor factor	+	+		
Humoral immunity	normal	↓		
Monocyte effector function	normal	↓		
Autocytotoxicity	+			
Other				
Familial occurrence	−	+	−	−
Hyperlipidemia	+	+++		

observed accumulation of histiocytes is the prominent pathological finding, there is no evidence that this accumulation is neoplastic except in malignant histiocytosis. Thus, if the prominent cells in the other childhood histiocytoses represents a reaction (whether normal or abnormal) and not the fundamental disease process, then therapy must be directed at the etiological process and not at the finding of a histiocytic infiltrate. The first implication of this concept is that cytotoxic chemotherapy, while resulting in transient clinical and pathological responses, may not be the ultimate therapy for these diseases. It is conceivable that these transient responses are due to the effect of cytotoxic chemotherapy on the histiocytic accumulations without affecting the disease process itself, thereby providing a logical explanation for 'relapse'. Also, cytotoxic therapy is frequently immunosuppressive. Since disordered immune function has been observed in several of the histiocytoses, further treatment-induced immunosuppression may be harmful.

An example of the potential adverse effect of cytotoxic therapy is the virus-associated hemophagocytic syndrome, in which such treatment could logically be expected to result in a poor outcome by allowing viral dissemination. The extent to which these considerations are important in histiocytosis X is not known, although autopsy studies have frequently documented 'no residual disease', the presumed or proven cause of death being infection associated with an immunosuppressed state. Without clear evidence that intensive cytotoxic chemotherapy is altering the overall outcome of this disease, the finding of death from presumed side-effects of this therapy is of grave concern. It would therefore appear prudent to attempt to limit therapy of the non-malignant histiocytoses pending better knowledge of their etiologies and pathogenesis.

Acknowledgement

Portions of the author's work cited were supported by Clinical Research Grant 6-268 from the March of Dimes Birth Defects Foundation.

References

1 AMBRUSO, D. R., HAYS, T., ZWARTJES, W. J., TUBERGEN, D. G. and FAVARA, B. E. Successful treatment of lymphohistiocytic reticulosis with phagocytosis with epipodophyllotoxin VP 16-213. *Cancer*, **45**, 2516–2520 (1980)

2 AVERY, M. E., McAFEE, J. G. and GUILD, H. G. The course and prognosis of reticuloendotheliosis (eosinophilic granuloma, Schuller-Christian disease and Letterer-Siwe disease). *American Journal of Medicine*, **22**, 636–652 (1957)

3 BASSET, F. and NEZELOF, C. L'Histiocytose X microscopie électronique. Culture in vitro et histoenzymologie: discussion à propos de 21 cas. *Revue Française de'Études Cliniques et Biologiques*, **14**, 31–45 (1969)

4 BIRBECK, M. S., BREATHNACH, A. S. and EVERALL, J. D. An electron microscopic study of basal melanocytes and high level clear cells (Langerhans' cell) in vitiligo. *Journal of Investigative Dermatology*, **37**, 51–64 (1961)

5 BISHOP, J. W., MARSH, W. L. and KOENIG, H. M. Hemophagocytic syndrome in kawasaki disease. *Clinical Research*, **28**, 111A (1980)

6 DANESHBOD, K. and KISSANE, J. M. Idiopathic differentiated histiocytosis. *American Journal of Clinical Pathology*, **70**, 381–389 (1978)

7 ELEMA, J. D. and POPPEMA, S. Infantile histiocytosis X (Letterer-siwe disease). *Cancer*, **42**, 555–565 (1978)

8 FARQUHAR, J. W. and CLAIREAUX, A. E. Familial haemophagocytic reticulosis. *Archives of Diseases of Children*, **27**, 519 (1952)

9 FREDERIKSEN, P. and THOMMESEN, P. Histiocytosis X. II. Histologic appearance correlated to prognosis and extent of disease. *Acta Radiologica Oncologica*, **17**, 10–16 (1978)

10 HUHN, D. and MEISTER, P. Malignant histiocytosis: morphologic and cytochemical findings. *Cancer*, **42**, 1341–1349 (1978)

11 HAMOUDI, A., NEWTON, W. and MANCER, K. Thymus morphology in 'histiocytosis X' (meeting abstract). *Laboratory Investigation*, **38**, 386 (1978)

12 KOMP, D. M., VIETTI, T. J., BERRY, D. H., STARLING, K. A., HAGGARD, M. E. and GEORGE, S. L. Combination chemotherapy and histiocytosis X. *Medical and Pediatric Oncology*, **3**, 267–273 (1977)

13 KOMP, D. M., MAHDI, A. E., STARLING, K. A., EASLEY, J., VIETTI, T. J., BERRY, D. H. and GEORGE, S. L. Quality of survival in histiocytosis X: a southwest oncology group study. *Medical and Pediatric Oncology*, **8**, 35–40 (1980)

14 LADISCH, S., POPLACK, D. G., HOLIMAN, B. and BLAESE, R. M. Immunodeficiency in familial erythrophagocytic lymphohistiocytosis. *Lancet*, **1**, 581–583 (1978)

15 LADISCH, S., POPLACK, D. G., HOLIMAN, B. and BLAESE, R. M. Patterns of immunodeficiency in two forms of childhood reticuloendotheliosis. *XVII Congress of the International Society of Hematology*, 746 (1978)

16 LADISCH, S., POPLACK, D. G., HOLIMAN, B. and BLAESE, R. M. Immunodeficiency in the childhood histiocytoses. *Pediatric Research*, **13,** 746A (1979)

17 LADISCH, S., HO. W., MATHESON, D., PILKINGTON, R. and HARTMAN, G. Treatment of familial erythrophagocytic lymphohistiocytosis (FEL) by repeated blood exchange. *Pediatric Research*, **14,** 536 (1980)

18 LADISCH, S. (Unpublished observations)

19 LAHEY, M. E. Prognosis in reticuloendotheliosis in children. *Journal of Pediatrics*, **60,** 664–671 (1962)

20 LAHEY, M. E. Histiocytosis X: an analysis of prognostic factors. *Journal of Pediatrics*, **87,** 184–189 (1975)

21 LAHEY, M. E., HEYN, R. M., NEWTON, W. A., SHORE, N., SMITH, W. B., LEIKEN, S. and HAMMOND, D. Histiocytosis X: clinical trial of chlorambucil. *Medical and Pediatric Oncology*, **7,** 197–203 (1979)

22 LAHEY, M. E., SMITH, B. and HEYN, R. Immunologic studies in histiocytosis X (meeting abstract). *Proceedings of the American Association for Cancer Research*, **20,** 436 (1979)

23 LEIKEN, S., PURUGANAN, G., FRANKEL, A., STEERMAN, R. and CHANDRA, R. Immunologic parameters in histiocytosis X. *Cancer*, **32,** 796–802 (1973)

24 LICHTENSTEIN, L. Histiocytosis X: integration of eosinophilic granuloma of bone, 'Letterer-Siwe' and 'Schuller-Christian disease' as related manifestations of a single nosologic entity. *Archives of Pathology*, **56,** 84–102 (1953)

25 LIEBERMAN, P. H., JONES, C. R. and FILIPPA, D. A. Langerhans cell (eosinophilic) granulomatosis. *Journal of Investigative Dermatology*, **75,** 71–72 (1980)

26 LILLEYMAN, J. S. The treatment of familial erythrophagocytic lymphohistiocytosis. *Cancer*, **46,** 468–470 (1980)

27 MANOHARAN, A., CATOVSKY, D., LAMPERT, I. A., Al-MASHADHANI, GORDON-SMITH, E. C. and GALTON, D. A. G. Histiocytic medullary reticulosis complicating chronic lymphocytic leukemia: malignant or reactive? *Scandinavian Journal of Haematology*, **26,** 5–13 (1981)

28 McCLURE, P. D., STRACHAN, P. and SAUNDERS, E. F. Hypofibrinogenemia and thrombocytopenia in familial hemophagocytic reticulosis. *Journal of Pediatrics*, **85,** 67–70 (1974)

29 MOZZICONACCI, P., NEZELOF, C., ATTAL, C., GIRARD, F. and PHAM-HUU-TRUNG. Familial lymphohistiocytosis. *Archives Française de Pediatrie*, **22,** 385–408 (1965)

30 NEWTON, W. A. and HAMOUDI, A. B. A histiologic classification with clinical correlation. *Perspectives in Pediatric Pathology*, **1,** 251–283 (1973)

31 NEZELOF, C., DIEBOLD, N. and ROUSSEAU-MERCK, M. F. Ig surface receptors and erythrophagocytic activity of the histiocytosis X cell in vitro. *Journal of Pathology*, **122,** 105–113 (1977)

32 NEZELOF, C., FRILEUX-HERBET, F. and CRONIER-SACHOT, J. Disseminated histiocytosis X: analysis of prognostic factors based on a retrospective study of 50 cases. *Cancer*, **44,** 1824–1838 (1979)

33 NEZELOF, C. Histiocytosis X: a histological and histogenetic study. *Perspectives in Pediatric Pathology*, **5,** 153–178 (1979)

34 OBERMAN, H. A. Idiopathic histiocytosis: a clinicopathologic study of 40 cases and review of the literature on eosinophilic granuloma of bone, Hand-Schuller-Christian disease and Letterer-Siwe disease. *Pediatrics*, **28,** 307–327 (1961)

35 OSBAND, M. E., LIPTON, J. M., LAVIN, P., LEVEY, R., VAWTER, G., GREENBERGER, J. S., McCAFFREY, R. P. and PARKMAN, R. Histiocytosis X; demonstration of abnormal immunity, T-cell histamine H2-receptor deficiency, and successful treatment with thymic extract. *New England Journal of Medicine,*, **304,** 146–153 (1981)

36 POPLACK, D. G. and BLAESE, R. M. The mononuclear phagocytic system. In *Immunologic Disorders in Infants and Children*, edited by E. R. Stiehm and V. A. Fulginiti, 109–126. Philadephia, W. B. Saunders (1980)

37 PERRY, M. C., HARRISON, E. C., BURGERT, E. O. and GILCHRIST, G. S. Familial erythrophagocytic lymphohistiocytosis. *Cancer*, **38,** 209–218 (1976)

38 RILKE, R., CARBONE, A., MUSUMECI, R., PILOTTI, S., De LENA, M. and BONADONNA, G. Malignant histiocytosis: a clinicopathologic study of 18 consecutive cases. *Tumori*, **64,** 211–227 (1978)

39 RISDALL, R. J., McKENNA, R. W., NESBIT, M. E., KRIVIT, W., BALFOUR, H. H., SIMMONS, R. L. and BRUNNING, R. D. Virus-associated hemophagocytic syndrome. *Cancer*, **44,** 993–1002 (1979)

40 SHAPIRO, D. N. and HUTCHINSON, R. J. Familial histiocytosis in offspring of two pregnancies after artifical insemination. *New England Journal of Medicine*, **304,** 757–759 (1981)

41 SLATER, J. M. and SWARM, O. J. Eosinophilic granuloma of bone. *Medical and Pediatric Oncology*, **8,** 151–164 (1980)

42 THOMMESEN, P., FREDERIKSEN, P. and JORGENSEN, F. Histiocytosis X: IV. Immunologic response assessed by lymphocyte transformation tests. *Acta Radiologica Oncologica*, **17,** 524–528 (1978)

43 TOOGOOD, I. R. G., ELLIS, W. M. and EKERT, H. Prognostic criteria, treatment and survival in disseminated histiocytosis X. *Australian Paediatric Journal*, **15,** 91–95 (1979)

44 THORBECKE, G. J., SILBERBERG-SINAKIN, I. and FLOTTE, T. J. Langerhans cells as macrophages in skin and lymphoid organs. *Journal of Investigative Dermatology*, **75,** 32–43 (1980)

45 WARNKE, R. A., KIM, H. and DORFAMN, R. F. Malignant histiocytosis (histiocytic medullary reticulosis): I. Clinicopathologic study of 29 cases. *Cancer*, **35,** 215–230 (1975)

46 WILLIAMS, J. W. and DORFMAN, R. F. Lymphadenopathy as the initial manifestation of histiocytosis X. *American Journal of Surgical Pathology*, **3,** 405–421 (1979)

47 WILSON, E. R., MALLUH, A., STAGNO, S. and CRIST, W. M. Fatal Epstein-Barr virus-associated hemophagocytic syndrome. *Journal of Pediatrics*, **98,** 260–262 (1981)

48 WOO, S. Y., KLAPPENBACH, R. S., McCULLARS, G. M., KERWIN, D. M., ROWDEN, G. and SINKS, L. F. Familial erythrophagocytic lymphohistiocytosis: treatment with vinblastine-loaded platelets. *Cancer*, **46,** 2566–2570 (1980)

49 ZUCKER, J. M., CAILAUX, J. M, VANEL, D. and GERARD-MARCHANT, R. Malignant histiocytosis in childhood: clinical study and therapeutic results in 22 cases. *Cancer*, **45,** 2821–2829 (1980)

7
Potential of bone marrow and fetal tissue transplantation in paediatrics

Jaak Vossen and Leonard J. Dooren

INTRODUCTION

The aim of grafting haematopoietic precursor cells from bone marrow or fetal tissues is to substitute for either deficient or malignant haemic cell lines in the recipient. When in the early 1950s stable radiation chimeras in experimental animals were obtained[156], clinical bone marrow transplantation followed quickly[24]. Sustained engraftment, however, was not obtained until the necessity of a match between donor and recipient for the major histocompatibility antigens was shown. Until then recipients of haematopoietic grafts did not survive, because of either failure of engraftment or severe graft-versus-host (GvH) reaction.

Clinical bone marrow transplantation using allogeneic donors genotypically identical for the major histocompatibility complex (MHC) was first successful in infants suffering from congenital severe combined immunodeficiency (SCID)[81, 148]. The clinical application of this mode of treatment was then extended to patients suffering from severe aplastic anaemia and acute leukaemia[25, 27, 244, 259]. Presently both clinical experience and therapeutic results are such that transplantation is no longer an experimental therapy for patients with these diseases. Cure following bone marrow transplantation has also been obtained for other diseases such as Wiskott–Aldrich syndrome, chronic granulomatous disease, and infantile malignant osteopetrosis, but for other haematological diseases, clinical experience is either very limited or absent. Therefore, this chapter will mainly deal with the potentials and hazards of bone marrow transplantation in infants and children suffering from severe combined immunodeficiency, severe aplastic anaemia and acute leukaemia in remission. Data on adult patients with the latter two diseases will also be included.

TRANSPLANTATION OF BONE MARROW CELLS
Selection of the donor

The donor has to be genotypically identical with the recipient for the major histocompatibility complex, that is for the serologically defined HLA-A, HLA-B and HLA-C antigens, and in the mixed lymphocyte culture (MLC, HLA-D) in order to obtain a sustained engraftment of the transplanted haematopoietic precursor cells and to reduce the risk for graft-versus-host disease. In practice the donor is either a sister or a brother of the recipient, and occasionally another member of the family, for example, in case of parental consanguinity[82,278]. In the favourable circumstance that more than one potential bone marrow donor is available, other polymorphic genetic markers and non-HLA histocompatibility antigens[114, 182, 217] can be taken into consideration. For still ill-understood reasons female bone marrow donors give worse results than male donors, irrespective of the sex of the recipient[26, 28, 98]. Therefore, male donors are preferred. For possibly relevant but as yet unidentifiable HLA-linked minor histocompatibility antigens, some additional information with respect to donor–recipient matching may be obtained by the typing of the red blood cell isoenzyme pattern for GLO_1[192] coded for by genes located in the vicinity of the HLA genes. Differences in ABO and other red blood cell antigens (except for MNSs, *see below*) do not correlate with graft-versus-host disease[36, 72]. However, in case circulating isohaemagglutinins are present in the recipient directed against A and/or B red blood cell antigens of the donor, plasmapheresis of the recipient shortly before transplantation is needed for prevention of adverse transfusion reactions and impairment of engraftment[188].

The potential donor should be fully informed about the bone marrow sampling procedure before he/she gives his/her consent for the donation. In case the potential donor is a younger child, the parents (or guardians) should give their informed consent. The donor must be physically, haematologically, immunologically and mentally fit.

Conditioning of the recipient

Infants suffering from severe combined immunodeficiency do not have an immunological allograft resistance, so that even very small numbers of white blood cells present in a single blood transfusion are not eliminated and may induce a lethal graft-versus-host disease[12, 117, 118]. A few patients with SCID, however, have some degree of allograft resistance as indicated *in vitro* by a significant response in the mixed lymphocyte culture[109, 227] and *in vivo* by the absence of graft-versus-host disease after transfusion of unirradiated blood. As a rule, no immunosuppressive pretreatment of a patient with SCID is necessary for a successful engraftment of bone marrow cells from a major histocompatibility complex genotypically identical bone marrow donor[26, 142].

In patients with severe aplastic anaemia sufficient marrow 'space' for the transplanted haematopoietic precursor cells is available, but in these patients the immunological allograft resistance must be suppressed. A supralethal dose of 800–1000 rad (8–10 Gy) total body irradiation, used originally, caused considerable complications and a poor survival prospect[244], and was changed to cyclophosphamide pretreatment on the basis of animal experiments[220, 255]. In many patients, however, who were sensitized by blood transfusions before grafting, no engraftment was obtained after pretreatment with cyclophosphamide alone. The tolerable dose of cyclophosphamide evidently abrogated the transplantation resistance to a lesser degree than the tolerable dose of total body irradiation. Different alternative

Table 7.1 Conditioning regimens and graft failure in patients transplanted for severe aplastic anaemia

Conditioning treatment	Total dose of drugs/radiation*	Graft failure or rejection EGBMT	IBMTR	Others (references)
Cyclophosphamide ± exposure to donor antigen before bone marrow transplantation	200 mg/kg body weight once, at day −1	45%	45%	50% (3/6) authors' own data
Cyclophosphamide + antithymocyte globulin (ATG) ± Procarbazine	200 mg/body weight 6 mg/kg body weight rabbit ATG, or 60 mg/kg body weight horse ATG 37.5–45 mg/kg body weight		13%	0% (0/16) authors own data
Cyclophosphamide ± total body irradiation	200 mg/kg body weight 300 rad			4% (1/26)[40]
Cyclophosphamide ± total body irradiation ± shielding of lungs	120 mg/kg body weight 800–1000 rad 400–500 rad			0% (0/27)[96]
Cyclophosphamide + infusion of donor buffy-coat cells after bone marrow transplantation	200 mg/kg body weight daily, at day +1, +2, +3 (+4, +5)	4%	4%	11% (3/27)[246]
Cyclophosphamide + total lymphoid irradiation (mantle + inverted Y fields + spleen)	200 mg/kg body weight 750 rad			0% (0/9)[205]

* 1 rad = 0.01 Gy.
EGBMT: European cooperative group for bone marrow transplantation[98].
IBMTR: International bone marrow transplant registry[28].

multiple-agent conditioning regimens have therefore been used, with a varying degree of success (*Table 7.1*). Also the combination with infusion of donor buffy-coat cells following bone marrow transplantation increased the success of engraftment in sensitized patients with severe aplastic anaemia[245,246], but resulted in a higher incidence of graft-versus-host disease in the hands of others[236]. Overall, conditioning with cyclophosphamide alone still seems preferable in non-transfused (non-sensitized) patients with severe aplastic anaemia, whereas a more intensive multiple-agent conditioning regimen should be preferred in (possibly) sensitized patients.

In patients with acute leukaemia in remission the aim of the conditioning for bone marrow transplantation is 3-fold: making 'space', abrogation of transplantation resistance, and eradication of remaining malignant cells. Therefore, a combination of cyclophosphamide (120 mg/kg body weight) and total body irradiation (for adults from 800–1000 rad, 8–10 Gy, according to the dose rate) is generally used. For children the same dose of cyclophosphamide is used together with a single irradiation dose of 700–800 rad (7–8 Gy), according to the size of the child, and given by a linear accelerator at a rate of 25 rad (0.25 Gy)/min. With this type of pretreatment, graft failures have been extremely rare.

Procedure of bone marrow transplantation

Bone marrow is taken from the donor under general anaesthesia by multiple punctures from the iliac crest. No complications of the bone marrow sampling from the donor have been found. Fat particles and small bone and tissue fragments are removed from the bone marrow aspirate by centrifugation, together with most of the red blood cells. The suspension is then filtered, which in the authors' experience does not lead to any significant cell loss. The bone marrow cell suspension prepared in this way can then safely be given intravenously without the use of a blood transfusion filter.

To obtain engraftment, a minimum number of nucleated bone marrow cells must be given, depending on the disease of the recipient, the genetic donor–recipient relationship, and the type of pretreatment of the recipient. In the MHC genotypically identical donor–recipient combination the required numbers of nucleated bone marrow cells per kg body weight are 5×10^6 or greater for patients with severe combined immunodeficiency disease, 3.0×10^8 or greater for patients with severe aplastic anaemia after cyclophosphamide conditioning, and 1.0×10^8 or greater for patients with severe aplastic anaemia and leukaemia after pretreatment including total body irradiation.

SUPPORTIVE CARE

Mitigation of adverse effects of conditioning

High doses of cytostatic drugs and total body irradiation given before bone marrow transplantation as a rule cause nausea and vomiting. Apart from parenteral fluid administration (*see below*), antiemetic drugs should be given: a combination of slight sedation, for instance with diazepam and chlorpromazine, gives the best results in the authors' experience. Haemorrhagic cystitis, caused by the urinary excretion of acrolein, a breakdown product of cyclophosphamide, can be prevented by the administration of 2-mercaptoethane sulphonate sodium which binds and inactivates this toxic substance in the urinary tract[32]. The sodium and water retention caused by high doses of cyclophosphamide[34, 220, 241] is counteracted by a single dose of furosemide (frusemide) halfway through the cyclophosphamide infusion. For dilution and rapid urinary excretion of toxic cytostatic drugs and their breakdown products, and of uric acid, the amount of parenteral fluid administration is increased to 50 per cent above the basic requirements. Allopurinol, for prevention of uric acid nephropathy, and bicarbonate for alkalinization of the urine are also given during the conditioning period.

Cardiomyotoxicity is another possible effect of high doses of cyclophosphamide and total body irradiation, the latter especially if preceded by high doses of anthracyclines. The combination of cranial irradiation, used after remission-induction in patients with acute lymphocytic leukaemia, and total body irradiation necessary for conditioning, leads to cumulative toxicity in the central nervous system. This may be prevented by spacing both irradiations by 6 months[147]. An acute veno-occlusive disease of the liver is seen in some patients and seems to be related to high dose chemoradiotherapy before bone marrow transplantation and not with graft-versus-host disease[231, 309]. For total body irradiation in patients with leukaemia, shielding of parts of the body is contraindicated, so that late irradiation effects (*see below*) cannot fully be prevented.

Parenteral nutrition and infusion of blood products

Because of nausea, vomiting, dysphagia, and anorexia, bone marrow recipients are given a central indwelling intravenous catheter. For parenteral nutrition hypertonic glucose and mixed aminoacid solutions are given, supplemented with requirements for water and electrolytes. If possible, lipid emulsions are not routinely administered during the first months after transplantation for fear of further lessening the defence capacities of the granulocytopenic recipient by blocking the remaining phagocytic capacity[67]. Supplements of trace elements and vitamins are given as such and by way of weekly infusions of fresh-frozen plasma.

Red blood cell and thrombocyte concentrates should have white blood cells removed by filtration[52] and fractional centrifugation[56] respectively. Granulocyte transfusions are only given in case of sepsis uncontrolled by antimicrobial treatment. All blood products given should be irradiated with 1500 rad (15 Gy) to prevent graft-versus-host disease.

Mitigation of graft-versus-host disease

On the basis of animal experiments[240] methotrexate is given after bone marrow transplantation to prevent or mitigate possible graft-versus-host disease (*see also*

Table 7.2 Graft-versus-host disease following allogeneic MHC identical bone marrow transplantation

Disease	Mitigation of graft-versus-host disease	Incidence of graft-versus-host disease Acute*	Incidence of graft-versus-host disease Chronic	Mortality due to graft-versus-host disease Acute	Mortality due to graft-versus-host disease Chronic	References
Severe combined immunodeficiency	none	20–35%	none§	5–10%		12, 26, 142
	T-cell depletion†	none§	none§			
Severe aplastic anaemia	methotrexate**	50–65%	20–40%	25–30%	5–10%	28, 98, 244, 250
	cyclosporin A††	30–50%	none§	15%		98, 128
	total lymphoid irradiation	30%	none§	10%		145
Acute leukaemia in relapse	methotrexate	50–60%	20–25%	35–45%	15%	27, 259
Acute leukaemia in remission	methotrexate	35–50%	30%	5–10%	5%	261, 262, 263, 315
	cyclosporin A	15–20%	5–13%	5%	none§	168, 198, 298, 315

* Moderate to severe graft-versus-host disease (grade II or more[257]).
† T-cell depletion by albumin gradient centrifugation[51].
§ None mentioned in the literature.
** 15 mg/m^2 body surface on day +1, and 10 mg/m^2 body surface on day +3, +6, +11 and weekly thereafter for 100 days.
†† 12.5–25 mg/kg body weight daily on days −1 → +5, and 12.5 mg/kg body weight daily thereafter for 6 months.

Table 7.2). Recently cyclosporin A, a potent and possibly more selective immunosuppressive drug[23, 162, 271] has been introduced in clinical bone marrow transplantation (*see also Table 7.2*). This drug seems to suppress graft-versus-host reaction considerably[197, 198] and more selectively[69], although the toxic side-effects in some patients are rather severe[99, 127]. Whereas methotrexate does not seem to have any adverse effect on engraftment, late rejections have been seen after discontinuing cyclosporin A[128].

Other methods used in an attempt to prevent graft-versus-host disease are pretreatment of the recipient by total lymphoid irradiation (TLI)[205, 232] and the elimination of mature T-lymphocytes from the bone marrow graft, for example, by albumin gradient centrifugation[51] or anti-T-cell antisera[169, 215].

Prevention of infectious complications

Infants with severe combined immunodeficiency are susceptible to infections with opportunistic microorganisms as *Pneumocystis carinii*, viruses, yeasts and bacteria, even before transplantation. Patients with severe aplastic anaemia or leukaemia have very low numbers of white blood cells for approximately 1 month after transplantation, during which period they are extremely susceptible to infections with endogenous and exogenous potentially pathogenic micro-organisms, especially bacteria and yeasts[43, 303]. For several months following transplantation the recipient's immune capacities are decreased and the chances for infections with viruses such as herpes simplex, h. zoster and cytomegalovirus (CMV), yeasts and fungi, and *Pn. carinii* are increased.

The authors prefer not to give regular granulocyte transfusions for the prevention of early infections[44, 304]. Apart from being laborious and expensive[218], such transfusions may cause fever and shivering in the patient, sensitization to HLA and white-cell-specific antigens, introduction of cytomegalovirus[305], lung infiltrates[249], and pneumopathy enhanced by amphotericin B in patients with Gram-negative bacteraemia[70, 310]. Moreover, one might think of possibly harmful allogeneic interactions between the transfused white blood cells and the transplanted lymphoid cell line precursors, resulting in an unwanted antigenic stimulation of the still unstable immune system. Instead the authors prefer to prevent infections by strict protective isolation and gastrointestinal decontamination of the patient.

For strict protective isolation, laminar cross-flow isolators are used for infants[149] and laminar down-flow isolators for older children[288] (*Figure 7.1*). The techniques for such gnotobiotic care of children have been described elsewhere[276, 277]. Gastrointestinal decontamination is given either as complete or selective. In complete decontamination all endogenous bacteria and yeasts are either eliminated or suppressed by high doses of non-absorbable antimicrobial drugs, given orally (for example, combinations of gentamicin, vancomycin and nystatin (Mycostatin) or amphotericin B[153, 200, 311] or combinations of polymyxin B/E, neomycin, cephaloridin and Mycostatin or amphotericin B[280, 289]). In selective gastrointestinal decontamination *Pseudomonas* sp., *Enterobacteria* spp., *Staphylococcus aureus*

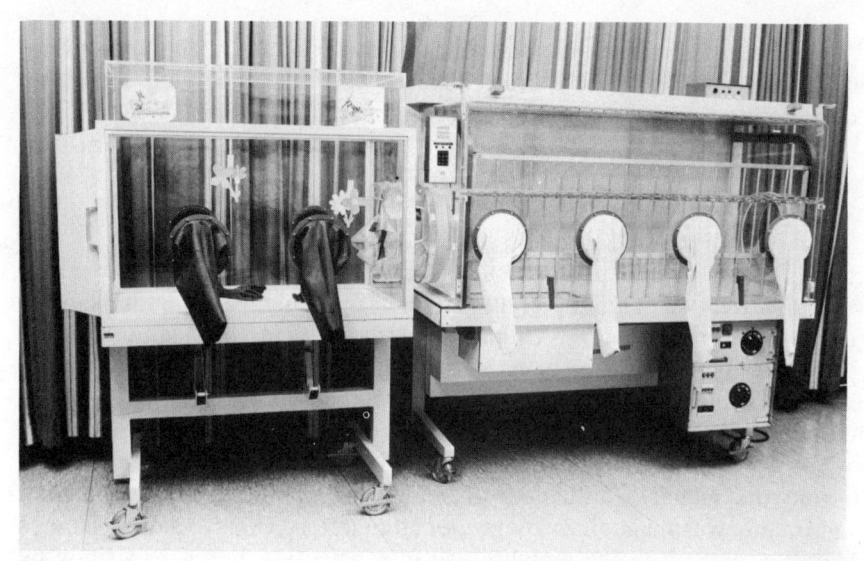

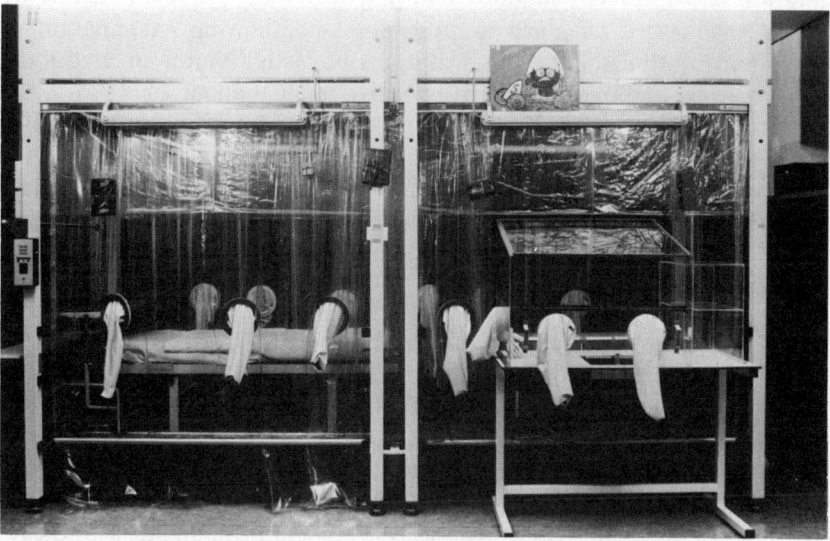

Figure 7.1 Laminar cross-flow (*above*) and down-flow (*below*) isolators, used for strict protective isolation of infants and older children respectively

and yeasts, the potentially pathogenic micro-organisms causing the majority of severe infections, are eliminated or suppressed, leaving the anaerobic micro-organisms unimpaired. In this way the colonization resistance against exogenous facultative aerobic potentially pathogenic micro-organisms is maintained[287, 290]. This is done by the oral administration of critical doses of the non-absorbable drugs polymyxin B/E and neomycin[61, 110] and/or by slightly increased doses (approximately 3/2 times the regular dose) of the absorbable drugs nalidixic acid and co-trimoxazole[285] for Gram-negative rods and cephradine for *Staphylococcus aureus*[254], in combination with mycostatin or amphotericin B[291]. The appropriate choice of the combination of these drugs depends on the antimicrobial sensitivity pattern of the endogenous potentially pathogenic micro-organisms.

Psychosocial support

Great care is given to the psychosocial support of patients and their family members, with strict programming of all activities and daily team-conferences for careful exchange of information. Guidance of the patient, his family and the team-members is supervised by an experienced clinical psychologist. In the authors' experience with some 50 infants and children, treated over a period of about 10 years, no important psychological or social harm to the patients and their parents, caused by the isolation procedure has been noted.

Apart from the negative influences of severe illness, normal developmental progress in infants was maintained by proper stimulation. Older children showed rapid adaptation and surprising mobility and play activities. Frequent visiting by the parents is encouraged as much as possible. On follow-up examination of children after leaving the isolator, no symptoms of lasting motor or emotional retardation were seen, and the children had positive feelings about their stay in the isolator. In some children a certain increase in verbal performance and power of concentration on the one hand, and some self-centredness, increased need for skin-to-skin contact, diminished zest for work, and some problems with social adaptability to children of the same age on the other hand, were seen during a period of several months after discharge[138].

FOLLOW-UP AFTER BONE MARROW TRANSPLANTATION

Haematological reconstitution and chimerism

The aim of the bone marrow cell grafting in patients with severe aplastic anaemia and with leukaemia is a full replacement of all haematopoietic cell lines of the recipient by those of the donor. Bone marrow transplantation in infants with severe combined immunodeficiency is only performed for immunological reconstitution, and no full take is aimed at.

It takes from 1–3 months after transplantation before the numbers of peripheral blood cells are normalized. An example of the haematological reconstitution in a boy with idiopathic severe aplastic anaemia is given in *Figure 7.2*. Generally an exponential increase in the numbers of white blood cells and the appearance of reticulocytes and young basophilic red blood cells in the peripheral blood are the first signs of recovery of the haematopoiesis. In almost every case a reticulocyte crisis can be seen. Despite this rapid normalization of the numbers of peripheral blood cells, and the normal appearance of the bone marrow on cytological examination as early as 4–6 weeks after transplantation, the numbers of committed haematopoietic precursor cells, counted as colony-forming units in culture (CFU-c)

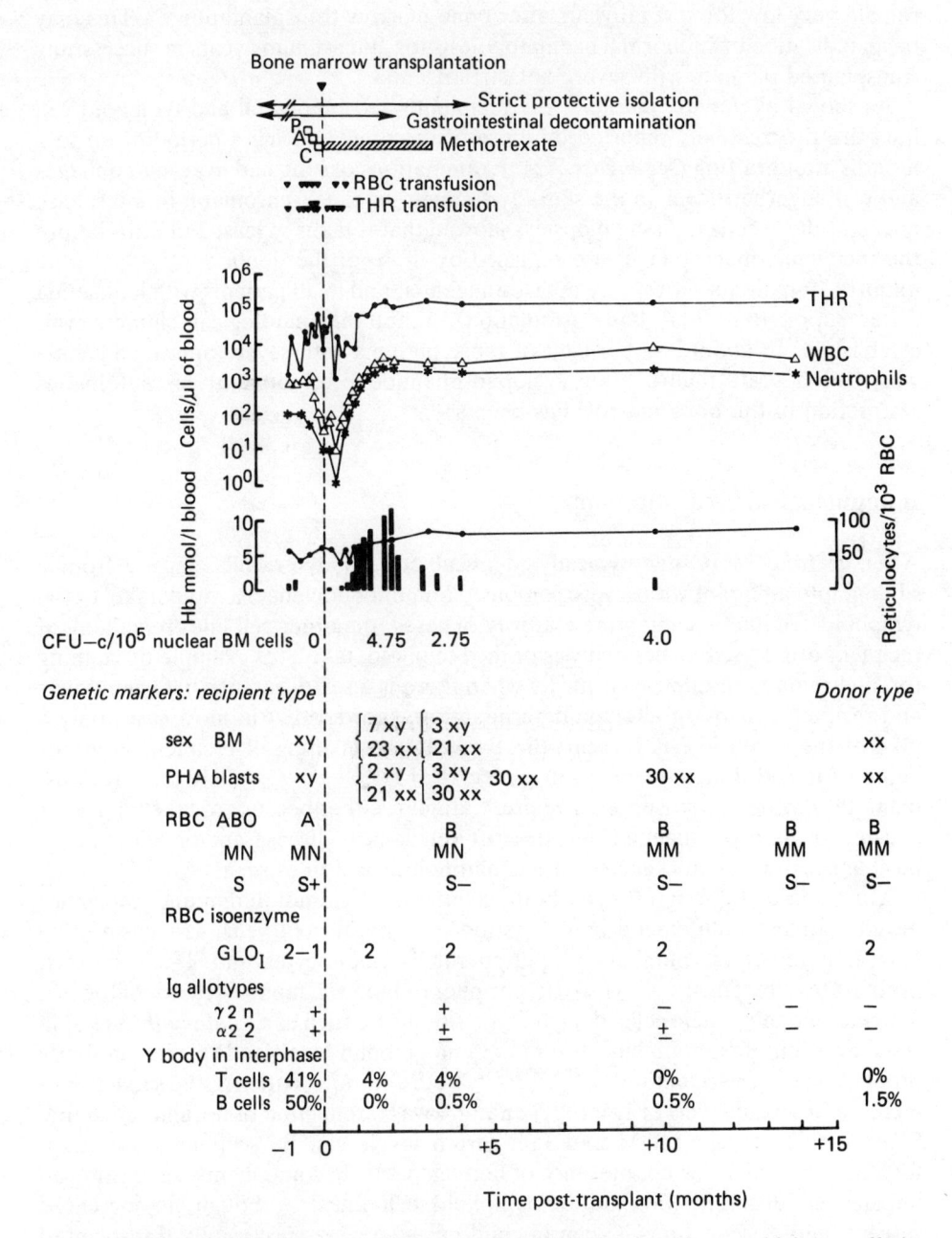

Figure 7.2 Haematological reconstitution and chimerism of a 10-year-old boy, suffering from idiopathic severe aplastic anaemia and transplanted with bone marrow cells from an MHC genotypically identical 7-year-old sister. BM = bone marrow; P = procarbazine; A = antithymocyte globulin; C = cyclophosphamide; THR = thrombocytes; PHA = phytohaemagglutinin

remain very low for several years after bone marrow transplantation[150]. This may be an indication of subnormal haematopoiesis for at least many years in successfully transplanted patients with severe aplastic anaemia.

As shown by genetic markers, the recipient's red blood cell and lymphoid cell lines are progressively replaced by those of the donor during a period of up to 3 months after grafting (*see Figure 7.2*). Examinations of lung and liver macrophages and of Langerhans cells in the skin, by staining for the Y-chromatin in interphase nuclei of those cells in tissue biopsies, showed that it takes at least 2 months before the recipient's macrophages are replaced by those of the donor[73, 140, 258]. In the majority of patients with severe aplastic anaemia, and in all patients with leukaemia (after supralethal total body irradiation), a full haematological chimerism is established. In about 3–9 per cent of those patients with severe aplastic anaemia who had a graft failure after cyclophosphamide pretreatment, an autologous restoration of the bone marrow has been seen[28, 98].

Immunological reconstitution

After grafting MHC genotypically identical bone marrow cells, mostly from a sibling, into an infant with severe combined immunodeficiency, a rapid 'take' of the lymphoid cell line is seen in the majority of cases, the other cell lines remaining of recipient origin[238]. Further analysis of the lymphoid 'take', for example by staining for Y-chromatin in interphase nuclei when there is a sex difference between donor and recipient, or by Ig allotype determination, showed that in most cases only a take of the T-cell line is present, the B-cell line remaining of recipient origin or being of mixed donor–recipient origin[108, 113, 175, 184, 278, 281]. Only after retransplantation with immunosuppressive pretreatment, either because of take failure, or because of aplastic anaemia due to graft-versus-host disease and/or alloimmune mechanisms, was a full take of all haematopoietic cell lines seen[165, 176, 184].

After successful engraftment both cellular and humoral immune capacities develop almost simultaneously in a period of 1 month to 1 year, as measured by several parameters: numbers of peripheral T-lymphocytes and T-cell subsets, proliferative responses *in vitro* of peripheral blood lymphocytes to mitogens, antigens and allogeneic cells, delayed type skin tests, such as *Candida albicans* skin test, rejection of skin implant, serum immunoglobulin levels and specific antibody production after vaccination[148, 204, 278, 282]. In the authors' patients, the sequence of increase in serum levels of IgM, IgG and IgA was a reflection of normal ontogeny. Some overshooting of IgM and IgG serum levels can be seen in most cases, together with the transient presence of homogeneous Ig components, suggesting an imbalanced differentiation of the lymphoid cell lines. Although no increased susceptibility to infections is seen in children, who were successfully transplanted during infancy for severe combined immunodeficiency, antibody-dependent (K-cell) and natural killing (NK-cell) activity appeared to be severely decreased in several of them[83, 282]. These *in vitro* functions are attributed to non-T-non-B lymphoid subpopulations. The reason for the lack of restoration of these cell lines, or its relationship with possible clinical symptomatology, is as yet not clear.

Long-term follow-up is needed to see whether such defects have any consequences in older age, like an increased susceptibility to (viral) infections or an increased incidence of malignancies.

The immunological reconstitution after bone marrow transplantation in patients with severe aplastic anaemia and leukaemia takes more time than in patients with severe combined immunodeficiency, that is more than 1 year in the majority of cases. Several factors, such as thymic involution, graft-versus-host disease or the drugs used for mitigating it, and infections may delay this immune reconstitution.

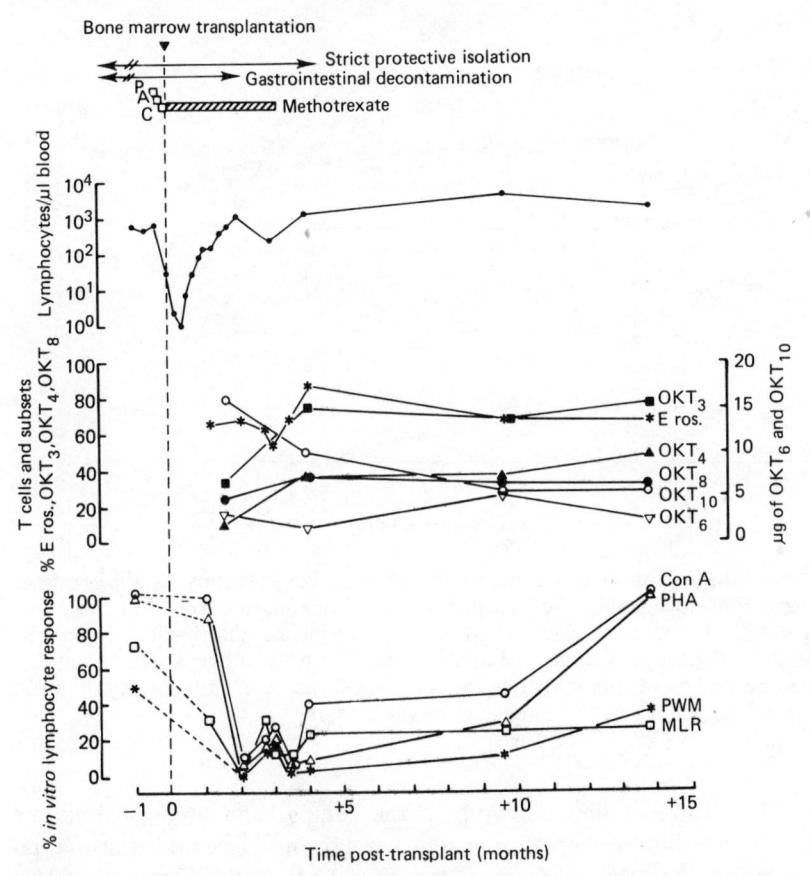

Figure 7.3 Reconstitution of cellular immunity of a 10-year-old boy, suffering from idiopathic severe aplastic anaemia and transplanted with bone marrow cells from an MHC genotypically identical 7-year-old sister. P, A, C = procarbazine, antithymocyte globulin and cyclophosphamide; OKT = monoclonal antibodies binding specifically to total peripheral T-cells (OKT$_3$), helper/inducer T-cells (OKT$_4$), cytotoxic/suppressor T-cells (OKT$_8$), stage II thymocytes (OKT$_6$) and all thymocytes (OKT$_{10}$)[209]. The binding of OKT$_6$ and OKT$_{10}$ is expressed as average antibody load per cell, that is, as mean fluorescence intensity in micrograph (μG) of the fluorescent population of cells[31]. (OKT antibodies were kindly supplied by Dr G. Goldstein, Ortho Pharmaceutical Laboratories, Raritan, NJ, USA). Con A, PHA, PWM, MLR: Concanavalin A, phytohaemagglutinin, pokeweed mitogen, mixed lymphocyte reaction. (After Vossen *et al.*[283])

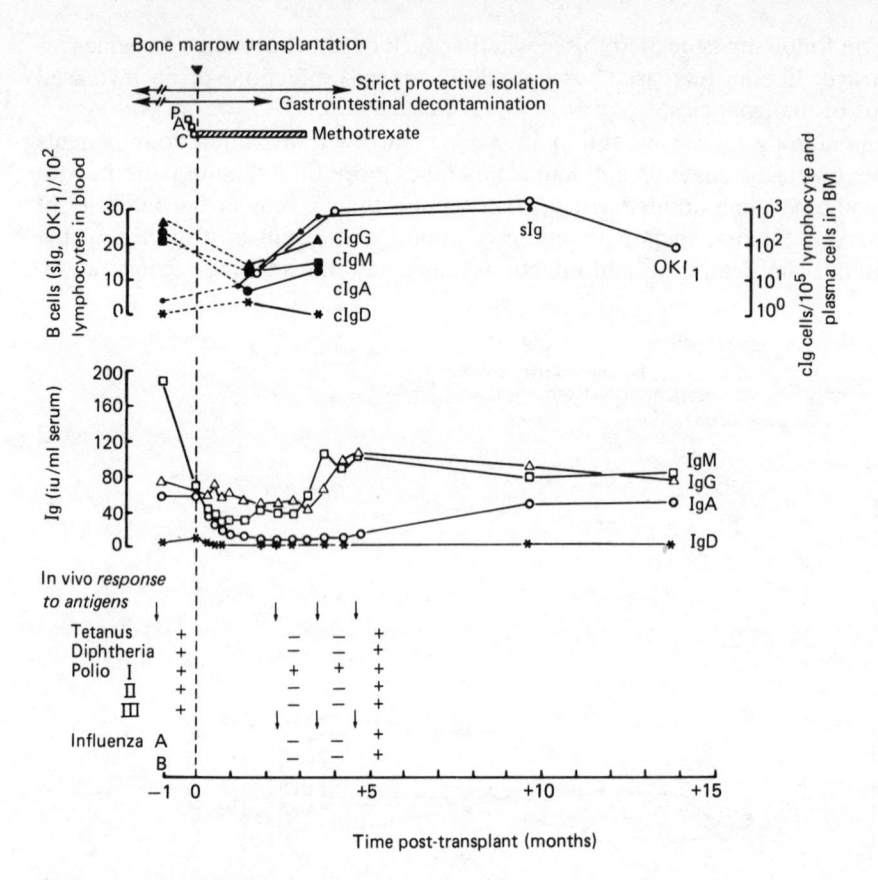

Figure 7.4 Reconstitution of humoral immunity of a 10-year-old boy, suffering from idiopathic severe aplastic anaemia and transplanted with bone marrow cells from an MHC genotypically identical 7-year-old sister. P, A, C = procarbazine, antithymocyte globulin and cyclophosphamide; OKI_1: monoclonal antibody binding to Ia antigens; sIg = lymphocytes with membrane-bound immunoglobulins; cIg = plasma cells with intracytoplasmic immunoglobulins; vertical arrow indicates date of vaccination

Figures 7.3 and *7.4* depict the follow-up of the cellular and humoral immune capacities in a boy with severe aplastic anaemia, following successful transplantation. Although the absolute numbers of peripheral blood lymphocytes and of E-rosetting T-lymphocytes returned to normal within a few months, the T-cell subset profile and the proliferative responsiveness *in vitro* of peripheral blood lymphocytes took much longer to normalize (*see Figure 7.3*). A longitudinal study of the immune reconstitution in several children transplanted for severe aplastic anaemia showed a great individual variability[31, 107, 123], but some trends could be seen. A reversed ratio of OKT_4^+ (helper/inducers T) to OK_8^+ (cytotoxic/suppressor T) lymphocytes and an increased relative number of immature T-cells (OKT_{10}^+) was noticed shortly after transplantation, but normalized progressively. The proliferative responsiveness of peripheral blood lymphocytes improved when 20 per cent or more of the E-rosetting T-lymphocytes were OKT_4^+ cells. In general the reactivity to antilymphocyte serum was restored initially, followed by the reactivity to phytohaemagglutinin and concanavalin A, and finally to pokeweed mitogen. No correlation was seen between the recovery of the proliferative responsiveness *in vitro* to different mitogens and to allogeneic cells. The responsiveness *in vitro* of peripheral blood lymphocytes to antigens behaved completely independently from the other reactions. Cell-mediated lymphocytolysis mostly became normal when the mixed lymphocyte culture response normalized.

Normalization of Ig levels in the serum took several months, and had the same sequence as in normal ontogeny (*see Figure 7.4*). In almost every patient transient restrictions in γ-globulins with formation of paraproteins were seen. In some of them such homogeneous components were seen simultaneously with a very high titre against cytomegalovirus, for instance, but in others no correlation with specific antibody formation was found. A sharp rise in serum IgE shortly after transplantation and possibly directed against antithymocyte globulin used for conditioning, described by Geha *et al.*[84] was not confirmed in the authors' patients. As a rule, antibody formation following vaccination or against (endogenous) herpetic viruses was seen from 3 months after transplantation onwards. Studies on the presence in the bone marrow of the different maturation stages of the B-cell line (the authors' own observations), and on the effect of peripheral T-lymphocytes on the pokeweed mitogen stimulated *in vitro* polyclonal B-cell activation, showed that the delay of humoral immune reconstitution was due both to a delay in maturation of B-cells and to a lack of T helper cells[8, 9, 58, 71, 160, 214, 224] (the authors' own observations).

K and NK-cell activity was greatly decreased in many patients with severe aplastic anaemia before bone marrow transplantation[154, 270] (the authors' own observations). NK-cell activity normalized within the second month after bone marrow transplantation; a very rapid normalization was found to be associated with graft-versus-host disease[270]. K-cell activity also became normal a few months following bone marrow transplantation[154] (the authors' own observations). Restoration of granulocyte function mostly paralleled their normalization in number in the peripheral blood[30, 253].

From the authors' limited experience with bone marrow transplantation in five children suffering from acute non-lymphocytic leukaemia and transplanted in first remission, it can be seen that the pattern of immune reconstitution was comparable to that in patients with severe aplastic anaemia following transplantation. Similar findings have been reported by others[62, 75, 171, 221].

Cellular and humoral immune responses and chemotactic activity of granulocytes have been found to be decreased in patients with acute graft-versus-host disease[42, 179, 306]. Immunosuppressive treatment and a poor general condition may contribute to this immunodeficiency. In chronic graft-versus-host disease the cellular immune responses are also very low, but the levels of immunoglobulins in serum and the production of antibodies are not always depressed; on the contrary high Ig levels even with production of autoantibodies can be found[224]. In patients with chronic graft-versus-host disease a long-lasting imbalance of T-cell subsets in the peripheral blood with a predominance of T-cells with suppressor phenotype has been reported[208]. However, the authors[31] and others[75, 88] found no suppressive effect of

T-cells on lymphocyte responses *in vitro* to mitogens, antigens and allogeneic cells in patients with generalized chronic graft-versus-host disease. However, Tsoi *et al.*[269] have found a suppressive effect in the mixed lymphocyte culture. Some investigators showed a prolonged suppressive effect of peripheral blood lymphocytes from these patients on the pokeweed mitogen-stimulated Ig production *in vitro*[160, 187, 224] (the authors' own observations).

With respect to the findings during immunological reconstitution in patients with severe combined immunodeficiency, severe aplastic anaemia and acute leukaemia, no clear-cut relationship has been found between the pattern of peripheral blood lymphocyte subsets and the responsiveness *in vitro* of these cells. Also no relationship could be shown between the lymphocyte responsiveness *in vitro* and the susceptibility of the patients to infections: apparently the findings *in vitro* have a low predictive value for the situation *in vivo*. From this it appears that much is still to be learned concerning the complex process of immune reconstitution after transplantation.

EARLY COMPLICATIONS FOLLOWING BONE MARROW TRANSPLANTATION

Failure of engraftment

As mentioned before, failure of engraftment is a particular problem in bone marrow transplantation of patients with severe aplastic anaemia, conditioned with cyclophosphamide alone, and is seen in 30–60 per cent of these cases[25, 94, 242]. On the one hand the likelihood of take is correlated with the number of transplanted bone marrow cells and the degree of lymphocyte-admixture of the graft (*see below*). On the other hand, take failure is related to immunological reactions of the recipient against the donor cells. The presence of HLA and non-HLA antibodies in the serum of the recipient, found either by serological tests or by antibody-dependent cell cytotoxicity were found to correlate positively with graft rejection[41, 74, 93, 97, 296, 297]. Both experimental and clinical data have shown that a single transfusion from a related donor sharing HLA antigens with the recipient, or multiple transfusions from unrelated donors, have detrimental effects on the chance of take[248]. A role of cell-mediated immunity, that is, T-lymphocyte-mediated or NK-cell-mediated cytotoxicity in the failure of engraftment, has not yet clearly been demonstrated. Some have found that the mixed lymphocyte culture–relative response index (MLC–RRI) of 2 per cent or more is related to rejection[166, 299], others have not[59]. Some indications for NK-cell-mediated rejection have been found in animals[146, 157] but not yet in man. The most sensitive *in vivo* estimate of allogeneic immunity against the graft is the survival time or increment of transfused random platelets[59], which appears to be related to the presence of lymphocytotoxins in serum and to the number of previous blood transfusions.

More severe immunosuppression (*see also Table 7.1*) either including total body irradiation or total lymphoid irradiation or using multiple-agent pretreatment with a combination of antithymocyte globulin (ATG), procarbazine and cyclophosphamide, gives sustained engraftment in almost all severe aplastic anaemia patients, irrespective of sensitization. Retransplantation after rejection is not possible in all patients, generally only in patients who have been nursed under gnotobiotic conditions[35], and has been successful in about 40 per cent of these patients, with about 20 per cent of long-term survivors[28, 98].

Graft-versus-host disease

Acute graft-versus-host disease is a severe and frequently lethal complication of allogeneic bone marrow transplantation, with lesions of the skin, the intestinal tract and the liver[308]. Skin exanthemata may be less or more extensive and vary from a measles-like eruption to epidermal necrolysis[95, 191]. Diarrhoea can be slight, moderate or severe and is sometimes associated with an irreversible pseudomembranous enteritis. Liver disease manifests itself by a cholestatic form of hepatitis. In HLA-identical sibling combinations the match is genotypically identical for the major histocompatibility complex loci. Despite this similarity, even in these combinations the graft-versus-host disease is considerable, but differs according to the type of the disease of the recipient (see Table 7.2).

Apart from histocompatibility, other factors have been found to influence the incidence of graft-versus-host disease. Recipients of a bone marrow graft from a female donor are significantly more prone to graft-versus-host disease[26, 28, 98]. A difference in the MNSs red blood cell group between donor and recipient was found to be correlated with an increased risk for graft-versus-host disease[235], but there were no differences in the ABO blood group[36, 72, 243]. The association between an increased NK-cell activity of the host and graft-versus-host disease is still not clear: Lopez et al.[155] found a positive correlation between a high NK–HSV$_1$ (NK activity against h. simplex$_1$ infected fibroblasts) of the recipient before transplantation and an increased risk of graft-versus-host disease, Tursz et al.[270] found an increased incidence of graft-versus-host disease in recipients in whom the NK–K$_{562}$ (NK activity against erythroleukaemia cell line K$_{562}$) rose rapidly following transplantation.

Animal experiments with mismatched donor–recipient combinations have shown that acute graft-versus-host disease can be divided into an early-onset (acute) type starting usually within 1 week after bone marrow transplantation and a late-onset (delayed) type starting after 3–4 weeks. The first type is due to the administration of mature immunocompetent T-lymphocytes with the graft, whereas the second type is caused by T-lymphocytes which develop from the grafted donor stem cells and T-cell precursors under host influence. The former type can be abrogated by eliminating mature T-lymphocytes from the graft, for example, by cell separation techniques[51, 210] or anti T-cell sera[169, 215], whereas the latter cannot. In the human situation one can expect an early-onset graft-versus-host disease when large numbers of bone marrow cells are transplanted, because immunocompetent lymphocytes are abundant in human marrow aspirate[15]. Therefore, the lowest possible cell number which gives a permanent take should be engrafted.

In order to mitigate the late-onset acute graft-versus-host disease different types of conditioning regimens or post-transplantation immunosuppression have been proposed, after a beneficial effect was found in experimental animals: bone marrow transplantation after total lymphoid irradiation[232], used in cases of severe aplastic anaemia only[205], administration of methotrexate up to 100 days after transplantation[240], and the administration of cyclosporin A up to 6 months after transplantation[197]. However, prevention of graft-versus-host disease by such measures is not complete and a recent retrospective evaluation of the transplant data of the European centres did not give a significant difference between the different regimens with respect to long-term survival[98].

Table 7.3 Gastrointestinal decontamination and acute graft-versus-host disease in children following bone marrow transplantation for severe aplastic anaemia

Gastrointestinal decontamination	n	Success of GID	n	Acute graft-versus-host disease* Early-onset	Late-onset	None	Donor Male	Female
Complete	9	yes	5	0	0	5	1	4
		no	4	1†	2	1	3	1
Selective	11	yes	8	1†	3	4	4	4
		no	3	2†	1	0	1	2

* Moderate to severe graft-versus-host disease (grade II or more[257]).
† Three patients had Fanconi's anaemia and one patient a familial non-Fanconi's anaemia.

In non-matched murine bone marrow chimeras delayed type of secondary disease, comparable with late-onset acute graft-versus-host disease in man, could be prevented or largely mitigated when the recipients were either germfree or made bacteria-free by complete gastrointestinal decontamination[119, 135], also when they were later reassociated with an anaerobic faecal flora[13]. A prospective study of the Seattle bone marrow transplantation team[45] concerning the potential beneficial effect of protective isolation combined with a suppression of the gut flora with non-absorbable antimicrobial drugs did not show significantly less graft-versus-host disease in patients under gnotobiotic conditions as compared with another group of patients. It should, however, be remarked that gastrointestinal decontamination proved to be effective only in nine out of 44 patients of the first group. A detailed microbiological investigation on the success of such gnotobiotic measures in 20 out of 24 children transplanted for severe aplastic anaemia in the authors' unit, who survived long enough to be at risk for graft-versus-host disease, showed the clear beneficial effect of a successful complete suppression of the intestinal microflora[284] (*Table 7.3*). Further investigations in this area are needed and may throw more light on the mechanisms involved.

Early infections

Infectious complications are a major cause of morbidity and mortality in transplant recipients. Many infants with severe combined immunodeficiency already suffer from infections at the time of diagnosis, for example candidiasis of mucous membranes and skin, Pn. carinii pneumonia, and viral infections. Several of these patients have died early post-transplantation due to such pre-existing infections[142, 233]. When immune reconstitution is successful, other infectious complications are very rare in these patients with severe combined immunodeficiency. Gnotobiotic techniques, such as protective isolation and gastrointestinal decontamination, are extremely useful when alternative therapeutic measures, for example, fetal tissue transplantations, are used and the waiting period for immune reconstitution is prolonged[233, 265, 279, 280].

In patients with severe aplastic anaemia or leukaemia, however, the pattern of infections following bone marrow transplantation is quite different. Roughly three episodes of an increased risk of infections can be seen: (1) an early period with severe granulocytopenia, up to 1 month after transplantation; (2) a middle period with immune deficiency and in some cases late-onset acute graft-versus-host disease, from 1 to 6 months after transplantation; and (3) a late period with immune deficiency and in some cases chronic graft-versus-host disease, after 6 months post-transplantation.

Infections during the first period are mainly due to bacteria, yeasts and fungi. Before 1976 especially, when many patients with end-stage leukaemia in relapse were transplanted, about 50 per cent of these patients developed septicaemia in the early post-transplantation period, which was lethal in up to half of them[43, 303]. Therapeutic granulocyte transfusions had little or no effect on these infections[303], but prophylactic granulocyte transfusions were effective in reducing these infectious complications[44], and gnotobiotic techniques such as protective isolation and gastrointestinal decontamination were even more effective[35, 45]. From the 24 children with severe aplastic anaemia, grafted so far in our unit and maintained in gnotobiotic conditions as described before, only one child died at 12 days after transplantation, before signs of engraftment were noticed, from a pre-existing uncontrollable *Klebsiella pneumoniae* septicaemia. Three others died later than 1 month after transplantation with bacteraemia in association with failure of take.

During the second period, many infections with bacteria and fungi are associated with late-onset acute graft-versus-host disease, and constitute a major cause of death and ultimate failure of the bone marrow grafting. The antimicrobial defence mechanisms of these hosts are severely depressed by bone marrow failure, immune deficiency, intestinal protein loss and a poor general condition. In this period also *Pn. carinii* infections and viruses like cytomegalovirus, h. simplex and h. zoster[7, 303], are seen, which are usually self-limiting. *Pn. carinii* pneumonia can be prevented by the prophylactic administration of co-trimoxazole[48, 129]. H. simplex and h. zoster infections can be treated successfully with acyclovir[167, 222, 226].

Also during this period after transplantation, interstitial pneumonia, another severe and often lethal complication, is seen in 20–50 per cent of the patients grafted for severe aplastic anaemia and leukaemia. The aetiological role of cytomegalovirus, h. simplex and *Pn. carinii* in this complication is not yet proven. Because the majority of grafted patients are carriers of these parasitic microorganisms, their presence in the lungs of about 45 per cent of the cases with interstitial pneumonia[172, 173, 303] could be explained as a mere coincidence. The propagation of these micro-organisms in the lungs might be the result of a general immunodeficiency or a local graft-versus-host reaction[19]. An increased incidence of interstitial pneumonia is seen in patients with graft-versus-host disease[173], diminished cellular immune capacity[307], multiple courses of cytostatic drugs (for example, for relapses of leukaemia)[259], and may be associated with radiation damage to the lungs[11]. However, this complication is far less frequently seen, that is, in less than 5 per cent of patients with comparable intensive chemoradiotherapy for refractory leukaemia, who received bone marrow from an identical twin, and in whom the chance for graft-versus-host disease is very low[64]. This finding argues in favour of a direct relationship between interstitial pneumonia and graft-versus-host disease. No satisfactory therapy is known for this complication.

In 20 out of 24 children with severe aplastic anaemia and in five out of five children with acute leukaemia, who were transplanted so far in the authors' unit and who lived long enough to be at risk for interstitial pneumonia, no signs of this complication were noticed. One possible explanation for the complete absence of this complication in these patients might be the prolonged (3–4 months) gnotobiotic care of the children, which includes the ultrafiltration of the inhaled air. The hypothesis of a possible pathogeneic role in interstitial pneumonia of an airborne challenge with (microbiotic) antigens is supported by the finding of the near-absence of pneumonia in leukaemic patients treated in strict protective isolation, as compared to control patients treated in the open ward[53, 153, 163, 170], whereas the incidence of other severe infections, such as sepsis, was found to be similar in both groups.

LATE COMPLICATIONS FOLLOWING BONE MARROW TRANSPLANTATION

Late rejection and recurrence of leukaemia

Late rejection after successful bone marrow transplantation is probably extremely rare. It has only been seen in some patients transplanted for severe aplastic anaemia, who have been treated with cyclosporin A after transplantation[128]. Recurrence of leukaemia has been seen in 10–50 per cent of patients who had transplantation for acute leukaemia in remission (*see below*). Almost all these relapses occurred within 2 years after the transplant[22, 37, 78]. In the majority of cases these relapses were in recipient cells and of the original type of leukaemia. Exceptionally, leukaemia recurred in donor cells[57, 66, 100, 174, 256]. Such findings would have important implications concerning the possible aetiology of leukaemia if proven irrefutably, but alternative explanations for these recurrences are possible[78].

Retransplantation following recurrent leukaemia, using bone marrow cells from the original donor, has been attempted in a small number of patients and has given prolonged remissions[161].

Chronic graft-versus-host disease

This disease, which affects up to 40 per cent of adult patients following bone marrow transplantation (*see also Table 7.2*) is less frequently seen in children. The clinical manifestations, in most cases starting later than 3 months after transplantation, are mainly lesions of the skin and mucous membranes. The skin lesions start in many cases as lichen planus-like scaling of the epidermis with disturbances of pigmentation, and may progress to systemic lupus erythematosus- or scleroderma-like lesions, which may generalize and become very disfiguring and debilitating[230]. In children, the generalized form is seen less frequently than localized scleroderma-like lesions[275]. The mucosal lesions may resemble the sicca or Sjögren syndrome[105], and can affect the digestive tract; the exocrine glands, and the liver are also affected[18].

In the majority of patients with chronic graft-versus-host disease a disregulation of the immune reactions is found with hyperimmunoglobulinaemia, circulating immune complexes, autoantibodies against red blood cells or lymphocytes[106,224], and IgM depositions in skin lesions[268,272]. Abnormalities were found in the T-cell subset profile and the profilerative response *in vitro* of peripheral blood lymphocytes of these patients. These findings, however, were not similar in all the patients and the relationship with the clinical symptoms is not clear. Impairment of thymic function has been suggested as a possible causative factor in chronic graft-versus-host disease[88,196,225], but this has not been proven.

Although the pathogenesis of chronic graft-versus-host disease is not yet known, viral infections, such as measles[65], h. simplex and h. zoster (the authors' own observations), and irradiation[314] may precipitate the skin lesions. Apart from local treatment and physiotherapy, prolonged immunosuppressive treatment with azathioprine and corticosteroids[250] has given the best results, leading to recovery in 70 per cent of patients.

Late infections

Apart from viral infections, especially h. zoster infection, bacterial infections after 6 months post-grafting were either relatively mild infections of the respiratory tract such as sinusitis or bacteraemias.

The latter infections were frequently caused by Gram-positive cocci, especially pneumococci, and were mostly seen in patients with chronic graft-versus-host disease[6]. Only occasionally did a patient die from such a late infection.

Late effects of conditioning of grafting

The massive doses of cytostatic drugs and irradiation given for conditioning and/or eradication of the disease may cause late effects after bone marrow transplantation. Judgement of their incidence and severity in paediatric patients is difficult, because for only a few patients grafted during childhood more than 10 years have elapsed after transplantation. On the basis of experiences so far several late complications may occur, although neither the incidence rate nor the time-lag can be predicted as yet.

The risk for such late effects will probably be greater when total body irradiation is used (with or without chemotherapy) than when chemotherapy only is used. The results of direct irradiation damage to the enamel of the teeth and the lens of the eyes may already be seen some years after irradiation as an increase in caries formation, and opacification of the lens leading to cataract formation. Some growth retardation may be expected as a result of a direct irradiation effect on cartilage-bone transformation. The gonads are extremely sensitive to irradiation, and spermatogenesis and follicle growth in particular are generally irreversibly damaged in all children receiving the doses of radiation used for conditioning, resulting in delay of puberty, infertility and sometimes in hypogonadism[228]. Cyclophosphamide has a less deleterious effect on the reproductive system[152,295]. Lung function may be impaired after bone marrow transplantation, but abnormal function is often already present, and the lung abnormalities probably have a multifactorial origin. Neurological sequelae are probably negligible, except when too short a period of time has elapsed between central nervous system prophylaxis with cranial and total body irradiation. A period of several months between the two irradiations is advised[147]. An increased risk of second malignancies may be expected because of the known carcinogenic potential of the drugs used for pretreatment. This was confirmed in canine radiation chimeras[49], but in humans only one case of an immunoblastic sarcoma after the transplant has been reported as yet[103]. Extensive monitoring and follow-up of long-term survivors of bone marrow transplantation is required to judge to what extent late effects may be expected and to find ways of prevention and treatment of these effects.

RESULTS OF CLINICAL BONE MARROW TRANSPLANTATION

Bone marrow transplantation and transplantation of fetal tissues for severe combined immunodeficiency

The results of transplantation of bone marrow cells and fetal tissues in patients with severe combined immunodeficiency are summarized in *Table 7.4*. When either an MHC genotypically identical, or an MHC genotypically haploidentical and HLA identical (related) donor was available, sustained immunological reconstitution was obtained in 37 out of 50 (74 per cent) of the patients described. MHC genotypically haploidentical but HLA haplo non-identical (related) donors have only been used in few patients: from nine mixed lymphocyte culture-negative combinations, four resulted in a successful reconstitution; from three mixed lymphocyte culture-positive combinations there was no success, and these patients died soon after transplantation[142,180]. At this point it should also be mentioned that at least two long-term survivors with severe combined immunodeficiency have been reported in the literature in whom the presence of HLA-A, HLA-B non-identical, mixed

Table 7.4 Results of bone marrow and fetal tissue transplantation in patients with severe combined immunodeficiency

Transplant type/match	Evaluable patients	Engraftment	Reconstitution in vitro T	Reconstitution in vitro B	Sustained reconstitution in vivo	References
Bone marrow cells						
1. Sibling						
HLA-A,B = /HLA D =	44 (56)*	42	41	38	32	102
2. Related						
HLA-A,B = /HLA D =	6 (10)	6	5	4	5	26, 109, 142, authors' own data
3. Related						
HLA-A,B ≠ /HLA D =	9 (11)	9	8	3	4	26, 142, 185
HLA-A,B = /HLA D ≠	3 (3)	3	2	1	0	142, 180
4. Unrelated						
HLA-A,B = /HLA D =	2 (2)	2	1	1	0	130 authors' own data
HLA-A,B ≠ /HLA D =	2 (2)	2	2	2	1	126, 183
HLA-A,B = /HLA D ≠	1 (1)	1	1	0	0	189
Fetal liver cells						
+ fetal thymus	21 (68)	12	8	5	2 (+4)†	184
– fetal thymus	31	7	7	3	1	
Fetal thymocytes + transfer factor	4 (4)	3	3	0	1	3, 112, 203, 229
Cultured thymic fragments	24 (24)	1§	1§	9	0 (+4)†	86, 124, 134, 176, 185, 264

*Total numbers of patients with severe combined immunodeficiency undergoing treatment are given between brackets.
† Alive for 2 years or more, but without immunological reconstitution.
§ Died at 4½ years of age from Pn. carinii pneumonia; graft lost[178].

lymphocyte culture-positive maternal cells could be proven as a result of maternofetal transfusion. In general, such patients die shortly after birth due to graft-versus-host disease[137]. The first of these children developed graft-versus-host disease with severe granulocytopenia and was fully reconstituted following retransplantation with bone marrow cells from the mother after conditioning[68, 176, 177]; the second child did not developed graft-versus-host disease and is still completely immunodeficient at more than 14 months of age and maintained in strict protective isolation[193, 234]. In both cases fresh maternal T-cells responded strongly in the mixed lymphocyte culture to patient's cells; no specific circulating suppressor cells mediating graft tolerance were found in these patients.

Taken together, it is clear from the above data that bone marrow transplantation from an MHC genotypically identical donor is the treatment of choice for infants with severe combined immunodeficiency. Because, however, more than half of these patients do not have such a donor, alternative modes for therapy have been sought. Although a bank of volunteer bone marrow donors has now been set up[132] it is not easy to find a suitable unrelated donor[252]. From the nine transplants from unrelated donors done so far (see Table 7.4)[90, 120, 125, 159] only one patient is alive with immune reconstitution after repeated grafts following conditioning[183]. This patient suffers from chronic graft-versus-host disease. All other patients died, mostly from graft-versus-host disease.

Fetal liver cells are capable of haematopoietic restoration without graft-versus-host disease in experimental animals[273]. However, fetal liver cell grafts usually failed to achieve sustained immunological reconstitution in severe combined immunodeficiency patients. Several cases have been reported in the literature with a reconstitution of mostly cellular immunity[1, 2, 33, 141, 185, 213, 264]. However, the decline of their immune capacities after 1 to 2 years and their ultimate death mostly due to infections has not always been made known. According to a recent inventory, only three out of 52 (6 per cent) severe combined immunodeficiency patients with fetal liver grafts are long-term survivors (see Table 7.4), two with full immune reconstitution[184, 267], and one with cellular immune reconstitution[33].

Intraperitoneal implantation of fetal thymocytes for immune reconstitution of patients with severe combined immunodeficiency has mainly been proposed by Ammann et al.[3]. Apart from four cases published by different authors (see Table 7.4), Ammann reported on four further evaluable cases[4], from which two had also received transfer factor and two had not. From the latter four patients, two showed a moderate T-cell reconstitution in vitro and were alive at 4½ and 8 years after treatment, the latter, however, with neurological impairment. A patient of Rachelefsky et al.[203] suffered from an encephalopathy more than 4 years after treatment. No B-cell reconstitution has ever been seen in any of these patients.

Because the addition of thymic factors or thymic-conditioned medium to peripheral blood lymphocytes or bone marrow cells of some severe combined immunodeficiency patients, and co-cultivation of thymic epithelium with peripheral blood lymphocytes of such patients resulted in an induction of E-rosette formation, increase of lymphocyte responsiveness in vitro and of T-cell dependent plaque-forming responses[89, 101, 186, 202], a possible role of the thymic epithelial cells or humoral products of these cells in the T-cell dysfunction of some severe combined immunodeficiency patients has been supposed. Administration of thymic factors, however, has never resulted in full and sustained immune reconstitution of severe combined immunodeficiency patients[5, 101, 164, 294]. The results of the implantation of cultured thymic fragments in patients with severe combined immunodeficiency are also disappointing (*see Table 7.4*). Mostly, only transient increases in serum IgM and sometimes IgG have been seen, sometimes with homogeneous components, and in some cases even with the development of a B-cell sarcoma[29, 136, 144]. Never has a full T-cell reconstitution *in vitro* been reported. No long-lasting immune reconstitution *in vivo* after a single implantation of thymic fragments has been seen. Apart from the patients described in *Table 7.4*, Gelfand[90] reported six other cases, and Fasth[63] and Kuis[151] each one other case of attempted reconstitution with cultured thymic fragments in severe combined immunodeficiency patients. Only one of these eight patients was a long-term survivor, that is 3 years after treatment, but without immunological reconstitution. All others died, mostly from viral infections. Hong[125] recently updated his results on implantations of cultured thymic fragments in severe combined immunodeficiency patients: of the 34 evaluable patients, treated so far in his department, eight are still alive, but only one of these is still alive three years after treatment. Several of these patients had repeated transplantations of thymic fragments. None of them is fully reconstituted. The only patient with severe combined immunodeficiency who had a complete T-cell reconstitution (*in vitro*) following thymic fragment implantation, proved to have an (accidental) take of donor T-cells[68, 176]. This patient, however, showed a progressive deterioriation of his immune capacities and died at age 4½ from pulmonary insufficiency[178].

Bone marrow transplantation for severe aplastic anaemia

The results of transplantation in patients with severe aplastic anaemia are given in *Table 7.5*. Except for 47 out of 74 patients transplanted in Seattle after 1975, the vast majority was refractory to conventional treatment before transplantation, and almost all of them were sensitized by blood transfusions. In those patients a long-term survival with full haematological reconstitution was achieved in about 45 per cent. The failures were mainly due to graft rejections and graft-versus-host disease, as discussed previously (*see also Tables 7.1* and *7.2*). A prospective study of the effect of early transplantation versus conservative treatment in patients with severe aplastic anaemia showed that an early transplant gave a significantly better long-term survival of about 60 per cent[38, 39]. Forty-seven non-sensitized patients transplanted in Seattle after 1975 resulted in a survival of 73 per cent[246, 247]. These results are superior to any other kind of treatment of severe aplastic anaemia. Also the results of bone marrow transplantation plus viable donor buffy-coat cells given after grafting, gave 20 out of 27 long-term survivors in Seattle[246]. From these data it

Table 7.5 Results of bone marrow transplantation in patients with severe aplastic anaemia

Bone marrow transplantation centres/cooperative groups	Transplant match	Evaluable patients All patients	Evaluable patients Children, or <20 years	Sustained engraftment/ haemopoietic restoration	Actuarial survival All patients	Actuarial survival Children, or <20 years	References
Seattle bone marrow transplantation team	allogeneic MHC =	73* 74†		52 63	43% 73%		246
	allogeneic MHC ≠ §	10		4	10%		116
IBMTR	allogeneic MHC =	144	100	107	44%	44%	28
EGBMT**	allogeneic MHC =	159		103	41%	no difference	98
Leiden Paediatrics††	allogeneic MHC =		24	20	54%		authors' own data

* Grafted before October, 1975.
† Grafted after October, 1975.
§ Genotypically identical for one HLA haplotype, sharing antigens of the other haplotype.
** Data on some patients also reported to IBMTR.
†† Data of majority of patients reported to IBMTR and to EGBMT.

should be concluded that early transplantation is the treatment of choice in non-sensitized patients with severe aplastic anaemia.

Apart from early transplantation in non-sensitized patients, other factors found to be associated with a higher survival rate were a male bone marrow donor, a younger age of the recipient and the absence of infections prior to grafting[28, 98]. Transplantation from MHC haploidentical donors has only been performed in a limited number of patients. The results have been disappointing with only a single long-term survivor (see Table 7.5).

Results of transplantation in patients with Fanconi's anaemia are less satisfactory: both the authors and others[95] lost four out of five patients from severe acute graft-versus-host disease, probably because the alkylating conditioning regimen causes severe necrolysis of the skin and gut mucosa on the basis of the defective DNA repair in these patients[17, 223].

Fetal liver cell transplants have been given to a limited number of patients with severe aplastic anaemia, who lacked a suitable bone marrow donor. In the largest series of patients reported in the literature, a survival of 1–2 years after treatment was seen in three out of 12 cases, without evidence of sustained engraftment[158]. Results of fetal liver cell transplantation in haematological disorders of man have been reviewed by Gale[79].

Bone marrow transplantation for acute and chronic leukaemia

Patients with end-stage acute leukaemia, refractory to cytostatic therapy, have a 10 per cent chance of long-term disease-free survival following allogeneic transplantation[27, 259]. The major causes of death were the high incidence of severe complications following transplantation, such as graft-versus-host disease (see also Table 7.2) and interstitial pneumonia, often associated with each other, and leukaemic relapse. Increase of the cytoreductive therapy before transplantation using multiple-drug schemes, did not improve the ultimate survival rate due to complications of cumulative toxicity[76, 260]. Except when an identical twin donor is available, in which case long-term disease-free survival can be obtained in a quarter of all cases[64], transplantation is no longer indicated in the treatment of acute leukaemia in relapse.

The results of bone marrow transplantation in patients with acute leukaemia in remission, that is of acute non-lymphocytic leukaemia in the first and subsequent remission, and of acute lymphocytic leukaemia mostly in second and subsequent remission, are given in Table 7.6. A long-term disease-free survival can be achieved in about half these patients. This is a significantly better result that can be expected with chemotherapy of these diseases in the same stage[133, 199]. Failures are mainly due to graft-versus-host disease and interstitial pneumonia in centres using methotrexate as graft-versus-host mitigation[78, 262, 315], and to an increased relapse rate in centres using cyclosporin A post-grafting[199, 298]. Relapses are much more frequent following bone marrow transplantation for acute lymphocytic leukaemia in second and subsequent remission, that is about 50 per cent[133, 261] as compared to transplantation for non-lymphocytic leukaemia mostly in first remission, that is less

Table 7.6 Results of bone marrow transplantation in patients with acute leukaemia in remission

Bone marrow transplantation centres/cooperative groups	ALL or A non-LL	Transplant match	Evaluable patients All patients	Evaluable patients Children, or <20 years	Sustained haematological remission	Actarial survival All patients	Actarial survival Children, or <20 years	References
Seattle bone marrow transplantation team	ALL	allogeneic MHC =	22*		9	35%		261
					9			133
	A non-LL	allogeneic MHC =	22*	24	12	55%	40%	37
			27†		12	44%		263
			26§		18	64%		263
	ALL/A non-LL	allogeneic MHC ≠ **	12		8	75%		116
UCLA bone marrow transplantation team	ALL	allogeneic MHC =	18			35%		80
	A non-LL	allogeneic MHC =	32			57%		
City of Hope bone marrow transplantation team	ALL	allogeneic MHC =	23 ⎫ 49			61%		21
	A non-LL	allogeneic MHC =	26 ⎭					
EGBMT	ALL	allogeneic MHC =	32		22	64%		315
	A non-LL	allogeneic MHC =	67		42	46%		
Royal Marsden bone marrow transplantation team††	A non-LL	allogeneic MHC =	39		28	55%		298
		allogeneic MHC ≠ **						
Leiden Paediatrics	A non-LL	allogeneic MHC	15	5	8	45%	100%	168 authors' own data

* Grafted before December 1977.
† Grafted after September 1978; total body irradiation with 1 × 1000 rad.
§ Grafted after September 1978; total body irradiation with 6 × 200 rad.
** Genotypically identical for one haplotype, sharing antigens of the other haplotype.
†† All centres used as a rule methotrexate post-grafting, except for Royal Marsden which used cyclosporin A.

than 10 per cent. This may be due to extramedullary seeding of lymphoblasts in the first group of patients. The relapse rate is smaller in allogeneic donor–recipient combinations than in identical twin combinations, probably due to an antileukaemic effect of the allogeneic graft[300]. This graft-versus-leukaemia effect was confirmed by a lower relapse rate in patients with graft-versus-host disease after bone marrow transplantation for leukaemia in comparison to patients without the disease[181, 302]. However, the ultimate survival rate in the former group was not increased[78], due to the adverse effects of graft-versus-host disease.

The results of transplantation in patients with chronic myeloid leukaemia in the acute phase have been extremely poor, with less than 10 per cent of long-term survivors[54, 78]. Only few transplants in patients with chronic myeloid leukaemia in the chronic phase have been reported: identical twin grafts and also allogeneic grafts seem to give at least as good results as in transplantation for acute leukaemia in first remission[78, 80, 219, 237].

As can be seen from *Table 7.6*, the actuarial survival after bone marrow transplantation for acute leukaemia in remission using a MHC genotypically haploidentical donor is also about 50 per cent, which is very promising. Only one successful transplant for acute leukaemia in remission using an unrelated phenotypically identical donor has been reported at this time[115].

No curative effect has been seen so far after autologous bone marrow transplantation in patients with leukaemia[78]. Autologous transplants have been used as haematopoietic rescue in patients with advanced solid tumours, resistant to conventional therapy, following aggressive combination radiochemotherapy, and may have potential beneficial effects[77].

FINAL REMARKS

Allogeneic bone marrow transplantation adds a powerful new dimension to the therapeutics of otherwise fatal diseases like severe combined immunodeficiency, severe aplastic anaemia, acute non-lymphocytic and chronic myeloid leukaemia, and offers possibilities for the treatment of other diseases. The applicability, however, is still limited and the results are adversely affected because of several major problems.

One major problem is graft-versus-host disease and the often associated interstitial pneumonia, which are obviously the most severe complications of allogeneic transplantation. Neither the use of an alternative conditioning therapy, such as total lymphoid irradiation, nor the administration of the new immunomodulating drug cyclosporin A, has been fully successful in preventing these complications in human transplantation, not even in the MHC genotypically identical donor –recipient combinations. Graft-versus-host disease has also not been prevented by depletion of the graft of T-lymphocytes, either by gradient separation[12] or by incubation of the bone marrow with absorbed anti-T-cell antisera[216] or with the monoclonal anti-T-cell antibody OKT$_3$[201]. Moreover, such depletion of the graft, either with gradient separation (the authors' own observations), or with anti-T-cell antisera[216], has caused take failures in human transplantation, even after conditioning with supralethal total body irradiation. As has been proven in the primate model, T-lymphocytes in the bone marrow graft eliminate residual allogeneic resistance in the host and thereby promote engraftment[292]. This is in accordance with the finding that additional transfusion of non-irradiated donor buffy-coat cells, containing many immunocompetent T-lymphocytes, promotes engraftment in sensitized patients[246]. A possible method to circumvent this decreased chance of take of T-cell depleted grafts is the use of more intensive conditioning treatment[286, 292, 293]. The latter, however, may increase the risk for interstitial pneumonia and other late effects. Altogether this poses the dilemma of the promotion of engraftment versus the increased risk for post-transplant complications and vice versa. Investigations ought to be done for the optimization of the conditioning regimens[111], of the quality and the quantity of the grafted cells[14] and of other measures aiming at the prevention of (late) rejection and the mitigation of graft-versus-host disease[16,50].

A second major problem is that allogeneic transplantation is still almost exclusively limited to the MHC genotypically identical donor–recipient combination. Transplants would be more common if the barrier of histocompatibility could be overcome, but in non-identical donor–recipient combinations the chance of take is decreased and the risk for graft-versus-host disease is increased considerably. Whereas MHC genotypically haploidentical (related) donors are generally available (parents, siblings), finding MHC phenotypically identical (unrelated) donors is difficult, and finding an unrelated donor–recipient combination, which is non-reactive in the mixed lymphocyte culture and in other tests for similarity, such as cell-mediated lymphocytotoxicity is often extremely difficult. In patients with leukaemia or severe aplastic anaemia long-term survival following transplantation of bone marrow cells from genotypically haploidentical (related) donors has only been obtained in recipients pretreated with an intensive conditioning regimen including total body irradiation. This is the case in recipients transplanted for leukaemia[116], but not in patients with severe aplastic anaemia, in whom a less intensive pretreatment is used (see Tables 7.5 and 7.6). This difference in outcome is as yet unexplained, but may be related to a difference in intensity of the conditioning regimen.

In patients with severe combined immunodeficiency, bone marrow transplantation is the treatment of choice. Under this diagnosis a heterogenous group of congenital deficiencies of cellular and humoral immunity are brought together: reticular dysgenesis[274]; X-linked and autosomal recessive severe combined immunodeficiency; combined immunodeficiency with immunoglobulins (Nezelof's type), or associated with adenosine deaminase (ADA) deficiency[91]; congenital T-cell deficiency associated with nucleoside phosphorylase (NP) deficiency[92]; combined immunodeficiency associated with lymphocyte membrane abnormalities like lack of HLA-expression (bare lymphocyte syndrome)[266] and the rare cases of membrane transport[85, 143, 312] and capping defects[87], and associated with familial reticulosis with eosinophilia (Omenn's disease)[47]. Neither the use of fetal tissues, nor of humoral factors like transfer factor or thymus-associated factors have given a significantly better survival than the natural course of the disease, provided some protection is given to the patients by avoiding viral contacts, substitution with immunoglobulins and prophylaxis with co-trimoxazole for Pn. carinii pneumonia.

Only in cases of congenital immunodeficiency associated with adenosine deaminase or nucleoside phosphorylase deficiency does enzyme replacement therapy by transfusion of N_2-stored, washed, irradiated red blood cells give some immunological restoration, which is erythrocyte dose-dependent[55, 194, 212, 239]. In adenosine-deaminase deficiency, instituting enzyme-replacement therapy has not always been successful[313], and a recent multi-institutional cooperative study has shown that a good clinical response is seen only in those patients who had some residual immunological function at the time of diagnosis[195].

For infants with severe combined immunodeficiency for whom a MHC genotypically identical bone marrow donor is not available, immune reconstitution should be tried by transplantation of bone marrow precursor cells from other donors, under optimal conditions for the prevention of graft-versus-host disease. The strategy for treatment might then be as follows. A genotypically haploidentical (related) donor, sharing other histocompatibility antigens with the recipient, should be searched for. It is still not clear whether in such a case a mixed lymphocyte culture-negative or a cell-mediated lymphocytotoxicity-negative donor should be preferred. If such a family donor is not available, an unrelated MHC phenotypically identical donor might be used as next best. In both cases the bone marrow should be depleted of mature T-cells, either by density gradient separation techniques[51] with extra E-rosette depletion[292], by lectin-binding techniques[211], or by monoclonal complement-binding antibodies[104]. A very low number of cells is transplanted and higher numbers of cells are gradually given only when no take is seen. A conditioning regimen, possibly including some form of irradiation, might be necessary. The patient is maintained in strict protective isolation and all potentially pathogenic micro-organisms are suppressed or eliminated by complete gastrointestinal decontamination before bone marrow transplantation and for at least 2 months following. Lastly, a graft-versus-host disease mitigating drug is administered following transplantation, such as methotrexate and/or cyclosporin A.

Inborn errors for which transplantation with healthy bone marrow cells might lead to correction of the disease, have recently been listed by Good[102] and Hobbs[122]. For each disease and for each individual patient the risk of bone marrow transplantation with its possible complications should be carefully weighed against the prospects of conventional treatment, but if a suitable donor is available bone marrow grafting may lead to complete cure of otherwise debilitating or lethal disorders. As an example transplantation has successfully been performed in individual patients with granulocytic disorders like Kostmann's disease, chronic granulomatous disease, and Chediak–Higashi syndrome[60, 206, 207]. Patients with Wiskott–Aldrich syndrome[139, 207] and malignant osteopetrosis[46] have also been reconstituted by allogeneic transplants, and biochemical improvement following successful allogeneic transplantation has been reported in a young child with Hurler's disease[121]. In all these disorders myeloablation with aggressive 'space-making' pretreatment such as total body irradiation or busulphan, is necessary to secure persistent allogeneic haematopoiesis, because otherwise only transient partial takes are seen[10, 190].

In congenital haemolytic anaemias, like thalassaemia major and sickle-cell anaemia, no successful engraftment has been reported until now. This is probably due to insufficient suppression of the hyperactive erythropoiesis in the attempted cases. However, congenital haemolytic anaemia in dogs can be treated by bone marrow transplantation following appropriate conditioning[301].

Fanconi's anaemia[223], Blackfan–Diamond anaemia[131], ataxia telangiectasia syndrome[251] and Bloom's syndrome[20], are severe, even eventually fatal haematological and immunological diseases associated with increased chromosome breakage. Although patients suffering from these diseases are potential candidates for bone marrow transplantation, the highly increased sensitivity of their nuclear DNA to cross-linking agents, such as cyclophosphamide and/or total body irradiation needed for the pretreatment, may lead to severe and even lethal toxic complications. Therefore the possibility of treating these patients by transplantation is still very limited, until conditioning regimens are developed which are specially adapted for them.

References

1 ACKERET, C., PLÜSS, H. J. and HITZIG, W. H. Hereditary severe combined immunodeficiency and adenosine deaminase deficiency. *Pediatric Research*, **10**, 67–70 (1976)

2 AIUTI, F., BUSINCO, L., FIORILLI, M., DE MARTINO, M. and VIERUCCI, A. Fetal liver transplantation in two infants with severe combined immunodeficiency. *Transplantation Proceedings*, **XI**, 230–234 (1979)

3 AMMANN, A. J., WARA, D. W., SALMON, S. and PERKINS, H. Permanent reconstitution of cellular immunity in a patient with sex-linked combined immunodeficiency. *New England Journal of Medicine*, **289**, 5–9 (1973)

4 AMMANN, A. J. First International Meeting on Congenital Immunodeficiencies, Tübingen, 1980 (personal communication)

5 ASTALDI, A., ASTALDI, G. C. B., WIJERMANS, P., DAGNA-BRICARELLI, F., KATER, L., STOOP, J. W. and VOSSEN, J. M. Experiences with thymosin in primary immunodeficiency disease. *Cancer Treatment Reports*, **62**, 1779–1785 (1978)

6 ATKINSON, K., STORB, R., PRENTICE, R. L., WEIDEN, P. L., WITHERSPOON, R. P., SULLIVAN, K., NOEL, D. and THOMAS, E. D. Analysis of late infections in 89 long-term survivors of bone marrow transplantation. *Blood*, **53**, 720–731 (1979)

7 ATKINSON, K., MEYERS, J. D., STORB, R., PRENTICE, R. L. and THOMAS, E. D. Varicella-zoster virus infection after marrow transplantation for aplastic anemia or leukemia. *Transplantation*, **29**, 47–50 (1980)

8 ATKINSON, K., GOEHLE, S., HANSEN, J., THOMAS, E. D. and STORB, R. Human T-cell subpopulations identified by monoclonal antibodies after bone marrow transplantation. *Experimental Hematology*, **9** (suppl. 9), 188 (1981)

9 BACIGALUPO, A., MINGARI, M. C., MORETTA, L., PODESTA, M., VAN LINT, M. T., PIAGGIO, G., RAFFO, M. R. and MARMONT, A. Imbalance of T-cell subpopulations and defective pokeweed mitogen-induced B-cell differentiation after bone marrow transplantation in man. *Clinical Immunology and Immunopathology*, **20**, 137–145 (1981)

10 BALLET, J. J., GRISCELLI, C., COUTRIS, C., MILHAUD, G. and MAROTEAUX, P. Bone-marrow transplantation in osteopetrosis. *Lancet*, **2**, 1137 (1977)
11 BARRETT, A., BARRETT, A. J. and POWLES, R. L. Total body irradiation and marrow transplantation for acute leukaemia. *Pathologie Biologie*, **27**, 357–359 (1979)
12 BEKKUM, D. W. VAN. Use and abuse of hemopoietic cell grafts in immune deficiency diseases. *Transplantation Reviews*, **9**, 3–53 (1972)
13 BEKKUM, D. W. VAN, ROODENBURG, J., HEIDT, P. J. and VAN DER WAAIJ, D. Mitigation of secondary disease of allogeneic mouse radiation chimeras by modification of the intestinal microflora. *Journal of the National Cancer Institute*, **52**, 401–404 (1974)
14 BEKKUM, D. W. VAN, LÖWENBERG, B. and VRIESENDORP, H. M. In *Immunological Engineering*, edited by D. W. Jirsch, 179. Lancaster, MTP Press (1978)
15 BEKKUM, D. W. VAN, WAGEMAKER, G. and VRIESENDORP, H. M. Mechanisms and avoidance of graft-versus-host-disease. *Transplantation Proceedings*, **XI**, 189–195 (1979)
16 BEKKUM, D. W. VAN In *Biology of Bone Marrow Transplantation*, edited by R. P. Gale and C. F. Fox, 175. New York, Academic Press (1980)
17 BERGER, R., BERNHEIM, A., GLUCKMAN, E. and GISSELBRECHT, C. *In vitro* effect of cyclophosphamide metabolites on chromosomes of Fanconi anaemia patients. *British Journal of Haematology*, **45**, 565–568 (1980)
18 BERNUAU, D., GISSELBRECHT, C., DEVERGIE, A., FELDMAN, G., GLUCKMAN, E., MARTY, M. *et al.* Histological and ultrastructural appearance of the liver during graft-versus-host disease complicating bone marrow transplantation. *Transplantation*, **29**, 236–244 (1980)
19 BESCHORNER, W. E., SARAL, R., HUTCHINS, G. M., TUTSCHKA, P. J. and SANTOS, G. W. Lymphocytic bronchitis associated with graft-versus-host disease in recipients of bone-marrow transplants. *New England Journal of Medicine*, **299**, 1030–1036 (1978)
20 BLOOM, G. E., PARK, S. G. and DIAMOND, L. K. Chromosome abnormalities in constitutional aplastic anemia. *New England Journal of Medicine*, **274**, 8–14 (1966)
21 BLUME, K. G., FORMAN, S. J., SPRUCE, W. E., WOLF, J. L., FARBSTEIN, M. J., SCOTT, E. P., FAHEY, J. L. *et al.* Bone marrow transplantation (BMT) for acute leukemia. *Experimental Hematology*, **9** (suppl. 9), 124 (1981)
22 BLUME, K. G., SPRUCE, W. E., FORMAN, S. J., WOLF, J. L., FARBSTEIN, M. J., SCOTT, E. P. and FAHEY, J. L. Bone-marrow transplantation for acute leukemia. *New England Journal of Medicine*, **305**, 101–103 (1981)
23 BOREL, J. F., FEURER, C., GUBLER, H. V. and STAHELIN, H. Biological effects of cyclosporin A; a new antilymphocytic agent. *Agents and Actions*, **6**, 468–475 (1976)
24 BORTIN, M. M. A compendium of reported human bone marrow transplants. *Transplantation*, **9**, 571–587 (1970)
25 BORTIN, M. M. Bone marrow transplantation from histocompatible, allogeneic donors for aplastic anemia. *Journal of the American Medical Association*, **236**, 1131–1135 (1976)
26 BORTIN, M. M. and RIMM, A. A. Severe combined immunodeficiency disease. *Journal of the American Medical Association*, **238**, 591–600 (1977)

27 BORTIN, M. M. and RIMM, A. A. Bone marrow transplantation for acute myeloblastic leukemia. *Journal of the American Medical Association*, **240**, 1245–1252 (1978)

28 BORTIN, M. M., GALE, R. P and RIMM, A. A. Allogeneic bone marrow transplantation for 144 patients with severe aplastic anemia. *Journal of the American Medical Association*, **245**, 1132–1139 (1981)

29 BORZY, M. S., HONG, R., HOROWITZ, S. H., GILBERT, E., KAUFMAN, D., DeMENDONCA, W. *et al*. Fatal lymphoma after transplantation of cultured thymus in children with combined immunodeficiency disease. *New England Journal of Medicine*, **301**, 565–568 (1979)

30 BROEK, P. J. VAN DEN, MEER, J. W. M. VAN DER, LEIJH, P. C. J., ZWAAN, F., BARSELAAR, M. VAN DEN and VAN FURTH, R. Functions of granulocytes after allogeneic bone marrow transplantation. *Blut*, **42**, 253–257 (1981)

31 BRUIN, H. G. DE, ASTALDI, A., LEUPERS, T., GRIEND, R. J. VAN DE, DOOREN, L. J., SCHELLEKENS, P. Th. A. *et al*. T lymphocyte characteristics in bone marrow-transplanted patients. II. Analysis with monoclonal antibodies. *Journal of Immunology*, **127**, 244–251 (1981)

32 BRYANT, B. M., FORD, H. T., JARMAN, M. and SMITH, I. E. Prevention of isophosphamide-induced urothelial toxicity with 2-mercaptoethane sulphonate sodium (mesnum) in patients with advanced carcinoma. *Lancet*, **2**, 657–659 (1980)

33 BUCKLEY, R. H., WHISNANT, J. K., SCHIFF, R. I., GILBERTSEN, R. B., HUANG, A. T. and PLATT, M. S. Correction of severe combined immunodeficiency by fetal liver cells. *New England Journal of medicine*, **294**, 1076–1081 (1976)

34 BUCKNER, C. D., RUDOLPH, R. H., FEFER, A., CLIFT, R. A., EPSTEIN, R. B., FUNK, D D. *et al*. High-dose cyclophosphamide therapy for malignant disease. Toxicity, tumor response, and the effects of stored autologous marrow. *Cancer*, **29**, 357–365 (1972)

35 BUCKNER, C. D., CLIFT, R. A., SANDERS, J. E. and THOMAS, E. D. The role of a protective environment and prophylactic granulocyte transfusions in marrow transplantation. *Transplantation Proceedings*, **X**, 255–257 (1978)

36 BUCKNER, C. D., CLIFT, R. A., SANDERS, J. E., WILLIAMS, B., GRAY, M., STORB, R. and THOMAS, E. D. ABO-incompatible marrow transplants. *Transplantation*, **26**, 233–238 (1978)

37 BUCKNER, C. D. Allogeneic marrow transplantation for patients with acute leukemia. *Transplantation Proceedings*, **XI**, 215–218 (1979)

38 CAMITTA, B. M., THOMAS, E. D., NATHAN, D. G., SANTOS, G., GORDON-SMITH, E. C., GALE, R. P. *et al*. Severe aplastic anemia: a prospective study of the effect of early marrow transplantation on acute mortality. *Blood*, **48**, 63–70 (1976)

39 CAMITTA, B. M., THOMAS, E. D., NATHAN, D. G., GALE, R. P., KOPECKY, K. J., RAPPEPORT, J. M. *et al*. A prospective study of androgens and bone marrow transplantation for treatment of severe aplastic anemia. *Blood*, **53**, 504–514 (1979)

40 CHAMPLIN, R., FEIG, S. and GALE, R. P. In *Fetal Liver Transplantation*, edited by G. Lucarelli, T. M. Fliedner and R. P. Gale, 210. Amsterdam, Excerpta Medica (1980)

41 CLAAS, F. H. J., ROOD, J. J. VAN, WARREN, R. P., WEIDEN, P. L., SU, P. J. and STORB, R. The detection of non-HLA antibodies and their possible role in bone marrow graft rejection. *Transplantation Proceedings*, **XI**, 423–426 (1979)

42 CLARK, R. A., JOHNSON, F. L., KLEBANOFF, S. J. and THOMAS, E. D. Defective neutrophil chemotaxis in bone marrow transplant patients. *Journal of Clinical Investigation*, **58**, 22-31 (1976)

43 CLARK, R. A., BUCKNER, C. D., FEFER, A., LERNER, K. G., NEIMAN, P. E., STORB, R. *et al.* Infectious complications of marrow transplantation. *Transplantation Proceedings*, **VI**, 389-393 (1974)

44 CLIFT, R. A., SANDERS, J. E., THOMAS, E. D., WILLIAMS, B. and BUCKNER, C. D. Granulocyte transfusions for the prevention of infection in patients receiving bone-marrow transplants. *New England Journal of Medicine*, **298**, 1052-1057 (1978)

45 CLIFT, R. A., BUCKNER, C. D. and THOMAS, E. D. In *Clinical and Experimental Gnotobiotics (Zbl. Bakt. Suppl. 7)*, edited by T. M. Fliedner, H. Heit, D. Niethammer and H. Pflierger, 255. Stuttgart, Gustav Fischer Verlag (1979)

46 COCCIA., P. F., KRIVIT, W., CERVENKA, J., CLAWSON, C., KERSEY, J. H. KIM, T. H. *et al.* Successful bone-marrow transplantation for infantile malignant osteopetrosis. *New England Journal of Medicine*, **302**, 701-708 (1980)

47 COHEN, A., MANSOUR, A., DOSCH, H. M. and GELFAND, E. W. Association of a lymphocyte purine enzyme deficiency (5'-nucleotidase) with combined immunodeficiency. *Clinical Immunology and Immunopathology*, **15**, 245-250 (1980)

48 DEEG, H. J., MEYERS, J. D., STORB, R., GRAHAM, T. C. and WEIDEN, P. L. Effect of trimethoprim-sulfamethoxazole on hematological recovery after total body irradiation and autologous marrow infusion in dogs. *Transplantation*, **28**, 243-246 (1979)

49 DEEG, H. J., STORB, R., PRENTICE, R., FRITZ, T. E., WEIDEN, P. L., SALE, G. E. *et al.* Increased cancer risk in canine radiation chimeras. *Blood*, **55**, 233-239 (1980)

50 DEEG, H. J., STORB, R., RAFF, R., WEIDEN, P. L., GRAHAM, T. C. and THOMAS, E. D. Resistance to allogeneic marrow grafts in dogs: effect of DLA matching, buffy coat cells, methotrexate (MTX), cyclosporin A (CyA) and fractionated total body irradiation (TBI). *Experimental Hematology*, **9** (suppl 9), 97 (1981)

51 DICKE, K. A. and BEKKUM, D. W. VAN. Allogeneic bone marrow transplantation after elimination of immunocompetent cells by means of density gradient centrifugation. *Transplantation Proceedings*, **III**, 666-668 (1971)

52 DIEPENHORST, P., SPROKHOLT, R. and PRINS, H. K. Removal of leukocytes from whole blood and erythrocyte suspensions by filtration through cotton-wool. *Vox Sanguinis*, **23**, 308-320 (1972)

53 DIETRICH, M., GAUS, W., VOSSEN, J., WAAIJ, D. VAN DER, and WENDT, F. Protective isolation and antimicrobial decontamination in patients with high susceptibility to infection. A prospective cooperative study of gnotobiotic care in acute leukemia patients. Part I: Clinical results. *Infection*, **5**, 107-114 (1977)

54 DONEY, K., BUCKNER, C. D., SALE, G. E., RAMBERG, R., BOYD, C. and THOMAS, E. D. Treatment of chronic granulocytic leukemia by chemotherapy, total body irradiation and allogeneic bone marrow transplantation. *Experimental Hematology*, **6**, 738-747 (1978)

55 DYMINSKI, J. W., DAOUD, A., LAMPKIN, B. C., LIMOUZE, S., DONOFRIO, J., COLEMAN, M. S. *et al.* Immunological and biochemical profiles in response to transfusion therapy in an adenosine deaminase-deficient patient with severe combined immunodeficiency disease. *Clinical Immunology and Immunopathology*, **14**, 307-326 (1979)

56 EERNISSE, J. G. and BRAND, A. Prevention of platelet refractoriness due to HLA antibodies by administration of leukocyte-poor blood components. *Experimental Hematology*, **9**, 77–83 (1981)

57 ELFENBEIN, G. J., BROGAONKAR, D. S., BIAS, W. B., BURNS, W. H., SARAL, R., SENSENBRENNER, L. L. et al. Cytogenetic evidence for recurrence of acute myelogenous leukemia after allogeneic bone marrow transplantation in donor hematopoietic cells. *Blood*, **52**, 627–636 (1978)

58 ELFENBEIN, G. J. and BELLIS, M. M. Paucity of helper T cells during early immune recovery after human marrow transplantation. *Experimental Hematology*, **9** (suppl. 9), 16 (1981)

59 ELFENBEIN, G., KALLMAN, C., BRAINE, H., BIAS, W., TUTSCHKA, P., KARP. J. et al. Analysis of factors related to bone marrow graft rejection in aplastic anemia: usefulness of measures of broad alloimmunity as predictors. *Transplantation Proceedings*, **XIII**, 1539–1543 (1981)

60 ELIN, R. J., REYNOLDS, H. Y., DURBIN, W. A., WOLFF, S. M. and KAZNIEROWSKY, J. A. Chediak–Higashi syndrome. Reversal of increased susceptibility to infection by bone marrow transplantation. *Blood*, **47**, 555–559 (1976)

61 EMMELOT, C. H. and WAAIJ, D. VAN DER. The dose range over which neomycin and polymyxin B can be applied for selective decontamination of the digestive tract in mice. *Journal of Hygiene (Cambridge)*, **84**, 331–340 (1980)

62 FASS, L., OCHS, H. D., THOMAS, E. D., MICKELSON, E., STORB, R. and FEFER, A. Studies of immunological reactivity following syngeneic or allogeneic marrow grafts in man. *Transplantation*, **16**, 630–640 (1973)

63 FASTH, A. First International Meeting on Congenital Immunodeficiencies, Tübingen (1980), personal communication

64 FEFER, A., CHEEVER, M. A., THOMAS, E. D., APPELBAUM, F. R., BUCKNER, C. D., CLIFT, R. A. et al. Bone marrow transplantation for refractory acute leukemia in 34 patients with identical twins. *Blood*, **57**, 421–430 (1981)

65 FENYK, J. R., WARKENTIN, Ph. I., GOLTZ, R. W., NESBIT, M. E., COCCIA, P. F., SMITH, C. M. et al. Sclerodermatous graft-versus-host disease limited to an area of measles exanthem. *Lancet*, **1**, 472–473 (1978)

66 FIALKOW, P. J., BRYANT, J. I., THOMAS, E. D. and NEIMAN, P. E. Leukaemic transformation of engrafted human marrow cells *in vivo*. *Lancet*, **1**, 251–255 (1971)

67 FISCHER, G. W., WILSON, S. R., HUNTER, K. W. and MEASE, A. D. Diminished bacterial defences with intralipid. *Lancet*, **2**, 819–820 (1980)

68 FLAD, H. D., GOLDMANN, S. F., NIETHAMMER, D., ULMER, A. J., COLOMBANI, J. and KLEIHAUER, E. In *Primary Immunodeficiencies*, edited by M. Seligmann and W. H. Hitzig, 435. Amsterdam, Elsevier/North-Holland Biomedical Press (1980)

69 FLIEDNER, V. E. VON, GRATHWOHL, A., JEANNET, M., NISSEN, C. and SPECK, B. Effect of cyclosporin A on immunological recovery after bone marrow transplantation. *Lancet*, **1**, 439 (1981)

70 FORMAN, S. J., ROBINSON, G. V., WOLF, J. L., SPRUCE, W. E. and BLUME, K. G. Pulmonary reactions associated with amphotericin B and leukocyte transfusions. *New England Journal of Medicine*, **305**, 584–585 (1981)

71 FRIEDRICH, W., O'REILLY, R. J., KOZINER, B., GEBHARD, D., GOOD, R. A. and EVANS, R. L. Human T cell subset development following marrow transplantation. *Experimental Hematology*, **9** (suppl. 9), 188 (1981)

72 GALE, R. P., FEIG, S., HO, W., FALK, P., RIPPEE, C. and SPARKES, R. ABO blood group system and bone marrow transplantation. *Blood*, **50**, 185–194 (1977)

73 GALE, R. P., SPARKES, R. S. and GOLDE, D. W. Bone marrow origin of hepatic macrophages (Kupffer cells) in humans. *Science*, **201**, 937–938 (1978)

74 GALE, R. P., CAHAN, M., FITCHEN, J. H., OPELZ, G. and CLINE, M. J. Pretransplant lymphocytotoxins and bone-marrow graft rejection. *Lancet*, **1**, 170–172 (1978)

75 GALE, R. P., OPELZ, G., MICKEY, M. R., GRAZE, P. R. and SAXON, A. Immunodeficiency following allogeneic bone marrow transplantation. *Transplantation Proceedings*, **X**, 223–227 (1978)

76 GALE, R. P. Current status of bone marrow transplantation in acute leukemia. *Transplantation Proceedings*, **XI**, 1920–1923 (1979)

77 GALE, R. P. Autologous bone marrow transplantation in patients with cancer. *Journal of the American Medical Association*, **243**, 540–542 (1980)

78 GALE, R. P. In *Biology of Bone Marrow Transplantation*, edited by R. P. Gale and C. F. Fox, 11. London, Academic Press (1980)

79 GALE, R. P. In *Fetal Liver Transplantation*, edited by G. Lucarelli, T. M. Fliedner and R. P. Gale, 268. Amsterdam, Excerpta Medica (1980)

80 GALE, R. P. Bone marrow transplantation for leukemia in remission. *Experimental Hematology*, **9** (suppl. 9), 125 (1981)

81 GATTI, R. A., ALLEN, H. D., MEUWISSEN, H. J., HONG, R. and GOOD, R. A. Immunological reconstitution of sex-linked lymphopenic immunological deficiency. *Lancet*, **2**, 1366–1369 (1968)

82 GEHA, R. S., MALAKIAN, A., LeFRANC, G., CHAYBAN, D. and SERRE, J. L. Immunologic reconstitution in severe combined immunodeficiency following transplantation with parental bone marrow. *Pediatrics*, **58**, 451–455 (1976)

83 GEHA, R. S. Origin of the antibody-dependent cytotoxic cell in man. *Clinical Immunology and Immunopathology*, **7**, 253–261 (1977)

84 GEHA, R. S., RAPPAPORT, J. M., TWAROG, F. J., PARKMAN, R. and ROSEN, F. S. Increased serum immunoglobulin E levels following allogeneic bone marrow transplantation. *Journal of Allergy and Clinical Immunology*, **66**, 78–81 (1980)

85 GEHRZ, R. C., McAULIFFE, J. J., LINNER, K. M. and KERSEY, J. H. Defective membrane function in a patient with severe combined immunodeficiency disease. *Clinical Experimental Immunology*, **39**, 344–348 (1980)

86 GELFAND, E. W., DOSCH, H. M., HUBER, J. and SHORE, A. *In vitro* and *in vivo* reconstitution of severe combined immunodeficiency disease (SCID) with thymic epithelium. *Clinical Research*, **25**, 358A. (1977)

87 GELFAND, E. W., OLIVER, J. M., SCHUURMAN, R. K., MATHESON, D. S. and DOSCH, H. M. Abnormal lymphocyte capping in a patient with severe combined immunodeficiency disease. *New England Journal of Medicine*, **301**, 1245–1249 (1979)

88 GELFAND, E. W., DOSCH, H. M., COHEN, A. and McCLURE, P. D. In *Biology of Bone Marrow Transplantation*, edited by R. P. Gale and C. F. Fox, 97. London, Academic Press (1980)

89 GELFAND, E. W., DOSCH, H. M., SHORE, A., LIMATIBUL, S. and LEE, J. W. W. In *Biological Basis of Immunodeficiency*, edited by E. W. Gelfand and H. M. Dosch, 39. New York, Raven Press (1980)

90 GELFAND, E. W. First International Meeting on Congenital Immunodeficiencies, Tübingen (1980), personal communication
91 GIBLETT, E. R., ANDERSON, J. E., COHEN, F., POLLARA, B. and MEUWISSEN, H. J. Adenosine-deaminase deficiency in two patients with severely impaired cellular immunity. *Lancet*, **2,** 1067–1069 (1972)
92 GIBLETT, E. R., AMMANN, A. J., SANDMAN, R., WARA, D. W. and DIAMOND, L. K. Nucleoside-phosphorylase deficiency in a child with severely defective T-cell immunity and normal B-cell immunity. *Lancet*, **1,** 1010–1013 (1975)
93 GLUCKMAN, E., GLUCKMAN, J. C., ANDERSEN, E., DEVERGIE, A. and J. DAUSSET. Lymphocytotoxic antibodies and bone marrow grafts from HLA-identical siblings. *Transplantation*, **26,** 284–286 (1978)
94 GLUCKMAN, E., DEVERGIE, A., BUSSEL, A. and BERNARD, J. In *Bone Marrow Transplantation in Europe*, edited by J. L. Touraine, 42. Amsterdam, Excerpta Medica (1979)
95 GLUCKMAN, E., DEVERGIE, A., SCHAISON, G., BUSSEL, A., BERGER, R., SOHIER, J. *et al.* Bone marrow transplantation in Fanconi anaemia. *British Journal of Haematology*, **45,** 557–564 (1980)
96 GLUCKMAN, E., DEVERGIE, A., GEROTTA, I., HORS, J., SASPORTES, M., BOIRON, M. *et al.* Bone marrow transplantation in 65 patients with severe aplastic anemia. *Blut*, **41,** 157–160 (1980)
97 GLUCKMAN, E., GLUCKMAN, J. C., ANDERSEN, E., GUILLET, J., DEVERGIE, A. and DAUSSET, J. Lymphocytotoxic antibodies after bone marrow transplantation in aplastic anemia. II. Non-HLA antibodies. *Transplantation*, **29,** 471–476 (1980)
98 GLUCKMAN, E., BARRETT, A. J., ARCESE, W., DEVERGIE, A. and DEGOULET, P. Bone marrow transplantation in severe aplastic anaemia: a survey of the European group for bone marrow transplantation (EGBMT). *British Journal of Haematology*, **49,** 165–173 (1981)
99 GLUCKMAN, E., DEVERGIE, A., LOKIEC, F., POIRIER, O. and BAUMELOU, A. Nephrotoxicity of cyclosporin A in bone-marrow transplantation. *Lancet*, **2,** 144–145 (1981)
100 GOH, K. and KLEMPERER, M. R. *In vivo* leukemic transformation: cytogenetic evidence of *in vivo* leukemic transformation of engrafted marrow cells. *American Journal of Hematology*, **2,** 283–290 (1977)
101 GOLDSTEIN, A. L., COHEN, G. H. and THURMAN, G. B. In *Control of Neoplasia by Modulation of the Immune System*, edited by M. A. Chirigos, 241. New York, Raven Press (1977)
102 GOOD, R. A., KAPOOR, N., PAHWA, R. N., WEST, A. and O'REILLY, R. J. In *Progress in Immunology IV*, edited by M. Fougereau and J. Dausset, 906. London, Academic Press (1980)
103 GOSSET, T. C., GALE, R. P., FLEISCHMAN, H., AUSTIN, G. E., SPARKES, R. S. and TAYLOR, C. R. Immunoblastic sarcoma in donor cells after bone-marrow transplantation. *New England Journal of Medicine*, **300,** 904–907 (1979)
104 GRANGER, S., JANOSSY, G., TIDMAN, N., ASHLEY, J., CRAWFORD, D. H., KOUBEK, K. *et al.* In *Leukemia Markers*, edited by W. Knapp, 419. London, Academic Press (1981)
105 GRATWOHL, A. A., MOUTSOPOULOS, H. M., CHUSED, Th. M., AKIZUKI, M., WOLF, R. O., SWEET, J. B. *et al.* Sjögren-type syndrome after allogeneic bone-marrow transplantation. *Annals of Internal Medicine*, **87,** 703–706 (1977)

106 GRAZE, P. R. and GALE, R. P. Chronic graft versus host disease: a syndrome of disordered immunity. *American Journal of Medicine*, **66**, 611–620 (1979)

107 GRIEND, R. J. VAN DE, ASTALDI, A., VOSSEN, J. M., DOOREN, L. J., SCHELLEKENS, P. Th. A., ZWAAN, F. E. et al. T lymphocyte characteristics in bone-marrow transplanted patients. 1. Changes in biochemical properties that correlate with the immunological reconstitution. *Journal of Immunology*, **126**, 636–640 (1981)

108 GRISCELLI, C., DURANDY, A., BALLET, J. J., PRIEUR, A. M. and HORS, J. T- and B-cell chimerism in two patients with severe combined immunodeficiency (SCID) after transplantation. *Transplantation Proceedings*, **IX**, 171–175 (1977)

109 GRISCELLI, C., DURANDY, A., VIRELIZIER, J. L. and BURIOT, D. In *Immunobiology of Bone Marrow Transplantation*, edited by S. Thierfelder, H. Rodt and H. J. Kolb, 403. Berlin, Springer Verlag (1980)

110 GUIOT, H. F. L. and FURTH, R. VAN. Partial antibiotic decontamination. *British Medical Journal*, **1**, 800–802 (1977)

111 HAGENBEEK, A. and MARTENS, A. C. M. The effect of fractionated versus unfractionated total body irradiation on the growth of the BN acute myelocytic leukemia. *International Journal of Radiation Oncology and Biological Biophysics*, **7**, 1079–1085 (1981)

112 HANEBERG, B., FRØLAND, S. S., FINNE, P. H., BAKKE, T., THUNOLD, S., MOE, P. J. et al. Fetal thymus transplantations in severe combined immunodeficiency. *Scandinavian Journal of Immunology*, **5**, 917–924 (1976)

113 HANSEN, G. S., DUPONT, B., FABER, V., JAKOBSEN, B. K., JUHL, F., NIELSEN, L. S. et al. Lymphocyte chimerism after bone-marrow transplantation. *Scandinavian Journal of Immunology*, **6**, 299–303 (1977)

114 HANSEN, J. A., CLIFT, R. A., THOMAS, E. D., BUCKNER, C. D., MICKELSON, E. M. and STORB, R. Histocompatibility and marrow transplantation. *Transplantation Proceedings*, **XI**, 1924–1929 (1979)

115 HANSEN, J. A., CLIFT, R. A., THOMAS, E. D., BUCKNER, C. D., STORB, R. and GIBLETT, E. R. Transplantation of marrow from an unrelated donor to a patient with acute leukemia. *New England Journal of Medicine*, **303**, 565–567 (1980)

116 HANSEN, J. A., CLIFT, R. A., MICKELSON, E. M., NISPEROS, B. and THOMAS, E. D. Marrow transplantation from donors other than HLA identical siblings. *Human Immunology*, **2**, 31–40 (1981)

117 HATHAWAY, W. E., GITHENS, J. H., BLACKBURN, W. R., FULGINITI, V. and KEMPE, C. H. Aplastic anemia, histocytiosis, and erythrodermia in immunologically deficient children – probable human runt disease. *New England Journal of Medicine*, **273**, 953–958 (1965)

118 HATHAWAY, W. E., BRANGLE, R. W., NELSON, Th. L. and ROECKEL, I. E. Aplastic anemia and alymphocytosis in an infant with hypogammaglobulinemia: graft-versus-host reaction? *Journal of Pediatrics*, **68**, 713–722 (1966)

119 HEIT, H., HEIT, W., KOHNE, E., FLIEDNER, T. M. and HUGHES, P. Allogeneic bone marrow transplantation in conventional mice: 1. Effect of antibiotic therapy on long term survival of allogeneic chimeras. *Blut*, **35**, 143–153 (1977)

120 HOBBS, J. R. First International Meeting on Congenital Immunodeficiencies, Tübingen, (1980), personal communication

121 HOBBS, J. R., BARRETT, A. J., CHAMBERS, D., JAMES, D. C. O., HUGH-JONES, K., BYROM, N. et al. Reversal of clinical features of Hurler's disease and biochemical improvement after treatment by bone-marrow transplantation. *Lancet*, **2**, 709–712 (1981)

122 HOBBS, J. R. Bone marrow transplantation for inborn errors. *Lancet*, **2**, 735–739 (1981)

123 HOLL, R. A., DOOREN, L. J., VOSSEN, J. M. J. J., ROOS, M. Th. L. and SCHELLEKENS, P. Th. A. Bone marrow transplantation in children with severe aplastic anemia. Reconstitution of cellular immunity. *Transplantation*, **32**, 418–423 (1981)

124 HONG, R., SCHULTE-WISSERMANN, H. and HOROWITZ, S. D. Thymic transplantation for relief of immunodeficiency diseases. *Surgical Clinics of North America*, **59**, 299–312 (1979)

125 HONG, R. First International Meeting on Congenital Immunodeficiencies, Tübingen, (1980), personal communication

126 HOROWITZ, S. D., BACH, F. H., GROSHONG, T., HONG, R and YUNIS, E. J. Treatment of severe combined immunodeficiency with bone-marrow from an unrelated, mixed-leucocyte-culture-non-reactive donor. *Lancet*, **2**, 431–433 (1975)

127 HOWS, J. M., PALMER, S., WANT, S., DEARDEN, C. and GORDON-SMITH, E. C. Serum levels of cyclosporin A and nephorotoxicity in bone marrow transplant patients. *Lancet*, **2**, 145–146 (1981)

128 HOWS, J. M., PALMER, S. and GORDON-SMITH, E. C. In *Bone Marrow Transplantation in Europe II*, edited by J. L. Touraine, E. Gluckman and C. Griscelli, 178. Amsterdam, Excerpta Medica (1981)

129 HUGHES, W. T., KUHN, Sh., CHAUDHARY, S., FELDMAN, S., VERZOSA, M., AUR, R. et al. Successful chemoprophylaxis for pneumocystis carinii pneumonitis. *New England Journal of Medicine*, **297**, 1419–1426 (1977)

130 HUGH-JONES, K. Third European Symposium on Bone Marrow Transplantation, Sankt Moritz (1979)

131 ISKANDAR, O., JAGER, M. J., WILLEMZE, R. and NATARAJAN, A. T. A case of pure red cell aplasia with a high incidence of spontaneous chromosome breakage: a possible X-ray sensitive syndrome. *Human Genetics*, **55**, 337–340 (1980)

132 JAMES, D. C. O. In *Bone Marrow Transplantation in Europe II*, edited by J. L. Touraine, E. Gluckman and C. Griscelli, 264. Amsterdam, Excerpta Medica (1981)

133 JOHNSON, F. L., THOMAS, E. D., CLARK, B. S., CHARD, R. L., HARTMANN, J. R. and STORB, R. A comparison of marrow transplantation with chemotherapy for children with acute lymphoblastic leukemia in second or subsequent remission. *New England Journal of Medicine*, **305**, 846–851 (1981)

134 JOLLER, P. W. and HITZIG, W. H. Cultured thymus epithelium transplantation in 4 children suffering from severe combined immunodeficiency (SCID). *Pediatric Research*, **15**, 1206 (1981)

135 JONES, J. M., WILSON, R. and BEALMEAR, P. M. Mortality and gross pathology of secondary disease in germfree mouse radiation chimeras. *Radiation Research*, **45**, 577–588 (1971)

136 JONES, J. F., SIEBER, Jr., O. F., FULGINITI, V. A., OCHS, H., SCHULTE-WISSERMAN, H. and HONG, R. Predominance of B-lymphocyte function after cultured thymus fragment therapy in severe combined immunodeficiency disease. *Clinical Immunology and Immunopathology*, **17**, 439–450 (1980)

137 KADOWAKI, J. I., ZUELZER, W. W., BROUGH, A. J., THOMPSON, R. I., WOOLLEY, P. V. and GRUBER, D. XX/XY lymphoid chimaerism in congenital immunological deficiency syndrome with thymic alymphoplasia. *Lancet*, **2**, 1152–1156 (1965)

138 KAMPHUIS, R. P. In *Clinical and Experimental Gnotobiotics (Zbl. Bakt. Suppl. 7)*, edited by T. M. Fliedner, H. Heit, D. Niethammer and H. Pflieger, 53. Stuttgart–New York, Gustav Fischer Verlag (1979)

139 KAPOOR, N., KIRKPATRICK, D., BLAESE, M. R., OLESKE, J., HILGARTNER, M. H., CHAGANTI, R. S. K. et al. Reconstitution of normal megakaryocytopoiesis and immunologic functions in Wiskott–Aldrich syndrome by marrow transplantation following myeloablation and immunosuppression with busulfan and cyclophosphamide. *Blood*, **57**, 692–696 (1981)

140 KATZ, S. I., TAMAKI, K. and SACHS, D. H. Epidermal Langerhans cells are derived from cells originating in bone marrow. *Nature*, **282**, 324–326 (1979)

141 KEIGHTLEY, R. G., LAWTON, A. R. and COOPER, M. D. Successful fetal liver transplantation in a child with severe combined immunodeficiency. *Lancet*, **2**, 850–853 (1975)

142 KENNY, A. B. and HITZIG, W. H. Bone marrow transplantation for severe combined immunodeficiency disease. *European Journal of Pediatrics*, **131**, 155–177 (1979)

143 KERSEY, J. H., FISH, L. A., COX, Sh. T. and AUGUST, Ch. S. Severe combined immunodeficiency with response to calcium ionophore: a possible membrane defect. *Clinical Immunology and Immunopathology*, **7**, 62–68 (1977)

144 KERSEY, J. H., FILIPOVICH, A. H., SPECTOR, B. D. and FRIZZERA, G. Lymphoma after thymus transplantation. *New England Journal of Medicine*, **302**, 301–302 (1980)

145 KERSEY, J. H., VALLERA, D. A., SODERLING, C., WARKENTIN, P., KIM, T., LEVITT, S. et al. In *Biology of Bone Marrow Transplantation*, edited by R. P. Gale and C. F. Fox, 29. London, Academic Press (1980)

146 KIESSLING, R., HOCHMAN, P. S., HALLER, O., SHEARER, G. M., WIGZELL, H. and CUDKOWICZ, G. Evidence for a similar or common mechanism for natural killer cell activity and resistance to hemopoietic grafts. *European Journal of Immunology*, **7**, 655–663 (1977)

147 KOGEL, A. J. VAN DER, BEKKUM, D. W. VAN and BARENDSEN, G. W. Tolerance of CNS to total body irradiation combined with chemotherapy applied for the treatment of leukemia. *European Journal of Cancer*, **12**, 675–677 (1976)

148 KONING, J. DE, BEKKUM, D. W. VAN, DICKE, K. A., DOOREN, L. J., ROOD, J. J. VAN and RÁDL, J. Transplantation of bone-marrow cells and fetal thymus in an infant with lymphopenic immunological deficiency. *Lancet*, **1**, 1223–1227 (1969)

149 KONING, J. DE, WAAIJ, D. VAN DER, VOSSEN, J. M., VERSPRILLE, A. and DOOREN, L. J. Barrier nursing of an infant in a laminar cross-flow bench. *Maandschrift voor Kindergeneeskunde*, **38**, 1–13 (1970)

150 KONING, J. DE, VEER-KORTHOF, E. T. VAN 'T and WEEL-SIPMAN, M. H. VAN In *Immunobiology of Bone Marrow Transplantation*, edited by S. Thierfelder, H. Rodt and H. J. Kolb, 381. Berlin, Springer Verlag (1980)

151 KUIS, W. First International Meeting on Congenital Immunodeficiencies, Tübingen, (1980), (personal communication)
152 KUMAR, R., McEVOY, J., BIGGART, J. D. and McGEOWN, M. G. Cyclophosphamide and reproductive function. *Lancet*, **1**, 1212–1214 (1972)
153 LEVINE, A. S., SIEGEL, S. E., SCHREIBER, A. D., HAUSER, J., PREISLER, H., GOLDSTEIN, I. M. *et al*. Protected environments and prophylactic antibiotics. A prospective controlled study of their utility in the therapy of acute leukemia. *New England Journal of Medicine*, **288**, 477–483 (1973)
154 LIVNAT, S., SEIGNEURET, M., STORB, R. and PRENTICE, R. L. Analysis of cytotoxic effector cell function in patients with leukemia or aplastic anemia before and after marrow transplantation. *Journal of Immunology*, **124**, 481–490 (1980)
155 LOPEZ, C., SORELL, M., KIRKPATRICK, D., O'REILLY, R. J. and CHING, C. Association between pre-transplant natural kill and graft-versus-host disease after stem-cell transplantation. *Lancet*, **2**, 1103–1106 (1979)
156 LORENZ, E., UPHOFF, D., REID, T. R. and SHELTON, E. Modification of irradiation injury in mice and guinea pigs by bone marrow injections. *Journal of the National Cancer Institute*, **12**, 197–201 (1951)
157 LOTZOVÁ, E. and POLLACK, S. B. The first direct evidence on the involvement of natural killer cells in bone marrow graft rejection. *Experimental Hematology*, **9** (suppl. 9), 16 (1981)
158 LUCARELLI, G., IZZI, Th., PORCELLINI, A., DELFINI, C., POLCHI, P., MORETTI, L. *et al*. In *Fetal Liver Transplantation*, edited by G. Lucarelli, T. M. Fliedner and R. P. Gale, 284. Amsterdam, Excerpta Medica (1980)
159 LUCAS, C. F. First International Meeting on Congenital Immunodeficiencies, Tübingen, (1980), personal communication
160 LUM, L. G., SEIGNEURET, M. C., STORB, R. F., WITHERSPOON, R. P. and THOMAS, E. D. In vitro regulation of immunoglobulin synthesis after marrow transplantation. I. T-cell and B-Cell deficiencies in patients with and without chronic graft-versus-host-disease. *Blood*, **58**, 431–439 (1981)
161 LUMLEY, H. S., POWLES, R., MORGENSTERN, G., CLINK, H. M., McELWAIN, T. J. In *Bone Marrow Transplantation in Europe II*, edited by J. L. Touraine, E. Gluckman and C. Griscelli, 24. Amsterdam, Excerpta Medica (1981)
162 MARKWICK, J. R., HOBBS, J. R., CHAMBERS, J. D. and PEGRUM, G. D. Timing of cyclosporin-A therapy for abrogation of HVG and GVH responses in rats. *Lancet*, **2**, 1037–1040 (1979)
163 MASAOKA, T., NAMIUCHI, S., KUBOTA, Y., SAIGO, K., UEDA, T., TAKUBO, T. *et al*. Exogenous infections during induction treatment of acute leukemia. Proceedings of the VIIth International Symposium on Gnotobiology, Tokyo, (in press)
164 MAWHINNEY, H., GLEADHILL, V. F. D. and McCREA, S. *In vitro* and *in vivo* responses to thymosin in severe combined immunodeficiency. *Clinical Immunology and Immunopathology*, **14**, 196–203 (1979)
165 MEUWISSEN, H. J., GATTI, R. A. TERASAKI, P. I., HONG, R. and GOOD, R. A. Treatment of lymphopenic hypogammaglobulinemia and bone-marrow aplasia by transplantation of allogeneic marrow. Crucial role of histocompatibility matching. *New England Journal of Medicine*, **281**, 691–697 (1969)

166 MICKELSON, E. M., CLIFT, R. A., FEFER, A., STORB, R., THOMAS, E. D., WARREN, R. P. et al. Studies of the response in mixed leukocyte culture of cells from patients with aplastic anemia to cells from HLA-identical siblings. *Transplantation*, **32**, 90–95 (1981)

167 MITCHELL, Ch. D., GENTRY, Sh. R., BOEN, J. R., BEAN, B., GROTH, K. E. and BALFOUR Jr., H. H. Acyclovir therapy for mucocutaneous herpes simplex infections in immunocompromised patients. *Lancet*, **1**, 1389–1392 (1981)

168 MORGENSTERN, G. R., LUMLEY, H., WATSON, J. G. and POWLES, R. In *Bone Marrow Transplantation in Europe II*, edited by J. L. Touraine, E. Gluckman and C. Griscelli, 156. Amsterdam, Excerpta Medica (1981)

169 MÜLLER-RUCHHOLTZ, W., WOTTGE, H. U. and MÜLLER-HERMELINK, H. K. In *Immunobiology of Bone Marrow Transplantation*, edited by S. Thierfelder, H. Rodt and H. J. Kolb, 153. Berlin, Springer-Verlag (1980)

170 NAGAO, T. Maintenance of aseptic environment and its clinical utility. *Proceedings of the VIIth International Symposium on Gnotobiology*, Tokyo, (in press)

171 NEELY, J. E., NEELY, A. N. and KERSEY, J. H. Immunodeficiency following human marrow transplantation: *in vitro* studies. *Transplantation Proceedings*, **X**, 229–231 (1978)

172 NEIMAN, P., WASSERMAN, P. B., WENTWORTH, B. B., KAO, G. F., LERNER, K. G., STORB, R. et al. Interstitial pneumonia and cytomegalovirus infections as complications of human marrow transplantation. *Transplantation*, **15**, 478–485 (1973)

173 NEIMAN, P. E., MEYERS, J. D., MEDEIROS, E., McDOUGALL, J. K. and THOMAS, E. D. In *Biology of Bone Marrow Transplantation*, edited by R. P. Gale and C. F. Fox, 75. London, Academic Press (1980)

174 NEWBURGER, P. E., LATT, S. A., PESANDO, J. M., GUSTASHAW, K., POWERS, M., CHAGANTI, R. S. K. et al. Leukemia relapse in donor cells after allogeneic bone-marrow transplantation. *New England Journal of Medicine*, **304**, 712–714 (1981)

175 NIELSEN, H., KOCH, Chr., MÜLLER-BERAT, N. and PHILIP, J. Y Chromatin as indicator of chimaerism following bone-marrow transplantation in severe combined immunodeficiency. *Scandinavian Journal of Immunology*, **2**, 327–331 (1973)

176 NIETHAMMER, D., GOLDMANN, S. F., FLAD, H. D., WERNET, P., STURSBERG, G., COLOMBANI, J. et al. In *Immunobiology of Bone Marrow Transplantation*, edited by S. Thierfelder, H. Rodt and H. J. Kolb, 391. Berlin, Springer Verlag (1980)

177 NIETHAMMER, D., GOLDMAN, S. F., FLAD, H. D., BIENZLE, U., DIETERLE, U., HAAS, R. J. et al. Nature of reconstitution with histoincompatible maternal marrow in a case of severe combined immunodeficiency with graft-versus-host disease following maternofetal transfusion. *Clinical Immunology and immunopathology*, **18**, 387–401 (1981)

178 NIETHAMMER, D. personal communication (1981)

179 NOEL, D. R., WITHERSPOON, E. P., STORB, R., ATKINSON, K., DONEY, K., MICKELSON, E. M. et al. Does graft-versus-host disease influence the tempo of immunologic recovery after allogeneic human marrow transplantation? An observation on 56 long-term survivors. *Blood*, **51**, 1087–1105 (1978)

180 OCHS, H. D. and WEDGWOOD, R. J. In *Fetal Liver Transplantation*, edited by G. Lucarelli, T. M., Fliedner and R. P. Gale, 257. Amsterdam, Excerpta Medica (1980)

181 ODOM, L. F., GITHENS, J. H., MORSE, H., SHARMA, B., AUGUST, Ch. S., HUMBERT, J. R. et al. Remission of relapsed leukaemia during a graft-versus-host reaction. A 'graft-versus leukaemia reaction' in man? *Lancet*, **2**, 537–540 (1978)

182 OPELZ, G., GALE, R. P., FEIG, S. A., WALKER, J., TERASAKI, P. I. and SAXON, A. Significance of HLA and non-HLA antigens in bone marrow transplantation. *Transplantation Proceedings*, **X**, 43–46 (1978)

183 O'REILLY, R. J., DUPONT, B., PAHWA, S., GRIMES, E., SMITHWICK, E. M., PAHWA, R. et al. Reconstitution in severe combined immunodeficiency by transplantation of marrow from an unrelated donor. *New England Journal of Medicine*, **297**, 1311–1318 (1977)

184 O'REILLY, R. J., KAPOOR, N. and KIRKPATRICK, D. In *Primary Immunodeficiencies*, edited by M. Seligman and W. H. Hitzig, 419. Amsterdam, Elsevier/North-Holland Biomedical Press (1980)

185 PAHWA, R., PAHWA, S., O'REILLY, R. and GOOD, R. A. In *Immune Deficiency*, edited by M. D. Cooper, A. R. Lawton, P. A. Miescher and H. J. Mueller-Eberhard, 121. Berlin, Springer Verlag (1979)

186 PAHWA, R. N., PAHWA, S. G. and GOOD, R. A. T-lymphocyte differentiation *in vitro* in severe combined immunodeficiency. Defects of stem cells. *Journal of Clinical Investigation*, **64**, 1632–1641 (1979)

187 PAHWA, S., FRIEDRICH, W., EVANS, R., O'REILLY, R. and GOOD, R. A. Humoral immune response *in vitro* after bone marrow transplantation (BMT). *Experimental Hematology*, **9** (suppl. 9), 189 (1981)

188 PALMER, S., HOWS, J. and GORDON-SMITH, E. C. In *Bone Marrow Transplantation in Europe II*, edited by J. L. Touraine, E. Gluckman and C. Griscelli, 120. Amsterdam, Excerpta Medica (1981)

189 PARK, B. H., BIGGAR, W. D., YUNIS, E. J. and GOOD, R. A. Recent advances in transplantation of incompatible marrow in infants with combined immunodeficiency. *Transplantation Proceedings*, **5**, 899–903 (1973)

190 PARKMAN, R., RAPPEPORT, J., GEHA, R., BELLI, J., CASSADY, R., LEVEY, R. et al. Complete correction of the Wiskott–Aldrich Syndrome by allogeneic bone-marrow transplantation. *New England Journal of Medicine*, **298**, 921–927 (1978)

191 PECK, G. L., HERZIG, G. P. and ELIAS, P. M. Toxic epidermal necrolysis in a patient with graft-versus-host reaction. *Archives of Dermatology*, **105**, 561–569 (1972)

192 POLLACK, M. S., YANG, S. Y., O'NEILL, G. J., O'REILLY, R., GROSSBARD, E., KAPOOR, N. et al. Bone marrow transplantation using typing for glyoxalase I as a tool in histocompatibility testing. *Transplantation*, **28**, 156–158 (1979)

193 POLLACK, M. S., KAPOOR, N., SORELL, M., MORISHIMA, Y., DUPONT, B. and O'REILLY R. J. Absence of demonstrable suppressor cell activity in a severe combined immunodeficiency patient with a sustained engraftment of DR-positive maternal T cells. *Transplantation Proceedings*, **XIII**, 270–272 (1981)

194 POLMAR, S. H., STERN, R. C., SCHWARTZ, A. L., WETZLER, E. M., CHASE, P. A. and HIRSCHHORN, R. Enzyme replacement therapy for adenosine deaminase deficiency and severe combined immunodeficiency. *New England Journal of Medicine*, **295**, 1337–1343 (1976)

195 POLMAR, S. H. In *Inborn Errors of Specific Immunity*, edited by B. Pollara, R. J. Pickering, H. J. Meuwissen and I. H. Porter, 343. New York, Academic Press (1979)

196 POTWOROWSKI, E., SEEMAYER, T., BOLANDE, R. and LAPP, W. Thymic stromal alterations in mice undergoing a chronic graft-versus-host reaction. *Zeitschrift für Immunologische Forschung*, **155**, 240–247 (1979)

197 POWLES, R. L., CLINK, H., SLOANE, J., BARRETT, A. J., KAY, H. E. M. and McELWAIN, T. J. Cyclosporin A for the treatment of graft-versus-host disease in man. *Lancet*, **2**, 1327–1331 (1978)

198 POWLES, R. L., CLINK, H. M., SPENCE, D., MORGENSTERN, G., WATSON, J. G., SELBY, P. J. *et al*. Cyclosporin A to prevent graft-versus-host disease in man after allogeneic bone-marrow transplantation. *Lancet*, **1**, 327–329 (1980)

199 POWLES, R. L., CLINK, H. M., BANDINI, G., WATSON, J. G., SPENCE, D., JAMESON, B. *et al*. The place of bone-marrow transplantation in acute myelogenous leukaemia. *Lancet*, **1**, 1047–1050 (1980)

200 PREISLER, H. D., GOLDSTEIN, I. M. and HENDERSON, E. S. Gastrointestinal 'sterilization' in the treatment of patients with acute leukemia. *Cancer*, **26**, 1976–1981 (1970)

201 PRENTICE, H. G., BLACKLOCK, H., JANOSSY, G., BRADSTOCK, K., GRANGER, S., GILMORE, M. J. M. L. *et al*. In *Bone Marrow Transplantation in Europe II*, edited by J. L. Touraine, E. Gluckman and C. Griscelli, 293. Amsterdam, Excerpta Medica (1981)

202 PYKE, K. W., DOSCH, H. M., IPP, M. M. and GELFAND, E. W. Demonstration of an intrathymic defect in a case of severe combined immunodeficiency disease. *New England Journal of Medicine*, **293**, 424–428 (1975)

203 RACHELEFSKY, G. S., STIEHM, E. R., AMMANN, A. J., CEDERBAUM, S. D., OPELZ, G. and TERASAKI, P. I. T-cell reconstitution by thymus transplantation and transfer factor in severe combined immunodeficiency. *Pediatrics*, **55**, 114–118 (1975)

204 RÁDL, J., DOOREN, L. H., EIJSVOOGEL, V. P., WENT, J. J. VAN and HIJMANS, W. An immunological study during post-transplantation follow-up of a case of severe combined immunodeficiency. *Clinical and Experimental Immunology*, **10**, 367–382 (1972)

205 RAMSAY, N. K. C., KIM, T., NESBIT, M. E., KRIVIT, W., COCCIA, P. F., LEVITT, S. H. *et al*. Total lymphoid irradiation and cyclophosphamide as preparation for bone marrow transplantation in severe aplastic anemia. *Blood*, **55**, 344–346 (1980)

206 RAPPEPORT, J. M., PARKMAN, R., NEWBURGER, P., CAMMITTA, B. M. and CHUSID, M. J. Correction of infantile agranulocytosis (Kostmann's syndrome) by allogeneic bone marrow transplantation. *American Journal of Medicine*, **68**, 605–609 (1980)

207 RAPPEPORT, J. M., PARKMAN, R., BELLI, J. A., CASSIDY, J. R. and LEVEY, R. Correction of congenital bone marrow disorders by allogeneic bone marrow transplantation following preparation with anti-human thymocyte serum and total body irradiation. *Transplantation Proceedings*, **XIII**, 241–244 (1981)

208 REINHERZ, E. L., PARKMAN, R., RAPPEPORT, J., ROSEN, F. S. and SCHLOSSMAN, S. F. Aberrations of suppressor T cells in human graft-versus-host disease. *New England Journal of Medicine*, **300**, 1061–1068 (1978)

209 REINHERZ, E. L. and SCHLOSSMAN, S. F. Current concepts in immunology. Regulation of the immune response – inducer and suppressor T-lymphocyte subsets in human beings. *New England Journal of Medicine*, **303**, 370–373 (1980)

210 REISNER, Y., O'REILLY, R. J., KAPOOR, N. and GOOD, R. A. Allogeneic bone marrow transplantation using stem cells fractionated by lectins: VI. *In vitro* analysis of human and monkey bone marrow cells fractionated by sheep red blood cells and soybean agglutinin. *Lancet*, **2**, 1320–1324 (1980)

211 REISNER, Y., KIRKPATRICK, D., DUPONT, B., KAPOOR, N., POLLACK, M. S., GOOD, R. A. *et al.* Transplantation for acute leukaemia with HLA-A and B nonidentical parental marrow cells fractionated with soybean agglutinin and sheep red blood cells. *Lancet*, **2**, 327–331 (1981)

212 RICH, K. C., MEJIAS, E. and FOX, I. H. Purine nucleoside phosphorylase deficiency: improved metabolic and immunologic function with erythrocyte transfusion. *New England Journal of Medicine*, **303**, 973–977 (1980)

213 RIEGER, Ch. H. L., LUSTIG, J. V., HIRSCHHORN, R. and ROTHBERG, R. M. Reconstitution of T-cell function in severe combined immunodeficiency disease following transplantation of early embryonic liver cells. *Journals of Pediatrics*, **90**, 707–712 (1977)

214 RINGDEN, O., WITHERSPOON, R. P., STORB, R. and THOMAS, E. D. The use of hemolysis in gel-assays to study polyclonal antibody secretion in bone marrow transplant recipients. *Blut*, **42**, 221–226 (1981)

215 RODT, H., NETZEL, B., NIETHAMMER, D., KÖRBLING, M., GÖTZE, D., KOLB, H. J. *et al.* Specific absorbed antithymocyte globulin for incubation treatment in human marrow transplantation. *Transplantation Proceedings*, **IX**, 187–191 (1977)

216 RODT, H., KOLB, H. J., NETZEL, B., HAAS, R. J., WILMS, K., GÖTZE, Ch. B. *et al.* Effect of antiT-cell globulin on GVHD in leukemic patients treated with BMT. *Transplantation Proceedings*, **XIII**, 257–261 (1981)

217 ROOD, J. J. VAN, LEEUWEN, A. VAN, GOULMY, E., TERMIJTELEN, A., BRADLEY, B. A., BRAND, A. *et al.* The importance of non-HLA systems and the feasibility of the use of unrelated donors in bone marrow transplantation. *Transplantation Proceedings*, **X**, 47–51 (1978)

218 ROSENSHEIN, M. S., FAREWELL, V. T., PRICE, T. H., LARSON, E. B. and DALE, D. C. The cost effectiveness of therapeutic and prophylactic leukocyte transfusions. *New England Journal of Medicine*, **302**, 1058–1062 (1980)

219 SANDERS, J. E., BUCKNER, C., STEWART, P. and THOMAS, E. D. Successful treatment of juvenile chronic granulocytic leukemia with marrow transplantation. *Pediatrics*, **63**, 44–46 (1979)

220 SANTOS, G. W., SENSENBRENNER, L. L., BURKE, Ph. J., COLVIN, M., OWENS, Jr., A. H., BIAS, W. B. *et al.* Marrow transplantation in man following cyclophosphamide. *Transplantation Proceedings*, **III**, 400–404 (1971)

221 SANTOS, G. W., ELFENBEIN, G. J., SHARKIS, S. and TUTSCHKA, P. J. In *Biological Basis of Immunodeficiency*, edited by E. W. Gelfand and H. M. Dosch, 293. New York, Raven Press (1980)

222 SARAL, R., BURNS, W. H., LASKIN, O. L., SANTOS, G. W. and LIETMAN, P. S. Acyclovir prophylaxis of herpes-simplex-virus infections. A randomized, double-blind, controlled trial in bone-marrow-transplant recipients. *New England Journal of Medicine*, **305**, 63–67 (1981)

223 SASAKI, M. S. and TONOMURA, A. A high susceptibility of Fanconi's anemia to chromosome breakage by DNA cross-linked agents. *Cancer Research*, **33**, 1829–1836 (1973)

224 SAXON, A., McINTYRE, R. E., STEVENS, R. H. and GALE, R. P. Lymphocyte dysfunction in chronic graft-versus-host disease. *Blood*, **58**, 746–751 (1981)

225 SEDDIK, M., SEEMAYER, T. A., KONGSHAVN, P. and LAPP, W. S. Thymic epithelial functional deficit in chronic graft-versus-host reactions. *Transplantation Proceedings*, **XI**, 967–969 (1979)

226 SELBY, P. J., JAMESON, B., WATSON, J. G., MORGENSTERN, G., POWLES, R. L., KAY, H. E. M. *et al.* Parenteral acyclovir therapy for herpesvirus infections in man. *Lancet*, **2**, 1267–1270 (1979)

227 SELIGMANN, M., GRISCELLI, C., PREUD'HOMME, J. L., SASPORTES, M., HERZOG, C. and BROUET, J. C. In *Immunodeficiency in Man and Animals*, edited by D. Bergsma, 154. Sunderland, Mass., Sinauer Associates (1975)

228 SHALET, S. M. and BEARDWELL, C. G. In *Topics in Paediatrics 1. Haematology and Oncology*, edited by P. H. Morris Jones, 125. Tunbridge Wells, Kent, Pitman Medical (1979)

229 SHEARER, W. T., WEDNER, H. J., STROMINGER, D. B., KISSANE, J. and HONG, R. Successful transplantation of the thymus in Nezelof's syndrome. *Pediatrics*, **61**, 618–624 (1978)

230 SHULMAN, H. M., SALE, G. E., LERNER, K. G., BARKER, E. A., WEIDEN, P. L., SULLIVAN, K. *et al.* Chronic cutaneous graft-versus-host disease in man. *American Journal of Pathology*, **91**, 545–570 (1978)

231 SHULMAN, H. M., McDONALD, G. B., MATTHEWS, D., DONEY, K. C., KOPECKY, K. J., GAUVREAU, J. M. *et al.* An analysis of hepatic.venocclusive disease and centrilobular hepatic degeneration following bone marrow transplantation. *Gastroenterology*, **79**, 1178–1191 (1980)

232 SLAVIN, S., FUKS, Z., KAPLAN, H. S. and STROBER, S. Transplantation of allogeneic bone marrow without graft-versus-host disease using total lymphoid irradiation. *Journal of Experimental Medicine*, **147**, 963–972 (1978)

233 SOLBERG, C. O., MATSEN, J. M., BIGGER, W. D., PARK, B. H., NIOSI, Ph. N. and GOOD, R. A. Infectious complications in patients with combined immunodeficiency diseases receiving bone marrow transplants. *Scandinavian Journal of Infectious Diseases*, **6**, 223–231 (1974)

234 SORELL, M., STEVENSON, R., KAPOOR, N., POLLACK, M. S., CHAGANTI, R. S. K., DUPONT, B. *et al.* Sustained chimerism without graft vs host disease (GVHD) in a patient with severe combined immunodeficiency (SCID) and intrauterine transfusion of maternal T cells. *Pediatric Research*, **13**, 455 (1979)

235 SPARKES, R. S., SPARKES, M. C., CRIST, M., YALE, C., MICKEY, M. R. and GALE, R. P. MNSs Antigens and graft versus host disease following bone marrow transplantation. *Tissue Antigens*, **15**, 212–215 (1980)

236 SPECK, B., GRATWOHL, A., NISSEN, C., RUGGERO, D., CORNU, P., BURRI, H. P. *et al.* Severe aplastic anemia: a prospective study on the value of different therapeutic approachs in 37 successive patients. *Blut*, **41**, 160–163 (1980)

237 SPECK, B., GRATWOHL, A., NISSEN, C., OSTERWALDER, B., MÜLLER, M., BURRI, H. P. et al. Further experience with cyclosporin A in allogeneic bone marrow transplantation. *Experimental Hematology*, **9** (suppl. 9), 124 (1981)

238 STIEHM, E. R., LAWLOR, Jr., G. J., KAPLAN, M. S., GREENWALD, H. L., NEERHOUT, R. G., SENGAR, D. P. S. et al. Immunological reconstitution in severe combined immunodeficiency without bone-marrow chromosomal chimerism. *New England Journal of Medicine*, **286**, 797–803 (1972)

239 STOOP, J. W., ZEGERS, B. J. M., KUIS, W., HEIJNEN, C. J., ROORD, J. J., DURAN, M. M., WADMAN, S. K. and STAAL, G. E. J. In *Primary Immunodeficiencies*, edited by M. Seligmann and W. H. Hitzig, 301. Amsterdam, Elsevier/North-Holland Biomedical Press (1980)

240 STORB., R., EPSTEIN, R. B., GRAHAM, T. C. and THOMAS, E. D. Methotrexate regimens for control of graft-versus-host disease in dogs with allogeneic marrow grafts. *Transplantation*, **9**, 240–246 (1970)

241 STORB, R., THOMAS, E. D., BUCKNER, C. D., CLIFT, R. A., JOHNSON, F. L., FEFER, A. et al. Allogeneic marrow grafting for treatment of aplastic anemia. *Blood*, **43**, 157–180 (1974)

242 STORB, R., PRENTICE, R. L. and THOMAS, E. D. Marrow transplantation for treatment of aplastic anemia. *New England Journal of Medicine*, **296**, 61–66 (1977)

243 STORB, R., PRENTICE, R. L. and THOMAS, E. D. Treatment of aplastic anemia by marrow transplantation from HLA identical siblings. *Journal of Clinical Investigation*, **59**, 625–632 (1977)

244 STORB, R., THOMAS, E. D., WEIDEN, P. L., BUCKNER, C. D., CLIFT, R. A., FEFER, A. et al. One-hundred-ten patients with aplastic anemia (AA) treated by marrow transplantation in Seattle. *Transplantation Proceedings*, **X**, 135–140 (1978)

245 STORB, R. Decrease in the graft rejection rate and improvement in survival after marrow transplantation for severe aplastic anemia. *Transplantation Proceedings*, **XI**, 196–198 (1979)

246 STORB, R. In *Immunobiology of Bone Marrow Transplantation*, edited by S. Thierfelder, H. Rodt and H. J. Kolb, 367. Berlin, Springer Verlag (1980)

247 STORB, R., THOMAS, E. D., BUCKNER, C. D., CLIFT, R. A., DEEG, H. J., FEFER, A. et al. Marrow transplantation in thirty 'untransfused' patients with severe aplastic anemia. *Annals of Internal Medicine*, **92**, 30–36 (1980)

248 STORB, R., TSOI, M., WITHERSPOON, R. P., SULLIVAN, K., LUM, L., DEEG, H. J. et al. Unique immunologic problems in human bone marrow transplant recipients *Transplantation Proceedings*, **XIII**, 1624–1627 (1981)

249 STRAUSS, R. G., CONNETT, J. E., GALE, R. P., BLOOMFIELD, C. D., HERZIG, G. P., McCULLOUGH, J. et al. A controlled trial of prophylactic granulocyte transfusions during initial induction chemotherapy for acute myelogenous leukemia. *New England Journal of Medicine*, **305**, 597–603 (1981)

250 SULLIVAN, K. M., SHULMAN, H. M., STORB, R. WEIDEN, P. L., WITHERSPOON, R. P., McDONALD, G. B. et al. Chronic graft-versus host disease in 52 patients: adverse natural course and successful treatment with combination immunosuppression. *Blood*, **57**, 267–276 (1981)

251 TAYLOR, A. M. R., HARNDEN, D. G., ARLETT, C. F., HARCOURT, S. A., STEVENS, S. and BRIDGES, B. A. Ataxia telangiectasia: a human mutation with abnormal radiation sensitivity. *Nature*, **258**, 427–429 (1975)

252 TERMIJTELEN, A., VOSSEN, J. M. J. J., NAUTA, J., VEER-KORTHOF, E. T. VAN 't and ROOD, J. J. VAN. Selection of unrelated bone marrow donors for two SCID and one Wiskott–Aldrich patient. *Blut*, **41**, 241–244 (1980)

253 TERRITO, M. C., GALE, R. P., CLINE, M. J. Neutrophil function in bone marrow transplant recipients. *British Journal of Haematology*, **35**, 245–250 (1977)

254 THIJM, H. A. and WAAIJ, D. VAN DER The effect of three frequently applied antibiotics on the colonization resistance of the digestive tract of mice. *Journal of Hygiene (Cambridge)*, **82**, 397–405 (1979)

255 THOMAS, E. D., STORB, R., FEFER, A., SLICHTER, Sh. J., BRYANT, J. I., BUCKNER, C. D. *et al.* Aplastic anemia treated by marrow transplantation. *Lancet*, **1**, 284–289 (1972)

256 THOMAS, E. D., BUCKNER, C. D., FEFER, A., NEIMAN, P., BRYANT, J. I., CLIFT, R. A. *et al.* Leukaemic transformation of engrafted human marrow cells *in vivo*. *Lancet*, **1**, 1310–1313 (1972)

257 THOMAS, E. D., STORB, R., CLIFT, R. A., FEFER, A., JOHNSON, F. L., NEIMAN, P. E. *et al.* Bone marrow transplantation (second of two parts). *New England Journal of Medicine*, **292**, 895–902 (1975)

258 THOMAS, E. D., RAMBERG, R. E., SALE, G. E., SPARKES, R. S. and GOLDE, D. W. Direct evidence for a bone marrow origin of the alveolar macrophage in man. *Science*, **192**, 1016–1018 (1976)

259 THOMAS, E. D., BUCKNER, C. D., BANAJI, M., CLIFT, R. A., FEFER, A., FLOURNOY, N. *et al.* One hundred patients with acute leukemia treated by chemotherapy, total body irradiation, and allogeneic marrow transplantation. *Blood*, **49**, 511–533 (1977)

260 THOMAS, E. D., BUCKNER, C. D., FEFER, A., SANDERS, J. E. and STORB, R. Efforts to prevent recurrence of leukemia in marrow graft recipients. *Transplantation Proceedings*, **X**, 163–165 (1978)

261 THOMAS, E. D., SANDERS, J. E., FLOURNOY, N., JOHNSON, L. F., BUCKNER, C. D., CLIFT, R. A. *et al.* Marrow transplantation for patients with acute lymphoblastic leukemia in remission. *Blood*, **54**, 468–476 (1979)

262 THOMAS, E. D., BUCKNER, C. D., CLIFT, R. A., FEFER, A., JOHNSON, F. L., NEIMAN, P. E. *et al.* Marrow transplantation for acute nonlymphoblastic leukemia in first remission. *New England Journal of Medicine*, **301**, 597–599 (1979)

263 THOMAS, E. D., BUCKNER, C. D., CLIFT, R. A., FEFER, A., HERSMAN, J., McGUFFIN, R. *et al.* Marrow transplantation for acute nonlymphoblastic leukemia in first remission using fractionated or single dose irradiation. *International Journal of Radiation Oncology and Biological Biophysics* (in press)

264 TOURAINE, J. L., BÉTUEL, H., BÉTEND, B., SOUILLET, G., HERMIER, M., EVRARD, A. *et al.* Fetal liver transplantation as an alternative to bone marrow transplantation in severe combined immunodeficiencies. *Blut*, **41**, 194–197 (1980)

265 TOURAINE, J. L., FREYCON, F., BÉTUEL, H., PHILIPPE, N., SOUILLET, G., SALLE, B. *et al.* Traitement des déficits immunitaires combinés sévères par greffe de moelle osseuse ou de foie foetal. *Nouvelle Presse Médicale*, **9**, 2215–2219 (1980)

266 TOURAINE, J. L. The bare-lymphocyte syndrome: report on the registry. *Lancet*, **1**, 319–321 (1981)

267 TOURAINE, J. L., PHILIPPE, N., BÉTUEL, N., SOUILLET, G., BÉTEND, B., SOUTEYRAND, P. et al. In *Bone Marrow Transplantation in Europe II*, edited by J. L. Touraine, E. Gluckman and C. Griscelli, 209. Amsterdam, Excerpta Medica (1981)

268 TSOI, M. S., STORB, R., JONES, E., WEIDEN, P. L., SHULMAN, H., WITHERSPOON, R. et al. Deposition of IgM and complement at the dermoepidermal junction in acute and chronic cutaneous graft-vs-host disease in man. *Journal of Immunology*, **120**, 1485–1492 (1978)

269 TSOI, M. S., STORB, R., DOBBS, S., SULLIVAN, K. M. and THOMAS, E. D. In *Biology of Bone Marrow Transplantation*, edited by R. P. Gale and C. F. Fox, 119. London, Academic Press. (1980)

270 TURSZ, T., DOKHELAR, M. C. and GLUCKMAN, E. Peripheral NK-cell activity after bone-marrow allograft. *Lancet*, **1**, 375 (1980)

271 TUTSCHKA, P. J., BESCHORNER, W. E., ALLISON, A. C., BURNS, W. H. and SANTOS, G. W. Use of cyclosporin A in allogeneic bone marrow transplantation in the rat. *Nature*, **280**, 148–151 (1979)

272 ULLMAN, S., SPIELVOGEL, R. L., KERSEY, J. H. and GOLTZ, R. W. Immunoglobulins and complement in skin in graft-versus-host disease. *Annals of Internal Medicine*, **85**, 205 (1976)

273 UPHOFF, D. E. Preclusion of secondary phase of irradiation syndrome by inoculation of fetal hematopoietic tissue following lethal total-body X-irradiation. *Journal of the National Cancer Institute*, **20**, 625–632 (1958)

274 VAAL, O. M. DE and SEYNHAEVE, V. Reticular dysgenesia. *Lancet*, **2**, 1123–1125 (1959)

275 VLOTEN, W. V. VAN, SCHEFFER, E. and DOOREN, L. J. Localized scleroderma-like lesions after bone marrow transplantation in man. *British Journal of Dermatology*, **96**, 337–341 (1977)

276 VOSSEN, J. M. and WAAIJ, D. VAN DER. Reverse isolation in bone marrow transplantation: ultra-clean room compared with laminar flow technique. I. Isolation systems. *European Journal of Clinical and Biological Research*, **17**, 457–461 (1972)

277 VOSSEN, J. M. and WAAIJ, D. VAN DER. Reverse isolation in bone marrow transplantation: ultra-clean room compared with laminar flow technique. II. Microbigical and clinical results. *European Journal of Clinical and Biological Research*, **17**, 564–574 (1972)

278 VOSSEN, J. M., KONING, J. DE, BEKKUM, D. W. VAN, DICKE, K. A., EYSVOOGEL, V. P., HIJMANS, W. et al. Successful treatment of an infant with severe combined immunodeficiency by transplantation of bone marrow cells from an uncle. *Clinical Experimental Immunology*, **13**, 9–20 (1973)

279 VOSSEN, J.M., DOOREN, L. J. and WAAIJ, D. VAN DER. In *Germfree Research*, edited by J. B. Heneghan, 97. London, Academic Press (1973)

280 VOSSEN, J. M. Ergebnisse der Antimikrobiellen Dekontamination von Patienten mit Schwerer Kombinierter Immuninsuffizienz. *Der Krankenhausarzt*, **50**, 348–361 (1977)

281 VOSSEN, J. M., SCHELLEKENS, P. Th. A. and DOOREN, L. J. Gradual establishment of split (autologous B, homologous T) immunological reconstitution following transplantations of stem-cell-enriched bone-marrow fractions in a patient with CID. *Pediatric Research*, **12**, 72 (1978)

282 VOSSEN, J. M., ASTALDI, A., GRIEND, R. J. VAN DE and DOOREN, L. J. In *Bone Marrow Transplantation in Europe II*, edited by J. L. Touraine, E. Gluckman and C. Griscelli, 218. Amsterdam, Excerpta Medica (1981)

283 VOSSEN, J. M., ASTALDI, A., BRUIN, H. G. DE and DOOREN, L. J. T-cell profile and reactivity *in vitro* during immune reconstitution following bone marrow transplantation. *Proceedings of the 29th Congress on Protides of the Biological Fluids*, edited by Peeters, H. 667–670. Brussels, Pergamon (1981)

284 VOSSEN, J. M., HEIDT, P. J., GUIOT, H. F. L. and DOOREN, L. J. Prevention of acute graft versus host disease in clinical bone marrow transplantation: complete versus selective intestinal decontamination. *Proceedings of the VIIth International Symposium on Gnotobiology*, Tokyo, (in press)

285 VRIES-HOSPERS, H. G. DE, WAAIJ, D. VAN DER, SLEIJFER, D. T., MULDER, H. N., NIEWEG, H. O. and SAENE, H. K. F. VAN. In *New Critera for Antimicrobial Therapy*, edited by D. van der Waaij and J. Verhoef, 117. Amsterdam, Excerpta Medica (1979)

286 VRIESENDORP, H. M., WAGEMAKER, G. and BEKKUM, D. VAN Engraftment of allogeneic bone marrow. *Transplantation Proceedings*, **XIII**, 643–648 (1981)

287 WAAIJ, D. VAN DER, BERGHUIS-DE VRIES, J. M. and LEKKERKERK-VAN DER WEES, J. E. C. Colonization resistance of the digestive tract in conventional and antibiotic-treated mice. *Journal of Hygiene (Cambridge)*, **69**, 405–411 (1971)

288 WAAIJ, D. VAN DER, VOSSEN, J. M. and KORTHALS-ALTES, C. In *Germfree Research*, edited by J. B. Heneghan, 31. London, Academic Press (1973)

289 WAAIJ, D. VAN DER and VOSSEN, J. M. Antibiotic decontamination in animals and in human patients. In *Proceedings of the First Intersectional Congress of IAMS*, edited by T. Hasewaga, **3**, 233 (1975)

290 WAAIJ, D. VAN DER and HEIDT, P. J. Intestinal bacterial ecology in relation to immunological factors and other defense mechanisms. *XIII Symposium for Swedish Nutrition Foundation*, 133–141 (1977)

291 WAAIJ, D. VAN DER, VOSSEN, J. M., HARTGRINK, C. A. and NIEWEG, H. O. In *New Criteria for Antimicrobial Therapy*, edited by D. van der Waaij and J. Verhoef, 135. Amsterdam, Excerpta Medica (1979)

292 WAGEMAKER, G., HEIDT, P. J., MERCHAV, S. and BEKKUM, D. W. VAN Abrogation of histocompatibility barriers to bone marrow transplantation in rhesus monkeys. *Experimental Hematology Today* (in press)

293 WALMA, E. P., VRIESENDORP, H. M. and KLAPWIJK, W. Fractionated total body irradiation (TBI) improves the takeability from lymphocyte depleted BM-grafts in DLA identical dogs. *Experimental Hematology*, **9** (suppl. 9), 99 (1981)

294 WARA, D. W. and AMMANN, A. J. Thymic cells and humoral factors as therapeutic agents. *Pediatrics*, **57**, 643–646 (1976)

295 WARNE, G. L., FAIRLEY, K. F., HOBBS, J. B. and MARTIN, F. I. R. Cyclophosphamide-induced ovarian failure. *New England Journal of Medicine*, **289**, 1159–1162 (1973)

296 WARREN, R. P., STORB, R., WEIDEN, P. L., MICKELSON, E. M. and THOMAS, E. D. Direct and antibody-dependent cell-mediated cytotoxicity against HLA-identical sibling lymphocytes. *Transplantation*, **22**, 631–635 (1976)

297 WARREN, R. P., STORB, R., WEIDEN, P. L., SU, P. J. and THOMAS, E. D. Lymphocyte-mediated cytotoxicity and antibody-dependent cell-mediated cytotoxicity in patients with aplastic anemia: distinguishing transfusion-induced sensitization from possible immune-mediated aplastic anemia. *Transplantation Proceedings*, XIII, 245–247 (1981)

298 WATSON, J. G., MORGENSTERN, G. R. and POWLES, R. In *Bone Marrow Transplantation in Europe II*, edited by J. L. Touraine, E. Gluckman and C. Griscelli, 8. Amsterdam, Excerpta Medica (1981)

299 WEIDEN, P. L; STORB, R., MICKELSON, E. M., WARREN, R. P. and THOMAS, E. D. Immune response to transplantation antigens in human marrow graft recipients. *Transplantation Proceedings*, X, 409–413 (1978)

300 WEIDEN, P. L., FLOURNOY, N., THOMAS, E. D., PRENTICE, R., FEFER, A., BUCKNER, C. D. *et al.* Antileukemic effect of graft-versus-host disease in human recipients of allogeneic-marrow grafts. *New England Journal of Medicine*, 300, 1068–1073 (1979)

301 WEIDEN, P. L., HACKMAN, R. C., DEEG, H. J., GRAHAM, Th. C., THOMAS, E. D. and STORB, R. Long-term survival and reversal of iron overload after marrow transplantation in dogs with congenital hemolytic anemia. *Blood*, 57, 66–70 (1981)

302 WEIDEN, P. L., SULLIVAN, K. M., FLOURNOY, N., STORB, R. and THOMAS, E. D. Antileukemic effect of chronic graft-versus-host disease. Contribution to improved survival after allogeneic marrow transplantation. *New England Journal of Medicine*, 304, 1529–1533 (1981)

303 WINSTON, D. J., GALE, R. P., MEYER, D. V. and YOUNG, L. S. Infectious complications of human bone marrow transplantation. *Medicine*, 58, 1–31 (1979)

304 WINSTON, D. J., HO, W. G., YOUNG, L. S. and GALE, R. P. Prophylactic granulocyte transfusions during human bone marrow transplantation. *American Journal of Medicine*, 68, 893–897 (1980)

305 WINSTON, D. J., HO, W. G., HOWELL, C. L., MILLER, M. J., MICKEY, R., MARTIN, W. J. *et al.* Cytomegalovirus infections associated with leukocyte transfusions. *Annals of Internal Medicine*, 93, 671–675 (1980)

306 WITHERSPOON, R., NOEL, D., STORB, R., OCHS, H. D. and THOMAS, E. D. The effect of graft-versus-host disease on reconstitution of the immune system following marrow transplantation for aplastic anemia or leukemia. *Transplantation Proceedings*, X, 233–235 (1978)

307 WITHERSPOON, R. P., STORB, R., MICKELSON, E. M., WEIDEN, P. L. and THOMAS, E. D. Association of interstitial pneumonia and diminished *in vitro* lymphocyte blastogenesis in human marrow graft recipients. *Transplantation*, 28, 412–414 (1979)

308 WOODRUFF, J. M., HANSEN, J. A., GOOD, R. A., SANTOS, G. W. and SLAVIN, R E. The pathology of the graft-versus-host reaction (GVHR) in adults receiving bone marrow transplants. *Transplantation Proceedings*, VIII, 675–684 (1976)

309 WOODS, W. G., DEHNER, L. P., NESBIT, M. E., KRIVIT, W., COCCIA, P. F., RAMSAY, N. K. C. *et al.* Fatal veno-occlusive disease of the liver following high dose chemotherapy. irradiation and bone marrow transplantation. *American Journal of Medicine*, 68, 285–290 (1980)

310 WRIGHT, D. G., ROBICHAUD, K. J., PIZZO, Ph. A. and DEISSEROTH, A. B Lethal pulmonary reactions associated with the combined use of amphotericin B and leukocyte transfusions. *New England Journal of Medicine*, **304**, 1185–1189 (1981)

311 YATES, J. W. and HOLLAND, J. F. A controlled study of isolation and endogenous microbial suppression in acute myelocytic leukemia patients. *Cancer*, **32**, 1490–1498 (1973)

312 YOUNT, W. J., UTSINGER, P. D., WHISNANT, J. and FOLDS, J. D. Lymphocyte subpopulations in X-linked severe combined immunodeficiency (SCID). Evidence against a stem cell defect. Transformation response to calcium ionophore A23187. *American Journal of Medicine*, **65**, 847–854 (1978)

313 ZIEGLER, J. B., LEE, Ch. H., WEYDEN, M. B. VAN DER, BAGNARA, A. S. and BEVERIDGE, J. Severe combined immunodeficiency and adenosine deaminase deficiency: failure of enzyme replacement therapy. *Archives of Disease in Childhood*, **55**, 452–457 (1980)

314 ZWAAN, F. E., JANSEN, J. and NOORDIJK, E. M. Graft-versus-host disease limited to area of irradiated skin. *Lancet*, **1**, 1081–1082 (1980)

315 ZWAAN, F. E. In *Bone Marrow Transplantation in Europe II.* edited by J. L. Touraine, E. Gluckman and C. Griscelli, 63. Amsterdam, Excerpta Medica (1981)

8
Antenatal diagnosis of inherited haematological disease

Bernadette Modell and Reuben S. Mibashan

INTRODUCTION

Antenatal diagnosis with selective termination of affected pregnancies is, for the present, the most practical way of controlling severe congenital disease. During the past 5 years reliable and acceptably safe methods have been developed for the antenatal diagnosis of the haemoglobinopathies and haemophilias, and a substantial demand for the services has been shown to exist. Because the birth of affected children can now be avoided, this advance has introduced a new element of responsibility for each birth, which properly belongs to the parents. The authors conclude that every effort should be made to identify women at risk of bearing children with thalassaemia major or haemophilia, in order to advise them of their risk and inform them of the possibility of antenatal diagnosis. The main practical relevance of this work for most haematologists is the additional importance it gives to the accurate diagnosis and counselling of heterozygotes.

Antenatal diagnosis has gradually entered clinical practice durng the past 20 years as the result of three basic observations: amniotic fluid sampling carries only small risk to the pregnancy[8,45], the cells in amniotic fluid are of fetal origin[74], and non-disjunction of chromosome 21 causes Down's syndrome[39].

Amniocentesis was used first for amniotic fluid bilirubin estimations in the diagnosis of rhesus haemolytic disease; next amniotic fluid cells grown in culture were used for the cytological diagnosis of fetuses with important chromosomal non-disjunctions, severe sex-linked inherited disease or inherited metabolic diseases; and more recently amniotic fluid has been used for the diagnosis of neural tube defects by amniotic fluid α-fetoprotein estimation. The most recent advance has been mid-trimester fetal blood sampling, which initially permitted the antenatal diagnosis of the haemoglobinopathies, and with improved obstetric methods has facilitated the reliable diagnosis of haemophilia. Fetal blood sampling cannot reliably be done before 18 weeks' gestation, and though amniocentesis is possible earlier it only yields sufficient fetal fibroblasts for cell culture at about 16 weeks. To establish the cells in culture takes time, so diagnostic results are rarely available before 19 weeks' gestation, and about 50 per cent of terminations for genetic reasons are after 20 weeks of pregnancy. This limits the conditions appropriate for control by antenatal diagnosis to a narrow range of very serious diseases.

The identification of pregnancies at risk is the first step in providing an antenatal diagnosis service. In general this has proved easier for non-hereditary congenital conditions (such as chromosomal non-disjunctions related to maternal age) or for neural tube defects (usually signalled by an elevated maternal plasma α-fetoprotein level) than it has for inherited diseases. This is due to the difficulty of accurate heterozygote diagnosis for most inherited conditions, because there is usually too much overlap between the normal and the heterozygote ranges even when the underlying biochemical abnormality is known. Thus for most inherited diseases couples at risk are only identified by producing an affected child, and antenatal diagnosis (if it is possible) can be offered only for subsequent pregnancies. The major inherited haematological diseases are exceptions to this general rule because in principle 100 per cent of heterozygotes for the haemoglobinopathies and the majority of women heterozygous for haemophilia are detectable prospectively.

Detecting and counselling couples who may produce children with inherited disease poses different problems according to the mode of inheritance. This chapter is concerned chiefly with sex-linked (haemophilia) and recessive inheritance (haemoglobinopathies).

Sex-linked inheritance of conditions such as haemophilia or Duchenne muscular dystrophy presents some useful features and some problems. A typical family history is the prime requirement for identifying possible female heterozygotes, though some will remain unsuspected if female transmission through several generations has occurred. Laboratory tests can help to establish the normal or heterozygous status of a potential carrier, but are by no means definitive because different degrees of Lyonization in the female lead to variable expression of the mutant gene. This entails a significant risk that heterozygotes may be misdiagnosed as normal. In addition, sex-linked inherited diseases that are lethal before reproductive age lose half their mutant genes in each generation, implying that if a significant incidence is maintained there must be a high rate of spontaneous mutation. This would lead to the new appearance of heterozygotes without a family history, and put in question the carrier status of the mother of a single affected boy. In practice this is more of a problem with Duchenne muscular dystrophy than with haemophilia, since even in the past many haemophilic males achieved reproductive age, and genetic studies have shown a high probability that the mother of a sporadic haemophiliac is a true heterozygote[24].

Before fetal blood sampling was available, a form of antenatal diagnosis for haemophilia could be done by fetal sexing and abortion of all male pregnancies. Since some uncertainty often remained about the carrier status of the mother, probably more than 50 per cent of the male fetuses aborted in the middle trimester were normal, a circumstance precluding this approach except for a strongly motivated minority. Precise antenatal diagnosis has introduced an entirely new option, and the indications for referring known or presumptive haemophilia carriers for antenatal diagnosis require active reassessment.

Though typical of recessive inherited diseases, the haemoglobinopathies are exceptional in several respects. They are very common, their biochemical basis is well understood, and heterozygotes can be diagnosed with certainty, so that prospective identification and genetic counselling of at-risk couples is possible. Antenatal diagnosis has therefore created the possibility of preventing haemoglobinopathies on a population scale, and public demand in the Mediterranean area has proved so high that in the first 3 years after introducing the service, the birth rate of infants with thalassaemia major dropped by 60 per cent in Southern Sardinia[11], approximately 50 per cent in Greece[41] and by over 70 per cent in Cyprus[7]. Social factors have proved to be very important in the acceptability of antenatal diagnosis as it is performed at present. For instance, the demand among at-risk Asians is much less than that among Cypriots[56], and though antenatal diagnosis for sickle cell disease is equally possible, the demand for it is much less than for thalassaemia. These observed differences have important implications in genetic counselling of heterozygotes for the haemoglobinopathies.

OBSTETRIC ASPECTS

Fetal blood sampling

This is currently necessary for the diagnosis of both haemoglobinopathies and haemophilia or related disorders in the fetus.

The best gestational age for fetal blood sampling is 18 weeks or more (i.e. fetal age 16 weeks or more) because the uterus has risen out of the pelvis enough to be accessible; the amniotic fluid volume is still large relative to the size of the fetus so there is room for manoeuvre; the placenta covers relatively less of the uterine wall than in earlier stages giving more scope for a successful entry; and the fetus is sufficiently large to withstand the 1 ml blood loss usually involved in fetal blood sampling. The upper age limit is 22–23 weeks because even where termination of pregnancy after 24 weeks is still legal, the increasing viability of the fetus makes it unacceptable.

Fetal blood has usually been obtained from the fetal vessels on the surface of the placenta rather than directly from the fetus. The main difficulty in fetal blood sampling from this site was the high probability of sample contamination by maternal blood; but preliminary experiments showed that pure fetal blood was not mandatory for antenatal diagnosis of haemoglobinopathies. Indeed samples mixed with as much as 95 per cent of maternal red cells can be dealt with successfully.

This led to the technique of amniocentesis being adapted to diagnostic fetal blood sampling by blind needling of the placenta. In routine amniocentesis the needle sometimes causes accidental bleeding from an anterior placenta into the amniotic fluid, which quite often contains fetal blood. Since in the great majority of such cases the fetus has come to no harm, it seemed reasonable to provoke fetal bleeding into the amniotic fluid to obtain red cells for haemoglobin studies. Though the first experimental efforts met with various degrees of success[12, 36], in diagnostic practice blind needling has given very reliable results[11, 18, 21], because the patient expects perseverance until a suitable sample is obtained. The main risk of placental aspiration is 6.5 per cent risk of immediate fetal death[4] due to exsanguination by the relatively large needle used without direct vision. The earliest fetal loss rate of 15 per cent[5,35] has improved with experience to around 3 per cent. Providing the fetus survives the procedure, there are few later complications of pregnancy; a prematurity rate of 5 per cent[4] is difficult to assess in this group of pregnant women. The absence of fetal abnormalities or severe complications of pregnancy in the first series of antenatal testing for haemoglobinopathies provided the clinical confidence necessary for the continuing development of improved fetal blood sampling methods.

Fetoscopy, a much more elegant procedure, has recently been fully reviewed[66]. The instrument shown in *Figure 8.1* is the Dyonics needlescope which is an endoscope with a 15 cm long shaft of 1.7 mm bore, containing light-conducting fibres for illumination and a crystalline viewing lens. It is inserted through a

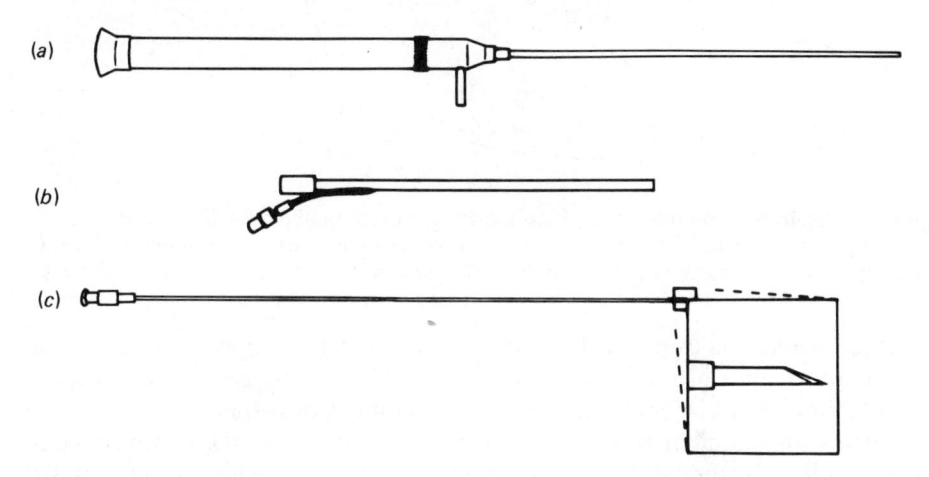

Figure 8.1 Fetoscope (Dyonics Needlescope) showing (*a*) fibre-optic endoscope, unconnected to light source. (*b*) Cannula, trocar withdrawn, with side channel for needle. (*c*) 21-gauge blood sampling needle with narrow 26-gauge tip. (From Mibashan *et al.*[48], courtesy of the Publishers, *Methods in Hematology: The Hemophilias* and Dr. C. H. Rodeck)

cannula with a side channel down which a 26 or 27 G needle can be passed for blood sampling. The fetoscope provides a clear view of a very small field. High quality real-time ultrasound guidance is essential for its successful insertion, which is made through a uterine area free of placenta (thus avoiding bleeding into the amniotic fluid) which also allows access to the cord insertion[46,67] or at least to a large fetal vessel on the surface of the placenta (*Figure 8.2*). Problems may arise from the rigidity of the instrument, from the tiny field of view restricting orientation, and from bleeding into the liquor amnii from the site of insertion or vessel puncture, which can obscure the procedure. The complications of fetoscopy differ from those of blind needling. There is a small risk (depending on the operator's experience) of intrauterine fetal death from retroplacental bleeding if the placenta is damaged during insertion, and problems may arise if the relatively large entry hole in the amniotic membranes fails to seal[65]. Leakage of liquor may ensue and rarely

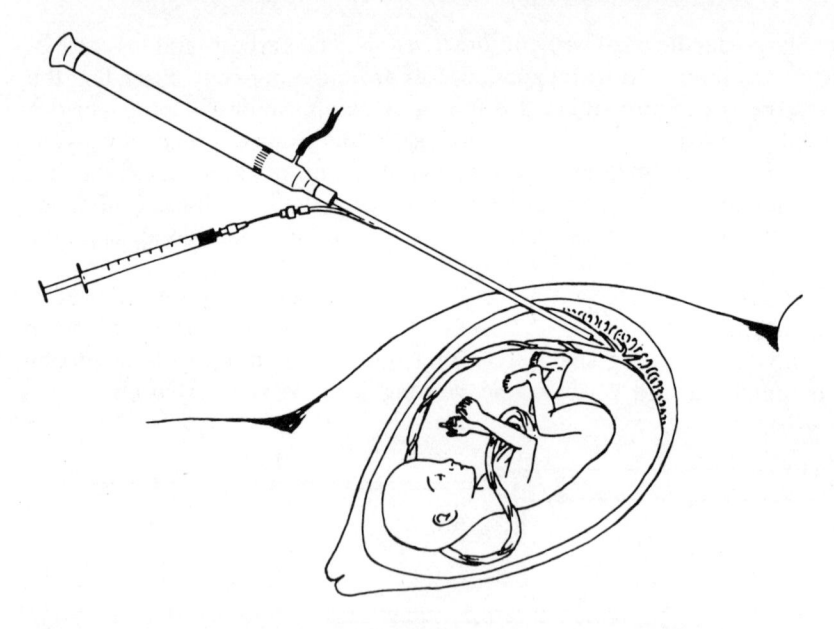

Figure 8.2 Aspiration of pure fetal blood from a vessel in the umbilical cord near its placental insertion (the fetal umbilicus is an alternative site). Diagrammatic. (From Mibashan et al.[48], courtesy of the Publishers, *Methods in Hematology: The Hemophilias*)

spontaneous abortion from two days to several weeks following the procedure. The 6 per cent incidence of premature labour[4, 67] may be slightly increased, but there are inadequate controls for comparison. The highest risk of spontaneous abortion is associated with a combination of bleeding into the liquor and the relatively large hole left in the membranes by the fetoscope[81]. Excessive bleeding can be avoided by sampling from an umbilical cord vessel near its placental insertion[67]; this approach, which is mandatory for the diagnosis of haemophilia, is associated with the lowest obstetric risk (less than 1 per cent in the series reported here; *see Table 8.8* on p. 187).

Obtaining high quality fetal blood samples regularly requires a naturally skilled operator, careful training and probably a year or more of regular weekly practice to maintain a high standard of performance. Providing these requirements are met, the fetal loss rate associated with fetoscopy can be kept at less than 3 per cent; but diagnostic fetal blood sampling on an occasional basis would carry an ineluctably greater risk.

Mid-trimester abortion

The main consideration determining the choice of method in terminating a pregnancy is protection of the mother's fertility. Suction termination under general anaesthesia cannot be done later than 12 weeks without risk of cervical injury. After 14 weeks' gestation the best method of termination is the induction of premature labour by introducing prostaglandins either directly into the amniotic cavity, or extra-amniotically by a catheter passed through the cervix. The average time from induction to delivery is 12–24 hours, and adequate analgesia can be given. Fetal death usually occurs before expulsion. Prostaglandins stimulate lactation, so suppressive treatment with hexoestrol or bromocryptine is required.

Hysterotomy is undesirable because the lower uterine segment, which heals well, is neither fully developed nor accessible at mid-trimester. The fetus is thus delivered through the upper segment entailing a significant risk of uterine rupture in subsequent pregnancies or termination. It also leaves a scar without the reward of a baby.

ANTENATAL DIAGNOSIS OF HAEMOGLOBINOPATHIES

Background

The common abnormal haemoglobins HbS and HbC are due to single amino-acid substitutions in the β-chain of adult haemoglobin (HbA, $\alpha_2\beta_2$); the hallmark of the thalassaemias is chain imbalance due to decreased synthesis of one or other globin chain. Haemoglobin E combines an amino-acid substitution with a form of β-thalassaemia[77]. Severe homozygous disorders of the α-chain (or theoretically, the γ-chain) cause intrauterine fetal death because they affect fetal haemoglobin (HbF, $\alpha_2\gamma_2$). Therefore the major haemoglobinopathies that present clinical problems in childhood are all disorders of the β-chain, and this section is relevant only to the β-thalassaemias and HbS, C and E.

In the β-thalassaemias the β-gene itself is usually present, but there is a family of thalassaemia mutations which either completely prevent (β^0) or greatly reduce (β^+) production of the β-chains. In the past few years the precise lesions in the DNA of the ε-γ-δ-β globin gene cluster that are responsible for most of the thalassaemias have been discovered (*Table 8.1*). The 1981 edition of *The Thalassaemia Syndromes* by D. J. Weatherall and J. B. Clegg gives an up-to-date review of this rapidly progressing field[82].

Antenatal diagnosis for haemoglobinopathies is limited to the severe abnormal haemoglobins and the β-thalassaemias, which are all β-gene disorders. The current image of the ε-γ-δ-β gene cluster is summarized in *Figure 8.3*. This concept is based on the recent deployment of gene mapping as described by Weatherall and Clegg[57].

All the non-α-genes are located in tandem on chromosome 16 in order of their activation in the fetus. The sections of DNA coding for each globin chain are separated by relatively long non-coding sections. The meaning of these intervening sequences is still only poorly understood, but they must be involved in gene switching. The coding sections themselves are each interrupted by two 'introns', one long and one short. These non-coding sequences are transcribed to nuclear messenger RNA but are spliced out before the message leaves the nucleus to direct globin chain synthesis in the cytoplasm. Detailed analysis of the DNA shows that

Table 8.1 Molecular basis of the well characterized β-haemoglobinopathies

Type of thalassaemia (or abnormal Hb)		Frequency	Molecular basis	+/−*	Reference†
Hereditary persistence of fetal haemoglobin (HPFH)	GγAγ type 1	All rare	Deletion of β + δ + 4kb of inter-γ-δ flanking DNA	+	79
	GγAγ type 2		Deletion of β + δ + 9kb of inter-γ-δ flanking DNA	+	
	Hb Kenya		Fusion of Aγ with β	+	
δβ-thalassaemia	GγAγ	All rare	Deletion of β + ½ δ	+	
	Gγ		Deletion of β, δ and Aγ genes	+	
	Gγ		Inversion of Aγ to δ segment + 2 deletions	+	
Hb lepore	Hollandia	All rare	50 δ-β fusion	+	
	Baltimore		86 δ-β fusion	+	
	Boston		116 δ-β fusion	+	
Normal A₂ β-thalassaemia, mild		Uncommon	Not known	−	
Normal A₂ β-thalassaemia, severe		Uncommon	?Coincidence of δ- and β-thalassaemia	−	
β⁰-thalassaemia mild: Indian		Rare	600 base pair deletion at 5′ end of gene	+	
β⁰-thalassaemia mild: British		Rare	Defective initiation of β mRNA synthesis	−	
β⁰-thalassaemia severe: Italian		Common	Abolition of splice site at start of large intron	+	Banks et al. (unpublished)
β⁰-thalassaemia severe: Italian, Greek		Common	β³⁹ Gln → stop (='nonsense') mutation	+	57
β⁰-thalassaemia severe: Chinese, Sardinian		Common	β¹⁷ Lys → stop (='nonsense') mutation	+	78
β⁰-thalassaemia severe: Ferrara		Common (locally)	Defective protein β-initiation factor	−	
β⁺-thalassaemia severe: Mediterranean		Common	Additional splice site generated in small intron	+	84
β⁺⁺-thalassaemia mild: Negro		Fairly common	Not known	−	10
HbE		Common (locally)	β²⁶ Glu → Lys (+ thalassaemia mutation?)	+	77
HbS		Common	β⁶ Glu → Val mutation	+	
HbC		Common (locally)	β⁶ Glu → Lys mutation	?	

* Indicates possibly now identifiable by molecular methods.
† If not in Weatherall and Clegg⁸².

many independent mutants can cause the phenotype of β-thalassaemia. For instance, two different single base substitutions in the introns lead to two of the common β-thalassaemias. One eliminates the first specific sequence recognized by the splicing enzyme so that, though nuclear messenger RNA is formed, splicing does not occur and no message reaches the cytoplasm. The result is an Italian β⁰-thalassaemia. In Cypriot β⁺-thalassaemia a mutation in the smaller intron generates an alternative splicing site so that only 10 per cent of nuclear messenger

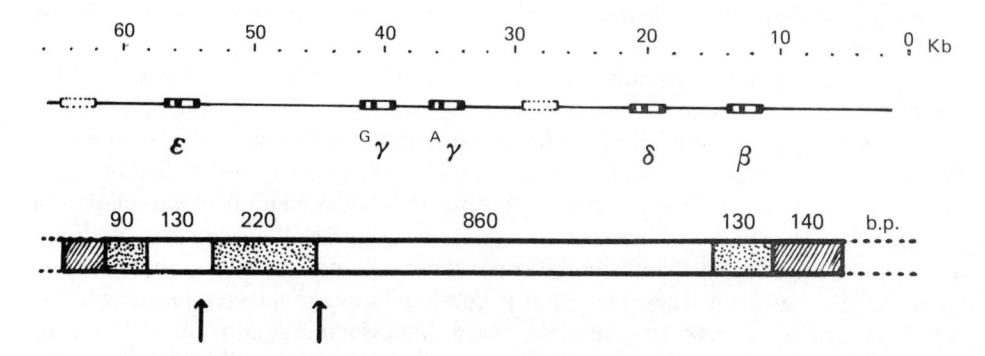

Figure 8.3 The current view of the structure of the ε-γ-δ-β gene cluster based on Efstradiadis et al.[17]. The upper part of the figure shows the genes are separated by long non-coding sections of DNA. These include two regions shown as dots where the DNA sequence resembles that of a globin gene, but no corresponding protein is produced. Each gene is divided into three coding sections (black) separated by two non-coding introns (white). The scale shows length in kilobases (Kb) = 1000 gene pairs. The lower part of the figure shows the structure of the β-globin gene in more detail. There is a non-coding leader section (striped), followed by a short coding section (dotted) of 90 base pairs (b.p.). This is followed by the first small intron (130 b.p.), a second coding section (220 b.p.), then the large intron followed by another coding section and a non-coding 'tail'. Sites of the known intron mutations producing a thalassaemia phenotype are shown by arrows.

RNA is correctly processed and reaches the cytoplasm. Two other common forms of β⁰-thalassaemia are generated by a single base substitution that produces a new 'stop' codon near the beginning of the messenger RNA so that only small polypeptide fragments are generated. Some rarer disorders such as the δβ-thalassaemias and hereditary persistence of fetal haemoglobin are caused by deletions of whole segments of coding and non-coding DNA. Precise understanding of these lesions now opens the way to improved methods of preventing the haemoglobinopathies, mentioned in the final discussion.

In both β-thalassaemia major and sickle cell disease intrauterine development is normal and the first symptoms appear between 3 months and 1 year of age. Thalassaemia major is predictably a very severe anaemia; more than 90 per cent of affected babies have classical 'thalassaemia major, i.e. are unable to maintain a haemoglobin of more than 7 g/dl and if untreated die of anaemia after 1–6 years of chronic illness. Regular blood transfusion to maintain the haemoglobin in the normal range preserves good health in the short term, but transfusional iron overload can lead to death from intractable heart failure between 16 and 22 years of age. It now seems that iron overload can be effectively controlled by nightly subcutaneous infusion of desferrioxamine, though many adolescents have considerable difficulty in accepting the treatment. A thalassaemic infant born today in a community capable of supplying its need for blood and drugs has a good prognosis, and the future prospects for cure by bone marrow transplantation or genetic engineering are bright. However, the treatment programme imposes such heavy strains on the family and the community that the improved prognosis seems to have increased rather than decreased the demand for antenatal diagnosis of thalassaemia[53].

Less than 10 per cent of children homozygous for β-thalassaemia have a milder syndrome, *thalassaemia intermedia*, and can survive with varying degrees of disability if left untransfused. Though a few such patients do very well, the majority of children with thalassaemia intermedia are chronically sick, and in Britain most are finally transferred to an intensive transfusion scheme combined with chelation therapy[54]. In most cases thalassaemia intermedia is due to the reduction of globin chain imbalance by the coincidental inheritance of one or more α-thalassaemia genes[34, 40, 83] so even when one child in the family has thalassaemia intermedia, there is usually a risk of classical severe thalassaemia major in subsequent pregnancies. At present it is not possible to predict the precise clinical picture that will follow from the inheritance of different types of α-thalassaemia together with two β-thalassaemia genes, and most couples seeking antenatal diagnosis for thalassaemia prefer to abort the pregnancy in all cases where homozygous β-thalassaemia is found.

Haemoglobin E thalassaemia is usually milder than typical homozygous β-thalassaemia[14]. Many patients survive untransfused into the second or third decade with varying degrees of disability and an Hb level of 6–9 g/dl, though there are more severe and milder cases. The treatment and the strains on the family can resemble those of thalassaemia intermedia and the indication for antenatal diagnosis is perceived by many at-risk couples to be similar.

The implications of homozygous sickle cell disease are less predictable. It causes a severe anaemia (Hb 7–8 g/dl), greatly increased susceptibility to infection in small children (probably due to poor or absent splenic function) and painful crises. Crippling and irreversible damage following infarction in bones, heart, brain or retina, though spectacular and distressing, are uncommon. The clinical picture varies with both genetic and environmental factors. In Saudi Arabia homozygous sickle cell disease is almost asymptomatic due to an associated genetic derepression of the γ genes so that a high protective level of fetal haemoglobin is present[62]. In Nigeria, by contrast, very few homozygous children survive their second birthday due to their susceptibility to infection. In Britain the majority of homozygotes survive at least into adolescence, and many have only mild or few painful crises[43]. Little treatment is available, apart from attention to hydration, nutrition, general care, antibacterial vaccines and prophylactic antibiotics in childhood. For those with intractable symptoms, maintenance blood transfusion and iron-chelation therapy can, as in thalassaemia, greatly improve the quality of life. This difference in the course of the disease, and in particular the absence of continual traumatic treatment as in thalassaemia major, makes it difficult to predict the prospects for couples at risk and for children with homozygous sickle cell anaemia. Consequently, the demand for antenatal diagnosis of sickle cell anaemia with present methods is much less than that for thalassaemia.

Laboratory diagnosis

Because the major haemoglobinopathies are disorders of adult haemoglobin synthesis, while fetuses make fetal haemoglobin, one might think antenatal diagnosis would be out of the question. However, Walker and Turnbull[80] showed in 1955 that the normal human fetus makes a small amount of adult haemoglobin and this was confirmed by Hollenberg et al.[25] in 1971. They and Cividalli et al.[15] measured the HbA synthesized by early fetuses obtained at hysterotomy terminations. Precise quantitation was aided by radioactive labelling of the haemoglobin and column chromatography which is still the main method used for antenatal diagnosis. *Figure 8.4* shows that after 16 weeks' gestational age the mean HbA synthesis found was 9.8 per cent (SD 1.72 per cent) so it was predicted that in thalassaemia trait about half the normal amount of HbA should be made, while in β^0-thalassaemia major, β-chain synthesis should be at most one-sixth of normal, i.e. 1.5 per cent HbA. In the β^0-thalassaemia major fetus there should of course be no HbA synthesis at all. The calculation, summarized in *Figure 8.5*, predicts real though narrow discrimination between β^+-thalassaemia major and β^0-thalassaemia trait, but considerable overlap between the values for β-thalassaemia trait and normal. A small preliminary study of fetuses at risk for thalassaemia was consistent with these predictions[13]. Pataryas and Stamatoyannopoulos[59] and Kan et al.[32] showed that β-chain mutants such as HbS and C could be identified as early as 11 weeks' gestation, and should also be diagnosable antenatally.

The first antenatal diagnoses for thalassaemia were performed in 1974[5, 33]. Information on the reliability and safety of the methods accumulated rapidly[5, 18, 21, 35, 41] and a regular antenatal diagnosis service is now available in many American, European and Australian centres[4] (*Figure 8.6*). The North American centres include Montreal, Toronto-Hamilton, Boston, Baltimore, New York, New Haven and San Francisco. The Australian ones are in Melbourne and Sydney.

Procedure

Once a couple is known to be at risk of producing a child with a major haemoglobinopathy, their risk and the problems associated with antenatal diagnosis should be discussed carefully with them. If they reject antenatal diagnosis, a neonatal diagnosis is offered and usually accepted. In fact the majority of those at risk for thalassaemia major choose antenatal diagnosis, while many at risk for sickle cell disease prefer a neonatal diagnosis. Fetal blood sampling is performed as

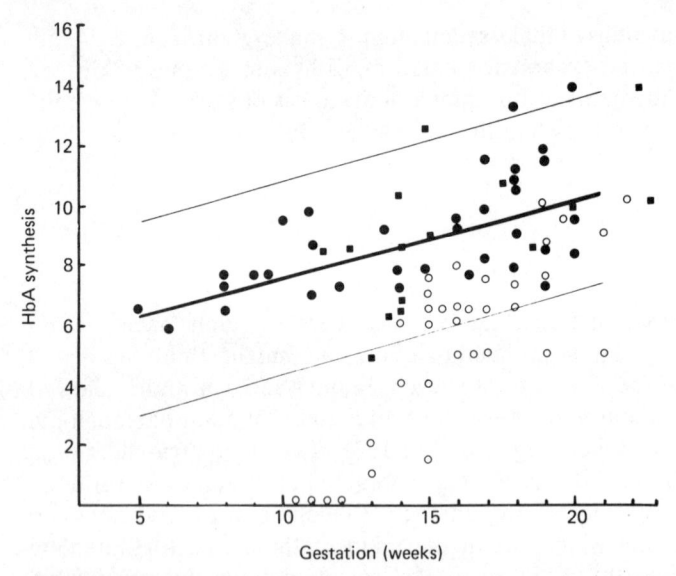

Figure 8.4 Haemoglobin A in the human fetus, in relation to gestational age. (○) Haemoglobin A present (Walker and Turnbull[80]). (■) Haemoglobin A synthesis observed by Kazazian *et al.*[38], and (●) by Cividalli *et al.*[15]. The regression line refers to the biosynthetic data of Cividalli and Kazazian *et al.* It does not refer to the accumulation of HbA mentioned by Walker and Turnbull since biosynthesis precedes accumulation. (From Modell and Berdoukas[54], courtesy of the Publishers, *The Clinical Approach to Thalassaemia*)

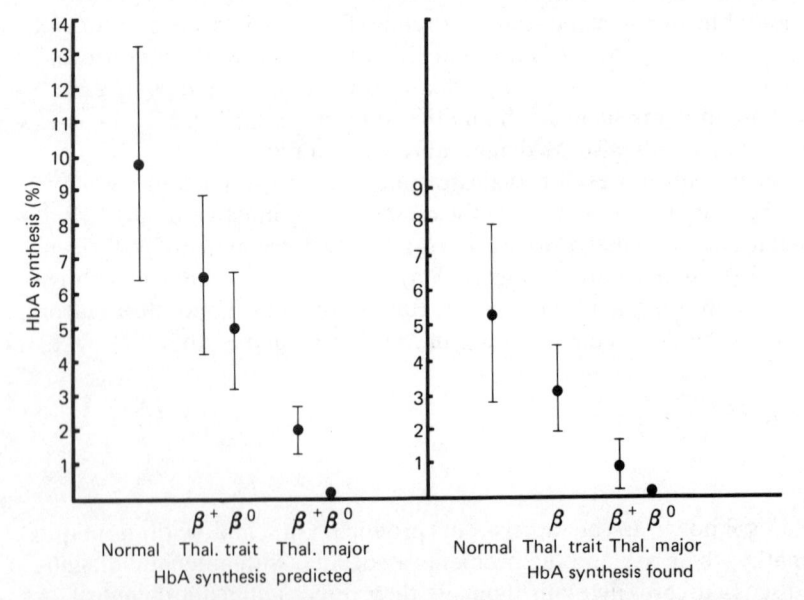

Figure 8.5 The left-hand part of the figure shows the predicted haemoglobin A synthesis in thalassaemia trait and two types of thalassaemia major predicted from the findings in normal fetuses. The right-hand side of the figure shows the actual values found at antenatal diagnosis, using a slightly different biochemical method.

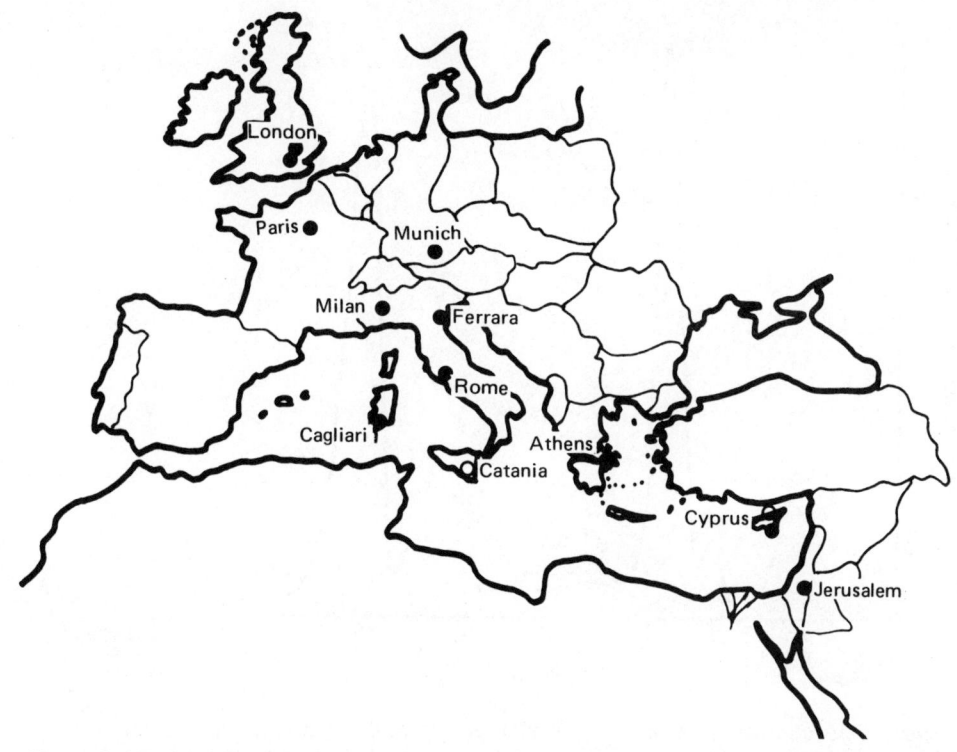

Figure 8.6 Existing and projected centres (1981) for antenatal diagnosis of haemoglobinopathies in Europe and the Mediterranean. The map shows that the method is spreading rapidly to endemic areas. (From Modell and Berdoukas[54], courtesy of the Publishers, *The Clinical Approach to Thalassaemia*)

above, the fetal red cells are incubated for 2 hours at 37°C in a medium containing [H^3]leucine, the newly synthesized globin chains are separated in 8 M urea on carboxymethyl cellulose (CMC) columns and measured by their radioactivity as shown in *Figure 8.7*. The biochemical results differ very slightly between laboratories. Those obtained by one of the authors (BM) are summarized in *Figure 8.5*. Fortunately it has proved possible to confirm the prediction of a narrow but real cut-off point between the upper limit of HbA synthesis in homozygous β$^+$-thalassaemia and the lower limit in β^0-thalassaemia trait, though in a few borderline cases confident discrimination has been possible only by repeating the whole procedure after a 2–3 week interval. The details of handling samples contaminated with maternal blood have been reviewed elsewhere[53].

Accuracy of results

The world data have been critically reviewed annually by Alter[3, 4, 6]. In 1979 there was a 2 per cent misdiagnosis rate – 1 per cent false positives and 1 per cent false

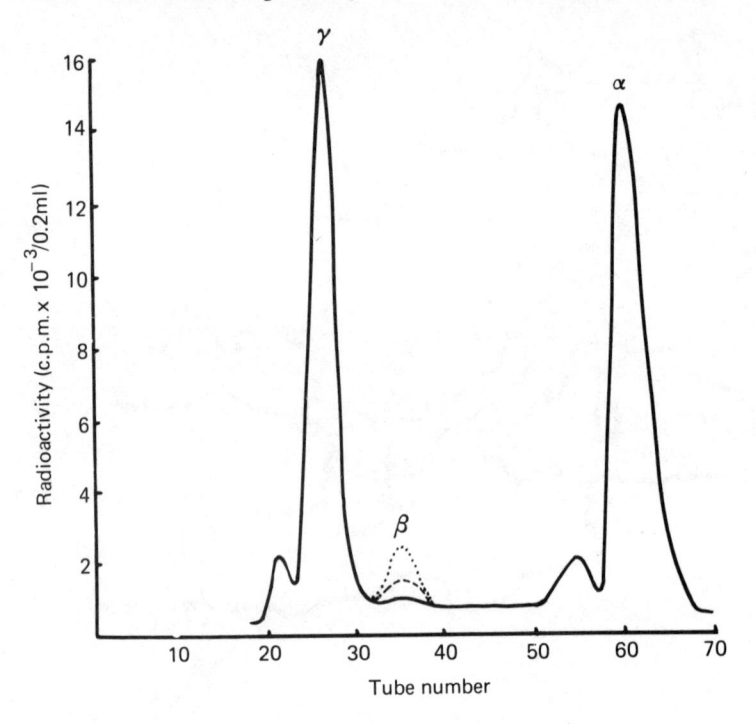

Figure 8.7 Composite globin chain elution pattern showing a typical result for a normal fetus (......), a fetus with β-thalassaemia trait (---), and a β⁺-thalassaemia major (—)

negatives – and a 7 per cent rate of fetal loss due to the obstetric procedure; these figures have improved, as already indicated, with growing experience and progressively better fetal blood samples. In our own series of 380 cases there have been 3 misdiagnoses[44]. Two (1 false positive and 1 false negative) were due to early uncertainty about the cut-off point for β⁺-thalassaemia major, and one false negative was probably due to a γ-mutant; a similar case has been reported by Furbetta *et al.*[21].

The diagnosis of *sickle cell anaemia* in the fetus is illustrated in *Figure 8.8*. This is simpler than that of thalassaemia major where problems arise in measuring accurately very small amounts of β-chain, whereas in homozygous sickle cell disease the total amount of β-chain present is close to normal, but its position on the elution pattern is shifted. The demand for antenatal diagnosis of homozygous sickle cell disease has been relatively low – only 6 in the authors' 380 cases, while 4 more were for HbS/β-thalassaemia. The authors have done only one antenatal diagnosis for HbE/thalassaemia due to its low incidence in Britain.

The laboratory method in use is cumbersome and difficult to set up in developing countries where it is most needed. A number of alternative methods have been developed but all still have similar limitations. The quantitative measurement of HbA separated by isoelectric focussing[16] is quick and elegant but requires completely pure samples of fetal blood and expensive equipment for measuring optical density. Separation of tetrameric haemoglobins on Biorex columns[9a, 25] is

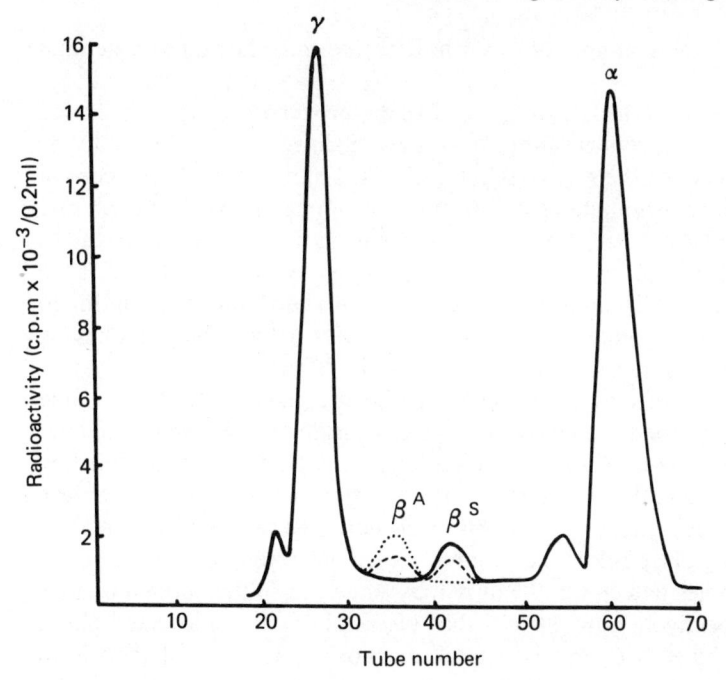

Figure 8.8 Composite figure showing the typical globin chain elution patterns for a normal fetus (......), a fetus with sickle cell trait (---), and a fetus with homozygous sickle cell disease (—)

quick and allows handling of contaminated samples because radioactivity can be counted; it is possible that in starting a new service this might be the method of choice. The most promising technical advance comes for the application of restriction enzyme methods of DNA analysis, discussed later, as these allow complete avoidance of protein studies.

However, the major task in setting up an antenatal diagnosis service is creating an organization to disseminate information and identify heterozygotes accurately, so that couples at risk are detected and referred for counselling before they produce affected children.

Who should be offered antenatal diagnosis?

In Britain, where β-thalassaemia occurs among two main ethnic groups, Cypriots and 'Asians', the uptake rate of antenatal diagnosis has differed markedly between the two groups. Only 2 per cent of Cypriots choose to continue an at-risk pregnancy without antenatal diagnosis, while nearly 50 per cent of 'Asian' at-risk couples choose to do so. The Cypriots are a uniform, well-informed group with 'middle-class' attitudes; it has proved possible, by analysing their reproductive behaviour, to obtain objective evidence on the effect of having an affected child in the family, and on the reaction of the community as a whole to the introduction of antenatal diagnosis[56].

In the years before they learnt of their risk, heterozygote couples behaved normally with regard to reproduction but once they realized their risk (usually by producing an affected child) the rate of pregnancies was halved, and 70 per cent of those that occurred were terminated for fear of thalassaemia major. The birth rate of unaffected children (which represents the biological viability of the group) fell to one per 50 married years, as a result of knowing the risk and access to contraception and elective termination of pregnancy. This behaviour, amounting to biological suicide, expresses quite unambiguously the destructive effect that having a child with severe chronic disease can exert on family life.

Since the introduction of antenatal diagnosis, the pregnancy rate in the same group of families has returned to slightly more than its original level. Nearly 100 per cent have been tested antenatally and termination has been requested only when the fetus was found to have thalassaemia major (or suffered intrauterine death as a result of the obstetric procedure). The number of married years (4.8) per healthy child produced is not greatly below the original pregnancy rate of one per 3 years. The behaviour of couples detected to be at risk by screening in the antenatal clinic and counselled prospectively now mirrors that of couples with an affected child, and nearly all who have had one antenatal diagnosis return for diagnosis in subsequent pregnancies. In short, these couples use antenatal diagnosis to achieve the family they wanted had they not been at risk. Cypriot parents who have produced a thalassaemic child since the introduction of antenatal diagnosis experience great distress at what they see as an avoidable catastrophe. They have marked difficulty in accepting their child's illness and treatment and show active interest in antenatal diagnosis for future pregnancies. Thus the introduction of such a service, while helping many, can make life *more* difficult for couples who are 'missed'.

The second large British group at risk for thalassaemia, the Asians, are themselves heterogeneous. There are three main groups: (1) Doctors and paramedical workers who tend to take advantage of antenatal diagnosis. (2) East African Asians, who are generally educated business people; about 70 per cent accept antenatal diagnosis. (3) The largest group are direct immigrants from rural areas of India and Pakistan; many are Muslims. They may find it difficult to understand the prediction of genetic disease, and even when they know what the disease means because they already have one or more affected children, may reject the idea of midtrimester termination of pregnancy as unnatural. Interestingly, this group is also least able to cope with the active treatment of the disease and though they bring the children for transfusion, may be unable to manage chelation therapy at home. What we have to offer both in the way of treatment and of prevention is inadequate for many of these families and better solutions must be found. Sickle cell anaemia also occurs in Britain in two contrasting populations, West Indians and West Africans. The very different social characteristics have been described by Fourer[20] and Goody and Groothues[23] respectively. About half the counselled West African at-risk couples have requested antenatal diagnosis, but we have not yet received a single request for antenatal diagnosis from a West Indian couple.

However, even when antenatal diagnosis was not requested all couples were interested in a neonatal diagnosis, as they felt it would either relieve their anxiety or help them to protect an affected child during the dangerous early years.

Since the demand for antenatal diagnosis is so widespread, the authors believe that all at-risk couples should be detected and counselled sensitively and informatively.

ANTENATAL DIAGNOSIS OF THE HAEMOPHILIAS

Background

Haemophilia, like thalassaemia, is biochemically and clinically heterogeneous, but its geographic distribution is universal, with a population incidence in developed countries approximating 1 in 10 000[30]. Classical haemophilia A is characterized by reduced or absent plasma factor VIII coagulant activity (VIIIC). About one-sixth of patients have haemophilia B (Christmas disease) and lack factor IX clotting activity (IXC); clinically the two disorders are indistinguishable and show a range of clotting factor deficit which runs remarkably true in an affected kindred.

Clotting factor levels between 0 and 1-2 per cent of normal (which averages 100 units/dl) are associated with severe disease and frequent spontaneous bleeding; patients with higher values have moderate or mild haemophilia, which may be equally dangerous after injury.

Since the inheritance of both haemophilias is X-linked recessive, the chance that a pregnant carrier's male fetus will be affected is 1 in 2, with a clinical severity that is characteristic of that family's haemophilia. Factor VIII deficiency also occurs in von Willebrand's disease (vWd) as an autosomal trait, which in its rare homozygous form is also a grave bleeding disorder.

While modern replacement treatment has greatly improved the outlook for young haemophiliacs, the disease continues to take a heavy medical and economic toll. Painful disabling haemorrhages with their sequelae of arthropathy and neurovascular or organ damage still occur[9, 30]. Acquired resistance to therapy is a serious, unpredictable development in a small proportion of patients, and a more frequent complication is liver damage probably resulting from multiple exposures to viral antigens in the factor VIII or IX concentrates[85].

Accordingly some carriers, whether known or presumptive, are deeply averse to bearing a haemophilic son and take steps to avoid pregnancy or to terminate it if the fetus is male[42, 46, 48, 63]. Since half (or more) of the aborted males are normal, such mothers carry a heavy burden of guilt in addition to the trauma of abortion, and those who find this recourse unacceptable either deny themselves parenthood or pass each pregnancy in dread of its outcome. Antenatal diagnosis offers such parents the new-found option of restricting abortions to haemophilic fetuses only, and the possibility of bearing normal sons[19, 50].

Molecular basis of the haemophilias

The premise that haemophilia A and B and severe vWd might be recognized antenatally by measuring fetal clotting factors stemmed from their presence, independent of maternal levels, both in the newborn and in midterm fetuses[26, 58]. The practical obstacles to implementing this approach have lately been overcome by two major achievements. They are (1) a reliable obstetric technique, described above, for sampling pure fetal blood[67, 68, 73], and (2) performance of valid clotting factor assays on the samples so obtained[19, 27, 47, 49-51, 60, 61]. The nature of these clotting factors explains the laboratory techniques which measure them and the co-ordinated steps required for successful antenatal diagnosis.

Factor VIII circulates as a complex of two proteins of unequal size – a large multimer (VIII related antigen, VIIIRAg) linked to a low molecular weight portion which promotes coagulation (VIIIC)[60]. While VIIIC activity is deficient in both haemophilia A and von Willebrand's disease, only vWd displays a prolonged bleeding time, failure of the intrinsically normal platelets to adhere to vascular subendothelium, and impairment of ristocetin-induced platelet aggregation. These features are due to lack of plasma 'Willebrand factor' (WF), which is measured as factor VIIIRAg by rabbit antibodies in precipitating or other immunoassays, and as 'ristocetin cofactor' in a platelet-aggregating system.

Genetic studies indicate that factor VIIIC (reduced or abnormal in haemophilia A) is coded for by the X-chromosome, while the larger VIIIRAg/WF (which serves as a 'carrier' for VIIIC) is under separate autosomal control and is unaffected in haemophilia. The reduced VIIIC in vWd is conditioned by the VIIIRAg/WF deficiency, and correcting this alone (as when haemophilic plasma was infused in early studies) leads to a rise of circulating VIIIC also.

Plasma factor VIIIC is *measured* by its ability, compared with that of a standard VIIIC preparation, to shorten the clotting time of severely haemophilic plasma. This bioactivity is unstable at ordinary temperatures and (like another labile factor, VC) is degraded during clotting, after transient amplification. Incipient coagulation in imperfectly collected blood may thus cause falsely high or abnormally low results. An elegant immunoradiometric assay (IRMA) of the antigenic determinant of factor VIIIC (VIIIC antigen or VIIICAg) using human IgG antibodies which may arise against VIIIC activity has permitted measurement of the smaller coagulant piece by an alternative method[19, 60, 61]. There is good – but not complete – correlation between the functional (VIIIC) and IRMA (VIIICAg) techniques, and while the VIIICAg assay is more sensitive and robust, a small proportion of severe haemophiliacs with no detectable VIIIC activity are CRM+, i.e. have VIIICAg levels within the normal range[61]. Such patients (and fetuses) are only recognizable by the coagulant bioassay for VIIIC activity[46, 48, 52].

In summary, factor VIII comprises two discretely coded protein subunits. The large, multimeric molecule, VIIIRAg/WF, present alike in normal and haemophilic subjects, promotes platelet activities and is reduced or defective in vWd. It is linked to and acts as carrier for a smaller, clot-promoting molecule, VIIIC/CAg, which is abnormal or lacking in haemophilia A.

Factor IX is a vitamin K-dependent clotting factor which functions in the coagulation sequence as a catalyst of the activation of factor X in the thrombin-generating cascade. Factor IX coagulant activity (IXC) – with related factors – is reduced in vitamin K lack or in impaired hepatic synthesis, a degree of both being normal in the newborn and fetus[26, 58]. Recognition of severe haemophilia B *in utero* depends on distinguishing *physiologically* low plasma IXC from the more extreme *inherited* deficiency[46, 48, 50]. Immunoassays with rabbit antibodies have been insensitive at levels below 10–20 per cent of normal[24, 27], but an IRMA using human inhibitors of IXC has successfully measured very low levels of factor IX antigen both in patients and fetuses[27]. Since in some series up to one-third of severe haemophilia B kindred have significant levels of functionally defective IXAg, the IRMA can only be diagnostic in antigen-deficient (CRM−) haemophilia B[27, 47].

Steps in antenatal diagnosis

The 'patient' requires informed counselling based on the fullest genetic, clinical and laboratory knowledge of the particular bleeding state, its familial severity, and the likelihood of her being a heterozygote. The limitations of carrier testing (if she is not obligate) and the current risks and accuracy of the procedures are discussed factually and unhurriedly. The diagnostic steps include *ultrasound* assessment of fetal age, fetal *sexing* by amniocentesis (haemophilia A and B), *fetoscopy* for blood sampling and *assay* of the relevant fetal clotting factors. Confirmation of the results in the newborn or the abortus should be sought, and further supportive counselling of the patient must be ensured. The overall programme is summarized as follows:

(1) Motivation and counselling
(2) Genetic information
   (a) Factor and severity; (CRM+ or CRM−, if IRMA used)
   (b) Carrier status
   (c) Amniocentesis (15–16th week)
   (d) Male fetus (vWd both sexes)
(3) Fetoscopy (18–20th week)
   (a) Fetal blood sampling
   (b) Emergency sexing, rarely
(4) Assay of fetal factor VIII or IX
   (a) Coagulant
   (b) Immunoradiometric
(5) Continuation or termination
   (a) Confirm diagnosis
   (b) Predictive accuracy
   (c) Support and further counselling

Carrier detection

Knowledge that a woman is heterozygous may appear indispensable to this programme, yet certain recognition is only possible in some. Such *obligate* carriers are (1) all the daughters of a haemophiliac; (2) a woman who has more than once had a haemophilic son; (3) a woman with a haemophilic son and a proven haemophilic relative in her or her mother's family. (4) Recently a new criterion of an obligate carrier has emerged by extension of the last: a haemophiliac's relative whose male fetus is found to be haemophilic on antenatal testing.

Putative (potential) heterozygotes are exemplified by the daughters of a carrier: each of them has a 1 in 2 chance – like her sons – of inheriting the abnormal X-chromosome; but while the hemizygous male is easily identified, the possibly heterozygous relative of a haemophiliac can only be given a statistical estimate of her genotype, utilizing kinship analysis combined with haematologic studies.

Laboratory detection is predicated on the approximate halving of plasma VIIIC or IXC levels, which are X-controlled, during Lyonization in heterozygous females[24, 64]. Since the range of these factors – which average 100 units/dl in normals – is very wide, e.g. 50–200 u/dl, even their *half*-values in obligate carriers too frequently fall within the normal limits to be diagnostic.

By simultaneous immunoassay of plasma VIIIRAg – synthesized normally in haemophilia A – a significantly reduced ratio of circulating VIIIC to VIIIRAg can be detected. Given adequate reference data, a statistical likelihood of carriership can be derived from this ratio[1] and used with the pedigree assessment to reach a final *probability* that the individual is a heterozygote[24]. The IRMA counterpart (VIIICAg to RAg ratio) may be even more sensitive as an indicator of carrier status[61a]. While similar principles have been applied to haemophilia B, IXAg levels vary more in relation to IXC[24, 37] and carrier detection is more intricate.

Tests demonstrating *linkage* between haemophilia A and another genetic marker (a G-6-PD variant) offer a further refinement of carrier detection in a very small proportion of families; and direct gene identification by *DNA analysis* currently holds promise as the definitive approach (*see* 'Future perspectives' p. 189).

The practical *limitations* of carrier tests for haemophilia have been emphasized by those with most experience[24, 64]. A misclassification rate of 10–25 per cent is typical of many haemophilia A studies, only part of which is due to technical error. A proportion of heterozygotes – 6–15 per cent in large series – are currently undetectable because of skewed Lyonization favouring normal VIIIC synthesis[24, 64]. Few centres can point to as low a false-normal rate in carrier detection (3 per cent) as Seligsohn *et al.*[75]. Clearly one must avoid telling a possible carrier that her tests prove her to be normal – more especially, perhaps, since the advent of antenatal diagnosis.

Carrier testing is not infrequently delayed until pregnancy, when factor VIII values are known to be raised[1, 24, 64]. A recent controlled study has shown that single determinations of mid-term ratios of VIIIC or VIIICAg to VIIIRAg are comparable as heterozygote discriminants with these ratios in non-pregnant women[51, 76]. However, the timing requirements of antenatal diagnosis militate against undue delay over this exercise in pregnancy.

Assignment of carrier probability in the authors' own 74 cases at risk for haemophilia A, based on the above principles, has led to their classification as (1) obligate (25 cases), (2) strongly putative or 'probable', when their final odds of heterozygosity are greater than even ($P > 0.5$, 40 cases), (3) putative or 'possible', denoting a lesser likelihood, which in practice has been $P < 0.25$ (9 cases).

Laboratory diagnosis

Successful antenatal diagnosis of haemophilia was first reported in 1979[19, 49, 50]. This account centres on two years' experience of the group at King's College Hospital, London[48] including collaborative studies with colleagues in Cardiff and Malmö[47, 51, 52].

After the patient's clinical and laboratory data have been critically reviewed and care taken to ensure that she receives full genetic counselling, fetal sexing by amniocentesis (not applicable to autosomal disorders like vWd) is performed at 15–16 weeks under ultrasound guidance. A provisional fetoscopy date is booked at the same time. Great care must be taken at amniocentesis to avoid red cell leakage into the amniotic fluid, as subsequent fetal blood sampling may be jeopardized. If the fetus is male, the mother is admitted for fetoscopy at about 19 weeks.

Fetal blood sampling

The maternal factor VIII or IX clotting activity is always assayed prior to fetoscopy to exclude a dangerously low level occurring in a few heterozygotes; this is relevant particularly if a termination of pregnancy ensues. In practice, precautionary replacement with cryoprecipitate or plasma was only deemed necessary once in 80 patients[48].

Fetoscopic blood sampling is performed as described for thalassaemia, except that immediately before puncturing a fetal vessel at the umbilical cord insertion, the sampling needle is flushed with a sterile, isotonic citrate-saline solution to

Table 8.2 Red cell values of successive blood samples at one fetoscopy

Sample	RBC ($10^{12}/l$)	MCV (fl)	PCV
Maternal	4.13	85	0.35
Fetal 0	1.91	122	0.23*
1	3.05	121	0.37
2	3.08	121	0.37
3	3.07	120	0.37
4	3.08	121	0.37

*First aliquot diluted by solution in fetoscopy needle.
Note constant hematocrit of successive aliquots.

exclude amniotic fluid, which might initiate clotting during sampling or accelerate the assay times[50]. Serial amounts of 200–250 µl of pure fetal blood are then withdrawn into graduated 1 ml plastic syringes, using a new syringe for each aliquot of blood. The samples are delivered into tiny polystyrene tubes calibrated at 200 µl and containing accurate volumes of buffered-citrate anticoagulant[48] for duplicate bioassays of fetal VIIIC and IXC, VIIIRAg/WF and (as internal controls) VC and XC. The rest of each aliquot goes into EDTA for cell counts and into heparin if radiometric assays are performed. A combined cell counter and particle-size analyser (Coulter 'Channelyzer') shows immediately that there is no maternal blood present and that successive blood samples have a haematocrit in the expected range which stays constant from tube to tube, thus excluding even small amounts of extraneous dilution by amniotic fluid (*Table 8.2*). Four to five aliquots, i.e. up to 1 ml of fetal blood, are usually taken and, after a short wait on ice, the plasma is separated for laboratory assays.

TWIN PREGNANCY

Two of the mothers were pregnant with twins. In one case both were male, and pure fetal blood was obtained from both through a single uterine insertion and trans-septal sampling of the second twin[73]. Both were found to be normal. The second mother had one male and one female fetus. Only the male was tested, found to be affected, and selectively aborted by umbilical vascular air embolism. Of 3 twin pregnancies managed in this way[70], the unaffected fetus proceeded to a normal term delivery in 2 cases and a live pre-term birth in the third.

Normal fetal values

Control assays of plasma factors VIIIC, VIIIRAg and IXC were determined (as were VC and XC) at King's College Hospital in pure fetal blood from 40 non-haemophilic fetoscopies. Immunoradiometric assays (IRMA) of VIIICAg and IXAg were also performed in 20 of these plasmas by Peake and Bloom[60,61] and Holmberg[27,47] and their colleagues in Cardiff and Malmö (*Table 8.3*). Significant positive correlation between the levels of VIIIC and VIIIRAg supported the validity of the bioassays in these samples.

Both factors VIII and IX are appreciably lower at mid-term than in the newborn[58], but are distinguishable from severe haemophilic levels with ease in the case of factor VIII, and by a much smaller – though clear – margin in respect of factor IX. There is no significant relation to fetal age in the narrow gestational range studied.

Table 8.3 Normal plasma levels in 40 patients of fetal factors VIII and IX (average adult values = 100 u/dl)

	Gestation (weeks)	PCV	VIIIC (u/dl)	VIIICAg* (u/dl)	VIIIRAg (u/dl)	IXC (u/dl)	IXAg* (u/dl)
Mean	19.2	0.37	45†	23	57†	8.3	4.6
SD	1.7	0.03	12	8	13	1.7	1.6
Range	16–23	0.33–0.43	25–89	11–43	41–103	5.9–12.8	2.0–7.8

* VIIICAg and IXAg assays performed by Peake and Bloom[60,61] and Holmberg[27,47] (n = 20).
† Correlation coefficient 0.74 ($P<0.001$).

Fetal serum is considerably less satisfactory than carefully anticoagulated plasma for measurement of factor VIIICAg. The mean levels in 7 normal fetal plasmas was 18.6 u/dl (range 11–29), and in the serum after clotting 4.3 u/dl (range 2–7) (Peake and Mibashan, unpublished). In adults this difference is smaller[61].

Blood from 74 consecutive male fetuses at risk of having haemophilia A and 6 of haemophilia B has been examined at the time of writing (*see Tables 8.4–8.7*), and one fetus was investigated for severe von Willebrand's disease (vWd), a total of 81 fetuses tested. In 80 of the 81 cases, pure undiluted fetal blood was obtained, thus enabling (with one exception) antenatal diagnosis to be made on the same day and parental choice to be exercised on the sole basis of the VIIIC or IXC assay (plus VIIIWF in the relevant case). The increasing use of pure umbilical cord blood, suitably collected, would extend this facility.

Haemophilia A

Of the 74 fetuses tested, 27 were found to be *affected* (*Table 8.4*) and pregnancy was interrupted at the parent's request by extra-amniotic prostaglandin administration (25), abdominal hysterotomy (1) and selective feticide of a twin (1). Blood was

Table 8.4 Abnormal prenatal tests in 27 of 74 male fetuses at risk of haemophilia A

	Gestation (weeks)	PCV	VIIIC (u/dl)	VIIICAg (u/dl)	VIIIRAg (u/dl)	VC (%)	IXC (u/dl)
Mean	19.8	0.37	1*	0.1†	56	51§	8.9
SD	1.2	0.03			13	9	1.4

Carrier status: 11 obligate; 15 probable ($0.5 < P < 1.0$); 1 possible ($P < 0.25$).
*Excludes one mild case (6 u/dl).
†Excludes 4 CRM+ fetuses (immunoassay not relevant).
§Control fetal VC: mean 52% (SD 8); range 36–67% (n = 20).

obtained from 16 abortuses and the diagnosis was confirmed in all; in the remaining 11 (9 of which were terminated abroad) haemophilia had been diagnosed by concurring assays of both fetal VIIIC and VIIICAg.

CRM+ CASES

Coagulant and radiometric assays were concordant except for 4 fetuses (from 2 kindred) with CRM+ haemophilia. In them the IRMA alone would not have permitted recognition of the disease, thus highlighting the value of being able to measure factor VIIIC[51].

The other 47 fetuses at risk of haemophilia A proved to be *normal* (*Table 8.5*). One was found to have exencephaly and was aborted after counselling; a second pregnancy was terminated for other indications. Again the application of two assay methods ensured 100 per cent diagnostic accuracy: four carriers (from 3 kindreds) with severely affected relatives who were CRM+ with respect to VIIICAg, had fetuses considered normal by virtue of their VIIIC as well as VIIICAg levels, which exceeded those in their haemophilic relatives. While this assumption for VIIICAg seems reasonable, the normal bioassays helped to dispel the possibility of false-normal IRMA values.

By contrast, the potential fallibility of fetoscopic VIIIC assays is emphasized by the patient whose amniotic fluid was too turbid, 3 weeks after bleeding at amniocentesis, to permit clear vessel puncture, resulting in a 1:1.5 dilution of fetal blood in amniotic fluid. Fetal VIIIC assay was thus precluded, and the normal VIIICAg value, in a CRM⁻ kindred, correctly established the fetal diagnosis.

Table 8.5 Normal prenatal tests in 47 of 74 male fetuses at risk of haemophilia A (including one pair of twins)

	Gestation (weeks)	PCV	Fetoscopy VIIIC (u/dl)	VIIICAg (u/dl)	VIIIRAg (u/dl)	Newborn VIIIC (u/dl)	VIIICAg (u/dl)	VIIIRAg (u/dl)
Mean	19.8	0.36†	43†	24§	56	117	101	132
SD	1.4	0.03	10	9	11			
Range	16–24	0.30–0.42	29–81	11–46	36–83			

Carrier status: 14 obligate; 24 probable ($0.5 < P < 1.0$); 9 possible ($0 < P < 0.25$).
* Excludes 7 still pregnant and 2 unrelated terminations.
† Excludes 1 sample diluted 1:1.5 with amniotic fluid.
§ Includes 4 with CRM⁺ kindred.

In 75 subsequent fetoscopies for haemophilia, including several more instances of comparable turbidity, a technique for locally clarifying the amniotic fluid has enabled a clean vessel puncture to be made in all cases. With such blood sampling, the bioassay on its own is entirely reliable as a yardstick of fetal coagulant status; but until an operator routinely obtains free-flowing, undiluted fetal blood, antenatal diagnosis of haemophilia will require immunoradiometric assays, which will succeed in the great majority of cases, namely those who are CRM⁻ with fetal samples neither overdiluted nor clotted[29, 48, 52]. Ideally the patient's interests are best served by methods permitting the use of both assay systems.

Altogether, of 44 'haemophilia A' pregnancies intended to continue after testing, 38 non-haemophilic babies have so far been born (1981), including the twins, and 7 pregnancies are still progressing. Factor VIII levels of 25 infants are depicted in *Table 8.5*, while the other 13, of whom 11 are abroad, are reportedly all normal.

PREDICTIVE ACCURACY

The results of antenatal haemophilia A tests are analysed in the light of each woman's assigned carrier status in *Table 8.6*. For each category of carrier probability, the frequency of diagnosed haemophilia corresponds closely to statistical prediction. The analysis illustrates why the proportion of affected fetuses (27/74) is appreciably less than the 50 per cent expected if all the carriers had been

Table 8.6 Predictive accuracy of prenatal tests for haemophilia A

Type of carrier	Total number	Expected number of carriers	Haemophilic fetuses expected	Haemophilic fetuses observed
Obligate	25	25	12–13	11
Probable ($P \geq 0.5$)	40	20–40	10–20	15
Possible ($P < 0.25$)	9	0–2	0–1	1

obligate, and highlights the 'reprieve' rate among male fetuses of mothers who are unwilling to bear a haemophilic child. The table also carries a reminder that there is an inherent fallibility of around 10 per cent[24,64] in assigning a genotype as probably normal on the basis of heterozygote testing.

Haemophilia B

Six fetuses were at risk of severe haemophilia B, reflecting both its lower prevalence and an appreciation of the added constraints imposed by the normally low levels of fetal factor IX. Diagnosis was made on the basis of plasma IXC assays in pure fetal blood (Table 8.7) and confirmed retrospectively in the 4 cases who were CRM⁻ by a sensitive radiometric IXAg assay[27,47,71]. The first 4 fetuses had

Table 8.7 Six male fetuses at risk of haemophilia B

Patient	Carrier status	Weeks	PCV	Fetoscopy* IXC	IXAg†	Confirmed
1	++	20	0.32	12.3	5.4	Newborn
2	Obligate	19	0.35	7.9	3.6	Newborn
3	++	22	0.34	9.4	4.8	Newborn
4	++	20	0.38	6.6	2.0	Newborn
5	Obligate	20	0.39	<1.0	<0.1	Abortus
6	++	19	0.35	<1.0	<0.1	Abortus

++ Carrier status: probable ($0.5 < P < 1.0$)
* Control fetal IXC, mean 8.4 u/dl (6.2–12.3)
 (n = 20) IXAg, mean 4.6 u/dl (2.0–7.8)
 Fetal XC, VC, VIIIC, VIIIRAg normal.
† Patients 2 and 3 have CRM⁺ relatives, i.e. immunoassay not applicable.

normal plasma assays, confirmed by the birth of 4 normal boys. The remaining 2 were severely affected on both assays, and the diagnosis was confirmed in abortal blood.

There are two added reasons to include a coagulant assay for the effective antenatal diagnosis of haemophilia B, and to develop a fetoscopy technique which makes it possible: (1) factor IXAg is found in small amounts in amniotic fluid, requiring a correction to be applied to blood samples diluted with liquor amnii[27]; and (2) the prevalence of CRM+ haemophilia B, while geographically variable, exceeds 30 per cent in some large series[24,37]. Though only one of 18 severely affected Swedish patients was CRM+ by the sensitive IRMA, 2 of the first 6 diagnostic cases were in this category and depended on fetal IXC determinations for correct antenatal diagnosis.

von Willebrand's disease

The very severe form of this disorder, in which little or no plasma factor VIIIC/CAg and VIIIRAg/WF are present, is uncommon. A couple who were at risk because they already had one such child sought antenatal diagnosis[48]. The fetus was similarly affected, with VIIIC levels below 1 u/dl, VIIIWF below 1.5 u/dl, and VIIIRAg (Laurell) less than 3 u/dl; fetal levels of VIIICAg and VIIIRAg (IRMA) lower than 0.1 u/dl further corroborated the diagnosis, which was confirmed after abortion. The *exclusion* of severe vWd has previously been reported[28,72].

OTHER HERITABLE HAEMOSTATIC DISORDERS
Other disorders identified or excluded antenatally, or to which existing laboratory techniques can be applied in pure fetoscopic blood samples, include thrombocytopenia with absent radii, familial amegakaryocytic thrombocytopenia, Glanzmann's thrombasthenia and Bernard-Soulier thrombocytopathy; Wiskott-Aldrich syndrome and other haematological disorders may prove to be detectable if they are found to be expressed early enough. The rare, severe autosomal coagulation defects also appear currently amenable to antenatal diagnosis.

Outcome of pregnancy

Fetoscopic blood sampling entails potential risks, from failure of diagnosis to fetal loss. In one report of 41 antenatal tests for haemophilia A these complications occurred in 10 and 7 per cent respectively[29], but experience and technical progress are likely to improve the results of fetoscopy generally.

Table 8.8 summarizes the outcome of pregnancy in the 80 consecutive women who were investigated antenatally for haemophilia A, B and vWd at King's College Hospital. There were no operative complications, including maternal bleeding; only one carrier, whose factor VIIIC was less than 30 u/dl, received two precautionary infusions of cryoprecipitate following termination of pregnancy.

In 48 women the pregnancy was intended to continue after fetoscopy. The pregnancies of 2 women who had transient vaginal loss of amniotic fluid, and of another with uterine contractions for some weeks, went safely to term. There were no spontaneous abortions and no accidental fetal deaths. (In a larger group of women, mostly heterozygotes for β-thalassaemia major, the fetal mortality related

Table 8.8 Outcome of pregnancy after prenatal tests for haemophilia A, B and von Willebrand's disease

Number of pregnancies	80
Number of fetuses	81
Pure fetal blood obtained in	80
Termination	
Haemophilia and von Willebrand's disease	30
Other causes	2
Pregnancies continued	48
Normal deliveries	36
Not yet delivered	7
Preterm labour (includes 2 twin pregnancies)	5
Maternal complications	0
Accidental abortions	0
Incorrect diagnosis	0

to fetoscopy was 3 per cent, a figure which has fallen below 2 per cent in the last 200 cases at King's College Hospital). Five patients delivered prematurely (before 37 weeks), two of whom had twin pregnancies: this is a normal incidence of preterm labour and is less than in the thalassaemia group. Two neonates had slight orthopaedic anomalies (one mild hip dislocation, completely corrected, and one mild talipes); no similar abnormalities occurred in other fetoscopy patients.

Thirty-six healthy babies have so far been delivered at term and, with five well premature infants, are developing normally. One preterm female infant, survivor of a selectively terminated twin pregnancy, died of sepsis in another hospital. There have been no diagnostic errors.

Who should be offered antenatal diagnosis?

Because haemophilia lacks the ethnic concentrations of thalassaemia, and possibly because antenatal diagnosis for haemophilia is more recent, there is not yet sufficient evidence of a large-scale demographic response to this new reproductive option. The authors' experience with antenatal studies of many haemophilic families has helped to clarify some of the complex issues.

With rare exceptions, women at risk are known to be *related* to a severe haemophiliac; current methods of heterozygote detection are inapplicable to population screening. Occasionally a presumptive heterozygote is discovered who herself has moderate bleeding problems and no affected male relative; such women have great difficulty in accepting the implications of antenatal diagnosis without close knowledge of someone with the disease.

The haemophilia in question is generally *severe*, but serious complications in a moderate sufferer may influence his female relatives to avoid having a similar child. The *facts* must be ascertained and put in perspective when counselling. The right of the prospective parents to choose freely after being fully informed is cardinal, as it is to reject fetoscopy 'illogically' on learning that the fetus is male, or to keep the pregnancy if it is affected. It has become harder for the authors to concur with advice to have the fetus sexed and, if male, to terminate pregnancy on the grounds that fetal blood testing is still experimental, dangerous or fraught with further delay; fetoscopy can be planned ahead for 24 hours after the karyotype result, with a result the same day (bioassay) or in 1–3 days (radiometric methods). There is complete accuracy of diagnosis, and the fetal loss rate in experienced hands (as at King's College Hospital) is low – nil so far in haemophilic cases and 1–2 per cent in all patients.

Motivation and attitudes

Women who are impelled actively to seek antenatal diagnosis are usually extremely anxious to avoid a haemophilic son, and all patients who chose fetal blood sampling would otherwise not have had children or else aborted a male fetus. By contrast, many others with an equal degree of risk, including obligate carriers, seem less motivated to seek eugenic advice. They may be unfamiliar with the disease at close hand, or prepared to accept the risk; but more often the options of the past decade, centring on abortion after amniocentesis, have been too discouraging. The presentation of many putative carriers for assessment when already pregnant[24, 64, 76], far from reflecting disinterest, indicates their imperative need for information in compelling circumstances. The option of accurate and safe fetal blood testing has greatly helped motivated couples in an ethical quandary to make up their mind about mid-term abortion.

Place of carrier assessment

The technical refinements in detecting non-obligate heterozygotes made a major contribution to genetic counselling when the price demanded of potential carriers to avoid having haemophilic children was fetal sexing and the consequent loss of more than 50 per cent of normal fetuses. With the advent of specific antenatal diagnosis, this figure will be weighed against the risks of the new procedures on the one hand and the dependability of carrier assessment on the other.

While some women at risk are spurred to positive thought when faced with a statistical estimate, we should not lose sight of the falsely normal laboratory tests which are a feature of such studies both in non-pregnant[24, 64] and pregnant obligate carriers[51, 76]. This 6–15 per cent error rate (exceptionally 3 per cent[75]) entails a 3–7 per cent chance that the sister of a haemophiliac, who starts with 1:1 odds of being affected, will bear a haemophilic son despite normal laboratory values. This risk, though smaller for less close relatives, will not knowingly be ignored by families with access to an antenatal diagnosis centre where the fetal loss rate is less than 2 per cent and whose insistence on an unaffected baby is strong. There seems a clear case for discussing this option with all carriers who are sufficiently motivated to seek advice, bearing in mind that its availability is still relatively limited and social and economic factors will continue to be important constraints.

Scope of pure fetal blood assays

The increasing adoption of the Rodeck technique[48, 67] not only enables antenatal diagnosis to be offered to families with molecular variants of haemophilia requiring coagulant bioassays for recognition (i.e. CRM⁺ variants) but also extends its scope to other, if rarer, bleeding disorders in which clotting factors or blood platelets are at fault.

FUTURE PERSPECTIVES

The recent advances in molecular biology that have led to the sequencing of the DNA around the globin gene clusters open up a new range of possibilities in antenatal diagnosis for haemoglobinopathies. It is now theoretically possible to develop methods of analysing leucocyte DNA from peripheral blood samples for the accurate diagnosis of heterozygotes and homozygotes for the thalassaemias and HbS disease.

If red blood cells are no longer necessary for the diagnosis, fetal blood sampling could be replaced by amniocentesis which a wider range of obstetricians could perform. More importantly, since any fetal tissue can be used, it should be possible to do antenatal diagnosis in the first trimester on small trophoblast samples obtained through the cervix. This would greatly reduce the stresses associated with antenatal diagnosis, as mid-trimester abortion of affected fetuses could be replaced by suction termination of pregnancy under general anaesthesia before 12 weeks of gestation. It is likely that this will greatly increase the wish for antenatal diagnosis by those who now find themselves most in conflict over it, such as Asian families and couples at risk for homozygous sickle-cell disease.

Such a method could similarly be applied to any other condition once the relevant section of DNA can be identified by molecular methods. Compared with other chromosomes, the X chromosome can be studied relatively easily because of the large number of X-linked characteristics that are known; and since it occurs in only a single dose in males the problems implicit in studying heterozygotes do not exist. As the molecular anatomy of this chromosome will be the first to be understood, it is likely that precise heterozygote diagnosis and early antenatal diagnosis for sex-linked conditions such as haemophilia will also become available within the next few years.

References

1 AKHMETELI, M. A., ALEDORT, L. M., ALEXANIANTS, S., BULANOV, A. G., ELSTON, R. C., GINTER, E. K., GOUSSEV, A., GRAHAM, J. B. *et al.* Methods for the detection of hemophilia carriers: a memorandum. *Bulletin of the World Health Organisation*, **55**, 675–702 (1977)

2 ALEPOROU-MARINOU, U., SAKARELOU-PAPAPETROU, N., ANTSAKLIS, A., FESSAS, Ph and LOUKOPOULOS, D. Prenatal diagnosis of thalassaemia major in Greece: evaluation

of the first large series of attempts. *Annals of the New York Academy of Sciences*, **344**, 181–188 (1980)

3 ALTER, B. P. Prenatal diagnosis of hemoglobinopathies and other hematologic diseases. *Journal of Pediatrics*, **95**, 501–513 (1979)

4 ALTER, B. P. Prenatal diagnosis of haemoglobinopathies: a status report. *Lancet*, **2**, 1152–1155 (1981)

5 ALTER, B. P., MODELL, B., FAIRWEATHER, D. V. I., HOBBINS, J. C., MAHONEY, M. J. and FRIGOLETTO, F. D. Prenatal diagnosis of hemoglobinopathies. A review of 15 cases. *New England Journal of Medicine*, **295**, 1437–1443 (1976)

6 ALTER, B. P. and NATHAN, D. G. Antenatal diagnosis of haematologic disorders '1978'. In *Clinics in Haematology*, **7**, *Perinatal Haematology*, edited by B. E. Glader, 195–216. London, W. B. Saunders (1979)

7 ANGASTINIOTIS, M. A. and HADJIMINAS, M. G. Prevention of thalassaemia in Cyprus. *Lancet*, **1**, 369–370 (1981)

8 BEVIS, D. C. A. The composition of liquor amnii in haemolytic disease of the newborn. *Journal of Obstetrics and Gynaecology of the British Empire*, **60**, 244 (1953)

9 BIGGS, R. Recent advances in the management of hemophilia and Christmas disease. In *Clinics in Hematology*, **8**, *Congenital Coagulation Disorders*, edited by C. R. Rizza, 95–114. London, W. B. Saunders (1979)

9a BLOUQUIT, Y., BEUZARD, Y., VARNAVIDES, L., CHABRET, C., DUMEZ, Y., JOHN, P. N., RODECK, C. H. and WHITE, J. M. Antenatal diagnosis of haemaglobinopathies by Biorex chromatography of haemaglobin. *British Journal of Haematology*, **50**, 7–15 (1982)

10 BUSSLINGER, M. MOSCHONAS, N. and FLAVELL, R. A. β-thalassaemia: aberrant splicing results from a single point mutation in an intron. *Cell*, **27**, 289–298 (1981)

11 CAO, A., FURBETTA, M. and GALANELLO, R. Screening for thalassaemia. *Lancet*, **2**, 1189 (1980)

12 CHANG, H., HOBBINS, J. C., CIVIDALLI, G., FRIGOLETTO, F. D., MAHONEY, M. J. and KAN, W. Y. In utero diagnosis of hemoglobinopathies. Hemoglobin synthesis in fetal red cells. *New England Journal of Medicine*, **290**, 1067 (1974)

13 CHANG, H., MODELL, C. B., ALTER, B. P., DICKINSON, M. J., FRIGOLETTO, F. D., HUEHNS, E. R. and NATHAN, D. G. Detection of the β-thalassaemia gene in the first trimester fetus. *Proceedings of the National Academy of Sciences of the United States of America*, **72**, 3633–3637 (1975)

14 CHERNOFF, A. L., MINNICH, V., NA-NAKORN, S., TUCHINDA, S., CHANRIVAT, K. and CHERNOFF, R. R. Studies on Hemoglobin E. I. The clinical, hematologic and genetic characteristics of the hemoglobin E syndromes. *Journal of Laboratory and Clinical Medicine*, **47**, 455–488 (1956)

15 CIVIDALLI, G., NATHAN, D. G., KAN, Y. W., SANTAMARINA, B. and FRIGOLETTO, F. Relation of beta to gamma synthesis during the first trimester: an approach to prenatal diagnosis of thalassaemia. *Pediatric Research*, **8**, 553–560 (1974)

16 DUBART, A., GOOSSENS, M., BEUZARD, Y., MONPLAISIR, N., TESTA, U., BASSET, P. and ROSA, J. Prenatal diagnosis of hemoglobinopathies: comparison of the results obtained by isoelectric focusing of hemoglobins and by chromatography of radioactive globin chains. *Blood*, **56**, 1092–1099 (1980)

17 EFSTRADIADIS, A., POSAKONY, J. W., MANIATIS, T., LAWN, R. M., O'CONNELL, C. and SPRITZ, R. A. The structure and evolution of the human β-globin gene family. *Cell*, **21**, 653–668 (1980)
18 FAIRWEATHER, D. V. I., MODELL, B., BERDOUKAS, V., ALTER, B. P., NATHAN, D. G. and LOUKOPOULOS, D. Antenatal diagnosis of thalassaemia major. *British Medical Journal*, **1**, 350–353 (1978)
19 FIRSHEIN, S. I., HOYER, L. W., LAZARCHICK, J., FORGET, B. G., HOBBINS, J. A., CLYNE, L. P., PITLICK, F. A., MUIR, W. A., MERKATZ, I. R. and MAHONEY, M. J. Prenatal diagnosis of classic hemophilia. *New England Journal of Medicine*, **300**, 937–942 (1979)
20 FOUER, N. The Jamaicans; cultural and social change among migrants in Britain. In *Between Two Cultures*, edited by L. Watson. Oxford, Blackwell (1977)
21 FURBETTA, M., ANGIUS, A., XIMINES, A., FAIS, R., CAO, A. and VALENTI, C. Prenatal diagnosis of β-thalassaemia. Experience with 24 cases. *Journal of Medical Genetics*, **16**, 366–368 (1979)
22 FURBETTA, M., ANGIUS, A., XIMENES, A., ROSATELLI, C., SCALAS, M. T., TUVERI, T. et al. Difficulties in antenatal diagnosis of inherited haemoglobinopathies: γ-chain variants. *British Journal of Haematology*, **46**, 319–321 (1981)
23 GOODY, E. N. and GROOTHEUS, C. M. The West Africans: the quest for education. In *Between Two Cultures*, edited by L. Watson. Oxford, Blackwell (1977)
24 GRAHAM, J. B. Genotype assignment (carrier detection) in the hemophilias. In *Clinics in Hematology*, **8**, *Congenital Coagulation Disorders*, edited by C. R. Rizza, 115–146. London, W. B. Saunders (1979)
25 HOLLENBERG, M. D., KABACK, M. M. and KAZAZIAN, H. H. Adult haemoglobin synthesis by reticulocytes from the human fetus at mid-trimester. *Science*, **174**, 698–702 (1971)
26 HOLMBERG, L., HENRIKSSON, P., EKELUND, H. and ASTEDT, B. Coagulation in the human fetus. *Journal of Pediatrics*, **85**, 860–964 (1974)
27 HOLMBERG, L. GUSTAVII, B., CORDESIUS, E., KRISTOFFERSSON, A.-C., LJUNG, R., LÖFTBERG, I., STRÖMBERG, P. and NILSSON, I. M. Prenatal diagnosis of hemophilia B by an immunoradiometric assay of factor IX. *Blood*, **56**, 397–401 (1980)
28 HOYER, L. W., LINDSTEN, J., BLÖMBACK, M., HAGENFELDT, L., CORDESIUS, E., STRÖMBERG, P. and GUSTAVII, B. Prenatal evaluation of fetus at risk for severe von Willebrand's disease. *Lancet*, **2**, 191–192 (1979)
29 HOYER, L. W. and MAHONEY, M. J. Prenatal diagnosis of classic hemophilia. *XIV International Congress of the World Federation of Hemophilia*, Costa Rica (abstract) (1981)
30 JONES, P. Developments and problems in the management of hemophilia. *Seminars in Hematology*, **14**, 375–390 (1977)
31 JONES, R. W., OLD, J. M., TRENT, R. J., CLEGG, J. B. and WEATHERALL, D. J. A major rearrangement in the human β-globin gene cluster. *Nature*, **291**, 39–44 (1981)
32 KAN, Y. W., DOZY, A. M., ALTER, B. P., FRIGOLETTO, F. D. and NATHAN, D. G. Detection of the sickle gene in the human fetus. Potential for intrauterine diagnosis of sickle cell anemia. *New England Journal of Medicine*, **287**, 1–5 (1972)
33 KAN, Y. W., GOLBUS, M. A., TRECARTIN, R., FURBETTA, M. and CAO, A. Prenatal diagnosis of homozygous β-thalassaemia. *Lancet*, **2**, 790–791 (1975)

34 KAN, Y. W. and NATHAN, D. G. Mild thalassaemia: the result of interaction of alpha and beta thalassaemia genes. *Journal of Clinical Investigation*, **49**, 635–642 (1970)

35 KAN, Y. W., TRECARTIN, R. F., GOLBUS, M. A. and FILLY, R. A. Prenatal diagnosis of β-thalassaemia and sickle cell anaemia. Experience with 24 cases. *Lancet*, **1**, 269 (1977)

36 KAN, Y. W., VALENTI, C., CARNAZZA, V., GUIDETTI, R. and RIEDER, R. F. Fetal blood sampling *in utero. Lancet*, **1**, 79–80 (1974)

37 KASPER, C. K., ØSTERUD, B., MINAMI, J. Y., SHONICK, W. and RAPAPORT, S. I. Hemophilia B: characterization of genetic variants and detection of carriers. *Blood*, **50**, 351–366 (1977)

38 KAZAZIAN, H. H. and WOODHEAD, A. O. Adult hemoglobin synthesis in the human fetus. *Annals of the New York Academy of Sciences*, **241**, 691 (1974)

39 LEJEUNE, J., TURPIN, R. and GAUTIER, M. Le mongolisme, premier example d'aberration autosomique humain. *Annales de Genetique*, **1**, 41 (1959)

40 LOUKOPOULOS, D., LOUTRADI, A. and FESSAS, P. A unique thalassaemic syndrome: homozygous α-thalassaemia plus homozygous β-thalassaemia. *British Journal of Haematology*, **39**, 377–390 (1978)

41 LOUKOPOULOS, D., TASSIOPOULOU, A. and FESSAS, Ph. Screening for thalassaemia. *Lancet*, **2**, 1188–1189 (1980)

42 MAHONEY, M. J. Socioethical consequences of prenatal diagnosis for hemophilia. *XIV International Congress of the World Federation of Hemophilia*, Costa Rica (abstract) (1981)

43 MANN, J. R. Sickle haemoglobinopathies in England. *Archives of Disease in Childhood*, **56**, 676–683 (1981)

44 MATSAKIS, M., BERDOUKAS, V. A., ANGASTINIOTIS, M., MOUZOURAS, M., IANNOU, P., FERRARI, M. *et al*. Haematological aspects of antenatal diagnosis for β-thalassaemia in Britain. *British Journal of Haematology*, **46**, 185–197 (1980)

45 MEDICAL RESEARCH COUNCIL WORKING PARTY. An assessment of the hazards of amniocentesis. *British Journal of Obstetrics and Gynaecology*, **85**, Suppl. 2, 1–41 (1978)

46 MIBASHAN, R. S. and RODECK, C. H. Prenatal diagnosis of haemophilia A and Christmas disease. In *Unresolved Problems in Haemophilia*, edited by C. D. Forbes and G. D. O. Lowe. Lancaster, MTP (1982)

47 MIBASHAN, R. S., RODECK, C. H., HOLMBERG, L., THUMPSTON, J. K., WHITE, J. M., KRISTOFFERSSON, A.-C., GORER, R., NILSSON, I. M. and CAMPBELL, S. Prenatal diagnosis of haemophilia B by assay of fetal factor IXC and IXAg (IRMA). *Thrombosis and Haemostasis*, **46**, 167 (1981)

48 MIBASHAN, R. S., RODECK, C. H. and THUMPSTON, J. K. Prenatal diagnosis of the haemophilias. In *Methods in Haematology: The Haemophilias*, edited by A. L. Bloom, Edinburgh, Churchill Livingstone (in press)

49 MIBASHAN, R. S., RODECK, C. H., THUMPSTON, J. K., ADELMAN, M. I., SINGER, J. D., WHITE, J. M. and CAMPBELL, S. Prenatal plasma assay factors VIII and IX. *British Journal of Haematology*, **41**, 611–612 (1979)

50 MIBASHAN, R. S., RODECK, C. H., THUMPSTON, J. K., EDWARDS, R. J., SINGER, J. D., WHITE, J. M. and CAMPBELL, S. Plasma assay of fetal factors VIIIC and IX for prenatal diagnosis of haemophilia. *Lancet*, **2**, 1309–1311 (1979)

51 MIBASHAN, R. S., PEAKE, I. R., NEWCOMBE, R. G., THUMPSTON, J. K., GORER, R., FURLONG, R. A. and RODECK, C. H. Carrier detection of haemophilia A in pregnancy by measurement of factor VIIIC/RAg and VIIIAg/RAg ratios. *Thrombosis and Haemostasis*, **46**, 187 (1981)

52 MIBASHAN, R. S., PEAKE, I. R., RODECK, C. H., THUMPSTON, J. K., FURLONG, R. A., GORER, R., BAINS, L. and BLOOM, A. L. Dual diagnosis of prenatal haemophilia A by measurement of fetal factor VIIIC and VIIIC antigen (VIIICAg). *Lancet*, **2**, 994–997 (1980)

53 MODELL, B. The social consequences of introducing antenatal diagnosis for inherited disease. In *The Future of Prenatal Diagnosis*, edited by H. Galjaard. London, Churchill Livingstone (in press)

54 MODELL, B. and BERDOUKAS, V. A. *The Clinical Approach to Thalassaemia*. New York, Grune and Stratton (in press)

55 MODELL, B. and WARD, R. H. T. Antenatal diagnosis and haemoglobinopathies. In *Fetoscopy*, edited by I. Rocker and K. M. Laurence, 87–145. Amsterdam, Elsevier/North-Holland (1981)

56 MODELL, B., WARD, R. H. T. and FAIRWEATHER, D. V. I. Effect of introducing antenatal diagnosis on reproductive behaviour of families at risk for thalassaemia major. *British Medical Journal*, **1**, 1347 (1980)

57 MOSCHONAS, N., DE BOER, E., GROSSVELD, F. G. *et al*. Structure and expression of a cloned β^0 thalassaemia globin gene. *Nucleic Acids Research*, **9**, 4391–4401 (1981)

58 NOSSEL, H. L., LANZKOWSKY, P., LEVY, S., MIBASHAN, R. S. and HANSEN, J. D. C. A study of coagulation factor levels in women during labour and in their newborn infants. *Thrombosis et Diathesis Haemorrhagica*, **16**, 185–197 (1966)

59 PATARYAS, H. A. and STAMATOYANNOPOULOS, G. Hemoglobins in human fetuses: evidence for adult hemoglobin production after the 11th gestational week. *Blood*, **39**, 688–695 (1972)

60 PEAKE, I. R. and BLOOM, A. L. Immunoradiometric assay of procoagulant factor VIII antigen in plasma and serum and its reduction in hemophilia. *Lancet*, **1**, 473–475 (1978)

61 PEAKE, I. R., BLOOM, A. L., GIDDINGS, J. C. and LUDLAM, C. A. An immunoradiometric assay for procoagulant factor VIII antigen. Results in haemophilia, von Willebrand's disease and fetal plasma and serum. *British Journal of Haematology*, **42**, 269–281 (1979)

61a PEAKE, I. R., NEWCOMBE, R. G., DAVIES, B. L., FURLONG, R. A., LUDLAM, C. A. and BLOOM, A. L. Carrier detection in haemophilia A by immunological measurement of factor VIII related antigen (VIIIRAg) and factor VIII clotting antigen (VIIICAg). *British Journal of Haematology*, **48**, 651–660 (1981)

62 PEMBREY, M. E., WOOD, W. G., WEATHERALL, D. J. and PERRINE, R. P. Fetal haemoglobin production and the sickle gene in the Oases of Eastern Saudi Arabia. *British Journal of Haematology*, **40**, 415–429 (1978)

63 POWLEDGE, T. M. and FLETCHER, J. Guidelines for the ethical, social and legal issues in prenatal diagnosis. *New England Journal of Medicine*, **300**, 168–172 (1979)

64 RATNOFF, O. D. and JONES, P. K. The art of betting: which of a bleeder's female relatives is a carrier? *Annals of Internal Medicine*, **89**, 281–282 (1977)

65 ROCKER, I. Defect in fetal membranes after fetoscopy. *Lancet*, **1**, 716 (1978)

66 ROCKER, I. and LAURENCE, K. M. (Eds). *Fetoscopy*. Amsterdam, Elsevier/North-Holland (1981)

67 RODECK, C. H. Fetoscopy guided by real-time ultrasound for pure fetal blood samples, fetal skin samples and examination of the fetus *in utero*. *British Journal of Obstetrics and Gynaecology*, **87**, 449–456 (1980)

68 RODECK, C. H. and CAMPBELL, S. Sampling pure fetal blood by fetoscopy in second trimester of pregnancy. *British Medical Journal*, **2**, 728–730 (1978)

69 RODECK, C. H., KEMP, J. R., HOLMAN, C. A., WHITMORE, D. A., KARNICKI. J. and AUSTIN, M. A. Direct intravascular fetal blood transfusion by fetoscopy in severe Rhesus isoimmunisation. *Lancet*, **1**, 625–627 (1981)

70 RODECK, C. H., MIBASHAN, R. S., ABRAMOVIC, J. and CAMPBELL, S. Selective feticide of affected twin by fetoscopic air embolism. *Prenatal Diagnosis* (in press)

71 RODECK, C. H., MIBASHAN, R. S., HOLMBERG, L. *et al.* (Unpublished observations)

72 RODECK, C. H., MIBASHAN, R. S., PEAKE, I. R. and BLOOM, A. L. Prenatal diagnosis of severe von Willebrand's disease. *Lancet*, **2**, 637–638 (1979)

73 RODECK, C. H. and WASS, D. Sampling pure fetal blood in twin pregnancies by fetoscopy using a single uterine puncture. *Prenatal Diagnosis*, **1**, 43–49 (1981)

74 ROSA, P. A. and FAUARD, A. E. A new method of prenatal diagnosis of sex. *International Journal of Sexology*, **4**, 160 (1951)

75 SELIGSOHN, U., ZIVELIN, A., PEREZ, C. and MODAN, M. Detection of haemophilia A carriers by replicate factor VIII activity and factor VIII antigenicity determinations. *British Journal of Haematology*, **42**, 433–439 (1979)

76 THUMPSTON, J. K., MIBASHAN, R. S., RODECK, C. H., GORER, R. and NEWCOMBE, R. G. Carrier detection for hemophilia A in pregnancy. *XIV International Congress of the World Federation of Hemophilia*, Costa Rica (abstract) (1981)

77 TRAEGER, J., WOOD, W. G., CLEGG, J. B., WEATHERALL, D. J. and WASI, P. Defective synthesis of HbE is due to reduced levels of β^EmRNA. *Nature*, **288**, 497–499 (1980)

78 TRECARTIN, R. F., LIEBHABER, S. A., CHANG, J. C., LEE, K. Y., KAN, Y. W. and FURBETTA, M. β^0-thalassaemia in Sardinia is caused by a nonsense mutation. *Journal of Clinical Investigation*, **68**, 1012–1017 (1981)

79 TUAN, D., MURNAME, M. J., deRID, J. K. and FORGET, B. G. Heterogeneity in the molecular basis of hereditary persistence of fetal haemoglobin. *Nature*, **285**, 335 (1980)

80 WALKER, J. and TURNBULL, E. P. N. Haemoglobin and red cells in the human foetus III. Foetal and adult haemoglobin. *Archives of Disease in Childhood*, **300**, 102–114 (1955)

81 WARD, R. H. T., MODELL, B., FAIRWEATHER, D. V. I., SHIRLEY, I. M. and HETHERINGTON, C. P. Obstetric outcome and problems of mid-trimester fetal blood sampling for antenatal diagnosis. *British Journal of Obstetrics and Gynaecology* (in press)

82 WEATHERALL, D. J. and CLEGG, J. G. *The Thalassaemia Syndromes*, 3rd Ed. Oxford, Basil Blackwell (1981)

83 WEATHERALL, D. J., PRESSLEY, L., WOOD, W. G., HIGGS, D. R. and CLEGG, J. B. Molecular basis for mild forms of homozygous β-thalassaemia. *Lancet*, **1**, 527–529 (1981)

84 WESTWAWAY, D. and WILLIAMSON, R. An intron nucleotide sequence variant in a cloned β^+ thalassaemia globin gene. *Nucleic Acids Research*, **9,** 1777–1788 (1981)

85 WHITE, G. C., BLATT, P. M., McMILLAN, C. W., WEBSTER, W. P., LESESNE, H. R. and ROBERTS, H. R. Medical complications of hemophilia. *Southern Medical Journal*, **73,** 155–160 (1980)

9
Neonatal erythropoiesis: changes in oxygen transport and delivery
James A. Stockman, III

INTRODUCTION

It has been over half a century since Anselmino and Hoffman first observed that the oxygen affinity of human fetal blood was greater than that of maternal blood[4]. Some 15 years have elapsed since Benesch and Benesch[9], and Chanutin and Curnish[16] reported the modulating effects of organic phosphates such as 2, 3-diphosphoglycerate on hemoglobin's affinity for oxygen. With these as a basis, a fuller understanding of the events associated with oxygen unloading and oxygen delivery has evolved with respect to both term and preterm newborns.

This chapter will examine current concepts of those factors thought to be important in regulating oxygen transport in the newborn. Since the story actually begins before birth, a description of the events surrounding the development of erythropoiesis will initiate this discussion.

ERYTHROPOIESIS IN THE NEWBORN

Development of erythropoiesis

Erythropoiesis begins *in utero* by 14 days gestation. The yolk sac is the first site of red cell production. Erythropoiesis occurring in the yolk sac appears to be very different from that occurring later in pregnancy. The red cells are very macrocytic and are nucleated. This evolving population of red cell precursors does not appear to be under the control of erythropoietin, as is the case in later gestation[28]. These unique characteristics have led to the conclusion on the part of some that the erythroid precursors found in the yolk sac are primitive and eventually disappear rather than 'seeding' other areas where erythropoiesis later becomes prominent. The red blood cell precursors in the yolk sac are megaloblastic with abundant polychromatophilic cytoplasm and a fine nuclear chromatin pattern.

Normoblastic erythropoiesis occurs first in the liver, at about 5 weeks gestation, and continues throughout the remainder of gestation, diminishing gradually during the second trimester and ending totally by a few weeks after birth. The onset of bone marrow erythropoiesis occurs during the second trimester[33]. By the termination of pregnancy, almost all erythropoiesis is taking place in the bone marrow. Concomitant with the onset of marrow red cell production, the spleen is also a site of erythropoiesis, but as with the liver, this ceases shortly after birth[69].

Regulation of erythropoiesis in the fetus and newborn

Red cell production in all adult mammals is regulated by the hormone erythropoietin. There is ample evidence that hypoxia, the fundamental erythropoietic stimulus, exerts its influence on fetal erythropoiesis via the production and action of erythropoietin[25]. In many ways, the regulation of erythropoiesis in the human fetus resembles that in the adult. Evidence for this has been derived from a number of mammalian species. This evidence includes:

(1) the presence of erythropoiesis-stimulating activity in the cord blood, amniotic fluid and urine of normal and premature infants[26, 27]. In this regard, the level of erythropoietin activity has been found to be greater in anemic than normal fetuses;
(2) the suppression of erythropoiesis in some mouse fetuses by anti-erythropoietin antibodies administered to the mother[56];
(3) delivery of polycythemic lambs following prolonged exposure of ewes to high altitude[35];
(4) the enhanced rate of erythropoiesis in fetuses subjected to bleeding or hypoxia[42];
(5) the observation that placental insufficiency resulting in intrauterine hypoxia causes neonatal polycythemia[32];
(6) the stimulation of heme synthesis by fetal liver cells and yolk sac upon exposure to erythropoietin *in vitro*[17].

With respect to *in vitro* studies of erythropoiesis, Hassan *et al.*, comparing adult and umbilical cord blood samples, found increased numbers of erythroid progenitors in cord blood[31]. In addition, they compared the time of appearance of the maximum number of colonies of erythroid progenitor cells and found that in cord blood cultures, the maximum number appeared between days 7 and 9, whereas in adult blood cultures, the greatest number was visible around day 14. These investigators documented the importance of erythropoietin to erythroid colony growth in the newborn since no colonies were observed in the absence of erythropoietin.

Studies in our laboratories have demonstrated that there is an abundance of erythroid progenitor cells in the cord blood of newborns compared to the peripheral blood of adults[18]. In addition, it is apparent that very low (but not absent) concentrations of erythropoietin will support this growth. It has been suggested that this unusual sensitivity to the effects of erythropoietin is related to fetal hemoglobin synthesis and that its disappearance after the neonatal period may be related to the switch from fetal to adult hemoglobin production. Tchernia *et al.* have observed spontaneous erythroid colony formation in the human newborn cord blood if a culture medium using methyl cellulose is employed[64]. A comparison of erythroid cultures from newborns, normal adults, anemic adults and adults with polycythemia vera and myelofibrosis showed that endogenous erythroid colonies were also found in cultures of patients with polycythemia vera and myelofibrosis but not in cultures of normal cells and cells from anemic subjects. The physiological relevance of these endogenous colony-forming cells in newborn blood is unknown, although the similarities with diseases such as myelofibrosis suggest that they may be related to residual extramedullary erythropoiesis at birth

In the postnatal period, a marked decrease in erythropoietic activity occurs. Elevated levels of erythropoietin are found in cord blood at term, but if a bioassay is used, no erythropoietin can be detected in the blood or urine from the second day of life[39]. The decline in erythropoietic activity during the first week of life is probably due to improved oxygenation and cessation of erythropoietin production. The finding of erythropoietic inhibitors in plasma from the fourth day of life may, however, suggest that inhibitory mechanisms are involved in the suppression of erythropoiesis postnatally[59]. Studies on natives of high altitudes who have been brought down to sea level, a condition similar to the neonatal period, have also demonstrated the appearance of erythropoiesis inhibitors in plasma during a period with a surplus of oxygen and circulating hemoglobin[52]. The presence of inhibitors in the postnatal period has not, however, been found by all investigators[41]. Varying assay techniques may explain some of these differences. If such inhibitory substances do exist in the plasma of healthy newborn infants, they may be part of a

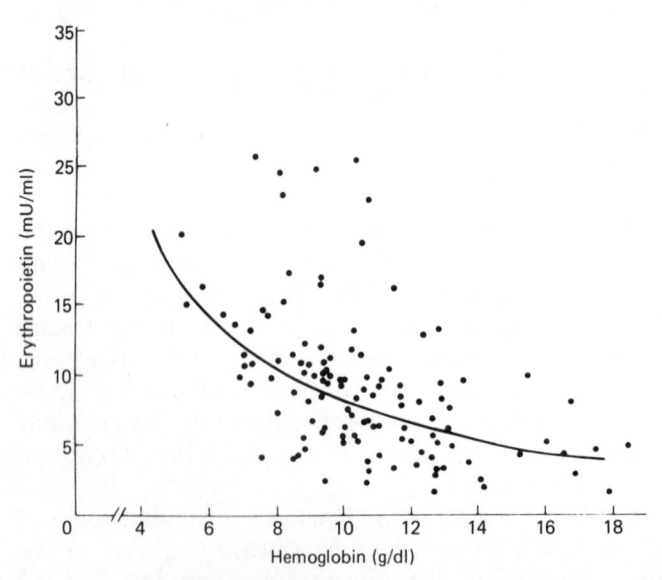

Figure 9.1 Changes in plasma erythropoietin in relation to hemoglobin levels in preterm infants born weighing less than 1500 g. (From Stockman *et al.*[63], courtesy of the Editor and Publishers, *New England Journal of Medicine*)

normal feedback mechanism which reflects the fact that adequate tissue oxygenation is occurring. This suppression of erythropoiesis is supported by studies on reticulocytes[57]; iron kinetics[29], and bone marrow[36].

The major site of erythropoietin production in the adult is the kidney[34]. There is certainly the possibility that a different site exists early in fetal development. There are no studies that have characterized any structural or functional differences in the erythropoietin of the fetus when compared to the adult.

There is no doubt about the ability of both term and preterm infants to produce erythropoietin. Whether quantitatively appropriate amounts can be made is a different question. It would be expected that during the first few weeks of life, because of the abundance of the hemoglobin present, erythropoietin production would cease and erythropoiesis would be suppressed. This is apparently what happens. Plasma erythropoietin by bioassay is absent after a few days of life but is measureable again at 2 to 3 months[39]. Using the more sensitive radioimmunoassay it may be seen that measurable values are obtained throughout early infancy[63] (*Figure 9.1*). The level of erythropoietin present roughly correlates with the inverse of the hemoglobin. The factors important in this fine modulation are related to the control of oxygen unloading and oxygen transport and are now discussed.

EXPECTED CHANGES IN HEMOGLOBIN

Cord hemoglobin levels vary relatively little in infants born prematurely compared with term infants. It has been suggested that in male infants maximum hemoglobin levels are achieved *in utero* by about 32 weeks gestation, while in girls a gradual rise in hemoglobin is found towards term[14].

In the day following birth, there is usually a rise in the hemoglobin level of as much as 5 percent or more. This is thought to represent a spontaneous decline in the plasma volume and the expected poor oral fluid intake, since there is no rise in the red cell mass itself. The hemoglobin will also rise if there has been any delay in clamping of the umbilical cord at the time of birth.

A progressive decline in the hemoglobin concentration begins by the second to third day of life. The rapidity of this decline is greater with increasing degrees of immaturity. The reason for this more accelerated decline may be related to the

Table 9.1 Normal hemoglobin levels (g/dl) in preterm infants of varying birthweights. The numbers in parentheses represent ranges. (From Williams *et al.*[68], courtesy of the Editor and Publishers, *New England Journal of Medicine*)

Birth weight (g)	2	4	Age (weeks) 6	8	10
800–1000	16.0 (14.8–17.2)	10.0 (6.8–13.2)	8.7 (7.0–10.2)	8.0 (7.1–9.8)	8.0 (6.9–10.2)
1001–1200	16.4 (14.1–18.7)	12.8 (7.8–15.3)	10.5 (7.2–12.3)	9.1 (7.8–10.4)	8.5 (7.0–10.0)
1201–1400	16.2 (13.6–18.8)	13.4 (8.8–16.2)	10.9 (8.5–13.3)	9.9 (8.0–11.8)	9.8 (8.4–11.3)
1401–1500	15.6 (13.4–17.8)	11.7 (9.7–13.7)	10.5 (9.1–11.9)	9.8 (8.4–12.0)	9.9 (8.4–11.4)
1501–2000	15.6 (13.5–17.7)	11.0 (9.6–14.0)	9.6 (8.8–11.5)	9.8 (8.4–12.1)	10.1 (8.6–11.8)

shorter red cell survivial of the tiny neonate[10]. The magnitude of the fall in hemoglobin is also inversely proportional to the gestational age. For example, hemoglobin levels as low as 7.0 g/dl are not unusual by 2 months of age in infants born weighing less than 1000 g[68]. *Table 9.1* illustrates the precise changes which are expected in preterm (less than 1500 g) infants who were otherwise well and had not experienced any unusual blood losses. *Table 9.2* indicates the changes observed over the first 12 weeks of life of term infants.

Table 9.2 Normal hematological values during the first 12 weeks of life in term infants as determined by an electronic cell counter. (From Matoth *et al.*[43], courtesy of the Editor and Publishers, *Acta Paediatrica Scandinavica*)

Age	No. of cases	Hb (g/dl) ± s.d.	RBC (×10^{12} /l ± s.d.)	PCV (± s.d.)	MCV (fl± s.d.)	MCHC (g/d ± s.d.)	Reticulocytes (% ± s.d.)
Days							
1	19	19.0 ± 2.2	5.14 ± 0.7	0.61 ± 0.074	119 ± 9.4	31.6 ± 1.9	3.2 ± 1.4
2	19	19.0 ± 1.9	5.15 ± 0.8	0.60 ± 0.064	115 ± 7.0	31.6 ± 1.4	3.2 ± 1.3
3	19	18.7 ± 3.4	5.11 ± 0.7	0.62 ± 0.093	116 ± 5.3	31.1 ± 2.8	2.8 ± 1.7
4	10	18.6 ± 2.1	5.00 ± 0.6	0.57 ± 0.081	114 ± 7.5	32.6 ± 1.5	1.8 ± 1.1
5	12	17.6 ± 1.1	4.97 ± 0.4	0.57 ± 0.073	114 ± 8.9	30.9 ± 2.2	1.2 ± 0.2
6	15	17.4 ± 2.2	5.00 ± 0.7	0.54 ± 0.072	113 ± 10.0	32.2 ± 1.6	0.6 ± 0.2
7	12	17.9 ± 2.5	4.86 ± 0.6	0.56 ± 0.094	118 ± 11.2	32.0 ± 1.6	0.5 ± 0.4
Weeks							
1–2	32	17.3 ± 2.3	4.80 ± 0.8	0.54 ± 0.083	112 ± 19.0	32.1 ± 2.9	0.5 ± 0.3
2–3	11	15.6 ± 2.6	4.20 ± 0.6	0.46 ± 0.073	111 ± 8.2	33.9 ± 1.9	0.8 ± 0.6
3–4	17	14.2 ± 2.1	4.00 ± 0.6	0.43 ± 0.057	105 ± 7.5	33.5 ± 1.6	0.6 ± 0.3
4–5	15	12.7 ± 1.6	3.60 ± 0.4	0.36 ± 0.048	101 ± 8.1	34.9 ± 1.6	0.9 ± 0.8
5–6	10	11.9 ± 1.5	3.55 ± 0.2	0.36 ± 0.062	102 ± 10.2	34.1 ± 2.9	1.0 ± 0.7
6–7	10	12.0 ± 1.5	3.40 ± 0.4	0.36 ± 0.048	105 ± 12.0	33.8 ± 2.3	1.2 ± 0.7
7–8	17	11.1 ± 1.1	3.40 ± 0.4	0.33 ± 0.037	100 ± 13.0	33.7 ± 2.6	1.5 ± 0.7
8–9	13	10.7 ± 0.9	3.40 ± 0.5	0.31 ± 0.025	93 ± 12.0	34.1 ± 2.2	1.8 ± 1.0
9–10	12	11.2 ± 0.9	3.60 ± 0.3	0.32 ± 0.027	91 ± 9.3	34.3 ± 2.9	1.2 ± 0.6
10–11	11	11.4 ± 0.9	3.70 ± 0.4	0.34 ± 0.021	91 ± 7.7	33.2 ± 2.4	1.2 ± 0.7
11–12	13	11.3 ± 0.9	3.70 ± 0.3	0.33 ± 0.033	88 ± 7.9	34.8 ± 2.2	0.7 ± 0.3

MCV = mean corpuscular volume.
MCHC = mean corpuscular hemoglobin concentration.

FUNCTIONAL BASIS FOR CHANGES IN OXYGEN TRANSPORT AND OXYGEN DELIVERY

Background

A series of factors are important in determining the actual amount of oxygen which is delivered to tissues. If the inspired gas mixture is deficient in oxygen, the amount transported may be deficient. If pulmonary function is abnormal or a pulmonary alveolar capillary block is present, arterial oxygen saturation will suffer. Arterial

Functional basis for changes in oxygen transport and oxygen delivery

oxygen content is made up of two variables, the hemoglobin concentration and the ability of that hemoglobin to bind oxygen, largely a characteristic of the hemoglobin–oxygen dissociation curve. The ability of blood to deliver oxygen to tissues is also a function of the cardiac output. The actual amount of oxygen released to tissues is a function again of the position of the hemoglobin–oxygen dissociation curve and the metabolic requirements of that tissue for oxygen. For neonates, not all of these variables are known, and judgements must often be made based on probabilities of certain circumstances being present.

The current understandings of those changes which are known to affect oxygen transport and delivery are discussed below.

Fetal hemoglobin and organic phosphates

The only truly significant function of the red blood cell is the transport of oxygen. The oxygen dissociation curve of blood reflects the affinity of hemoglobin for oxygen. If pulmonary function is normal, as blood circulates through the lung, there is a rise in oxygen tension in both adults and neonates from the 40 mmHg (40 Torr) of venous blood to the 100 mmHg (100 Torr) of arterial blood. These arterial tensions ensure a 95 percent saturation by oxygen of hemoglobin, and further increases in oxygen tension produce little additional rise in saturation. In the normal adult, when the oxygen tension has fallen to approximately 27 mmHg, 50

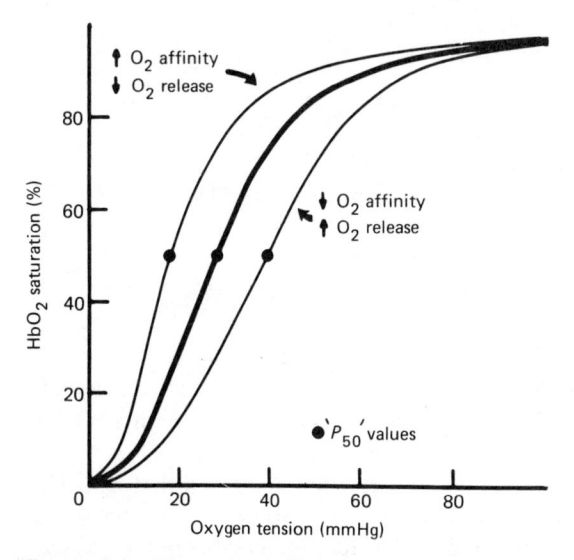

Figure 9.2 The oxygen dissociation curve of normal adult blood. The P_{50}, the oxygen tension at 50 percent oxygen saturation of hemoglobin, is approximately 27 mmHg (27 Torr). As the curve shifts to the right, the oxygen affinity of hemoglobin decreases and more oxygen is released at a given oxygen tension. With a shift to the left, the opposite occurs. A decrease in the pH or an increase in temperature decreases the affinity of hemoglobin for oxygen. (From Oski and Delivoria-Papadopoulos[49], courtesy of the Editor and Publishers, *Journal of Pediatrics*)

percent of the hemoglobin-bound oxygen has been released (P_{50}). In situations in which the hemoglobin–oxygen dissociation curve is shifted to the right, the affinity of hemoglobin for oxygen is reduced and more oxygen is released to tissues. Conversely, if the affinity of the hemoglobin for oxygen is increased, the oxygen tension must drop to lower than normal before the hemoglobin releases an equivalent amount of oxygen, and in this case the dissociation curve appears shifted to the left[48] (*Figure 9.2*).

A number of factors are known to alter hemoglobin's affinity for oxygen. These are listed below:

(1) Increased red cell , 3-DPG, increased P_{50}
    Adaptation to high altitude
    Hypoxemia associated with chronic pulmonary disease
    Hypoxemia associated with cyanotic heart disease
    Anemia
        secondary to iron deficiency
        secondary to chronic renal disease
        caused by sickle cell anemia
    Decreased red cell mass
    Chronic liver disease
    Hyperthyrodism
    Red cell pyruvate kinase deficiency
(2) Decreased red cell 2, 3-DPG, decreased P_{50}
    Septic shock
    Severe acidosis
    Following massive transfusions of stored blood
    Neonatal respiratory distress syndrome
(3) Increased P_{50}, no consistent alteration in red cell DPG
    Abnormal hemoglobins (Kansas, Seattle, Hammersmith, Tacoma, E)
    Vigorous exercise
(4) Decreased P_{50}, no consistent alteration in red cell DPG
    Abnormal hemoglobins (Kempsey, Philly, Chesapeake, J. Capetown, Yakima, Rainier)

The most important of the factors influencing hemoglobin affinity for oxygen are the fetal hemoglobin concentration and the red cell 2, 3-diphosphoglycerate (DPG) content.

Benesch and Benesch[9] and Chanutin and Curnish[16] demonstrated that a variety of organic phosphates, when added to adult hemoglobin in solution, had the ability to reduce the affinity of hemoglobin for oxygen. Of the organic phosphates tested, the compound 2, 3-diphosphoglycerate appeared to be the most potent modifier of hemoglobin function. In addition, of all the organic phosphates found in human erythrocytes, 2, 3-DPG is the highest in concentration (averaging 5 mmols/ml of red cells) and thus is quantitatively the most important with respect to modulating hemoglobin's affinity for oxygen.

Numerous investigators have examined the interaction of 2, 3-DPG with fetal hemoglobin in an attempt to determine why the fetal erythrocyte demonstrates a higher affinity for oxygen than the adult red cell. In 1930, Anselmino and Hoffman first observed that the oxygen affinity of human fetal blood was greater than that of maternal blood[4]. Fetal blood had a P_{50} value approximately 8 mmHg lower than that of adult blood. It became apparent that adult and fetal red cells dialyzed the same surrounding media to remove 2, 3-DPG manifest virtually identical oxygen affinities[3]. Freshly prepared lysates of fetal hemoglobin actually demonstrate a slightly lower affinity for oxygen than those of HbA[44]. This peculiarity was understood when it was demonstrated that the affinity of fetal hemoglobin for 2, 3-DPG was far less than that of adult hemoglobin. Deoxyhemoglobin, but not oxyhemoglobin, binds the highly charged 2, 3-DPG molecule. The deoxy form of fetal hemoglobin has a much smaller decrease in affinity with the addition of 2, 3-DPG than the deoxyhemoglobin form of HbA. This phenomenon can be partially explained by the insertion points of 2, 3-DPG on the hemoglobin molecule. The β-chain will bind anionic 2, 3-DPG at the highly charged histidine located at position 143[12]. Serine, a relatively neutral charged amino acid occupies this position on the γ-chain. From these studies, it appears that the major reason for the shift in the hemoglobin–oxygen equilibrium curve of the newborn infant to the left of that of the normal adult is the failure of fetal hemoglobin to bind 2, 3-DPG to the same degree as adult hemoglobin[13].

The decline of fetal hemoglobin in the newborn period appears to be strictly regulated. The switchover between HbF synthesis and HbA synthesis follows a sigmoid curve. Fetal hemoglobin synthesis is fairly constant until 30–32 weeks gestation, when a sharp fall-off occurs which reaches a plateau at about 52 weeks from conception; this is followed by a very gradual decline until adult levels are reached. It is important to realize that this switchover is based on post-conceptual age and is not related directly to the physical act of birth[6]. There are a few factors which are known to affect this normal decline in fetal hemoglobin. Included in these are the thalassemia syndromes and hereditary persistence of fetal hemoglobin. Although acute hypoxia produces no alterations of fetal hemoglobin, chronic intrauterine hypoxia may result in elevations of fetal hemoglobin[12]. The effects of hypoxia on fetal hemoglobin synthesis have been demonstrated in vivo as well[2, 65].

Unlike fetal hemoglobin, the level of red cell 2, 3-DPG gradually increases with gestation and at term its concentration within the infant's erythrocytes is similar to that of the normal adult[38]. The level may transiently fall during the first several days of life and then rise. By the end of the first week of life, in the term infant, the 2, 3-DPG levels are considerably higher than they are at birth[23].

It can be demonstrated in the adult red blood cell that hypoxia will cause 2, 3-DPG to rise rapidly[50]. This response appears to occur for two reasons. One is that an increase in deoxyhemoglobin causes increased binding of the 2, 3-DPG, which derepresses the synthesis of this organic phosphate. Secondly, hypoxia causes an intracellular pH rise as a consequence of absorption of protons by the deoxygenated hemoglobin molecule. This increase in intracellular pH results in an augmentation of the glycolytic mechanism by which 2, 3-DPG is produced. Newborn red cells are subject to these same mechanisms which control 2, 3-DPG synthesis, but the magnitude of the response is markedly diminished. In addition to all of this, 2, 3-DPG appears to be much less stable within the red blood cell of the neonate. Various theories have been proposed to account for this instability, but whatever the mechanism, the levels of red cell 2, 3-DPG decline six times more rapidly *in vitro* than in normal adult red cells[70].

Changes in oxygen affinity in the newborn and its effects on oxygen transport and delivery

In the term infant, the hemoglobin–oxygen equilibrium curve gradually shifts to the right and the P_{50} value approximates that of the adult by about 4 to 6 months of age[23]. Even during the first week of life, there is a significant rise in the P_{50} value, a reflection of the changes in red cell 2, 3-DPG mentioned previously[49] (*Figure 9.3*).

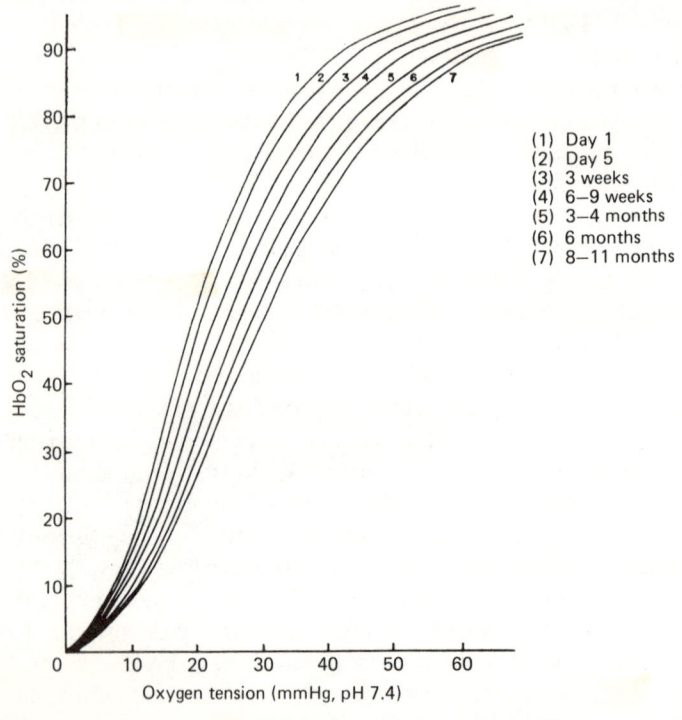

Figure 9.3 Oxygen equilibrium curves of blood from normal term infants at different postgestational ages. (From Oski and Delivoria-Papadopoulos[49], courtesy of the Editor and Publishers, *Journal of Pediatrics*)

The situation is somewhat different in the preterm infant. Since the switchover to adult hemoglobin synthesis appears to be programmed from conception, there may be little contribution to a rise in P_{50} caused by a fall in fetal hemoglobin. The red cell 2, 3-DPG is also lower in these infants. Clearly, the changes which do occur in the P_{50} reflect an interplay between the levels of HbA and red cell 2, 3-DPG. A precise correlation does not exist solely between the decrease in the oxygen affinity of the neonate's blood and the progressive decline in the concentration of fetal hemoglobin. Again, the first week of life in the term infant is illustrative of this point. The P_{50} rises by at least 1 mmHg (1 Torr) at the time when the percentage of fetal hemoglobin has not remarkably changed.

The sharp rise in the level of red cell 2, 3-DPG occurring during the first week of life returns to birth levels by 2 to 3 weeks, following which it remains relatively unchanged for the next 6 months. In adults, changes in oxygen affinity can usually be related to changes in the red cell 2, 3-DPG concentration. In contrast, when data from term and preterm infants were evaluated, it was observed that the position of the hemoglobin–oxygen affinity curve, as reflected in the P_{50}, was not directly related to the total red cell 2, 3-DPG alone[23].

Since the change in hemoglobin's affinity for oxygen correlates neither with the change in red cell DPG content alone nor with the decline in fetal hemoglobin alone, a unifying concept has emerged consisting of a 'functioning 2, 3-DPG fraction'[23, 47]. This 'functioning 2, 3-DPG fraction' is usually expressed in nmol/ml of red cells and is obtained by multiplying the red cell DPG content by the percentage of adult hemoglobin. This relation serves to explain why, during week 1 of life, infants with similar concentrations of fetal and adult hemoglobin may have many differences in their oxygen affinities.

Although hemoglobin's affinity for oxygen increasingly favors oxygen release to tissues as the infant moves on from the time of birth, the oxygen carrying capacity

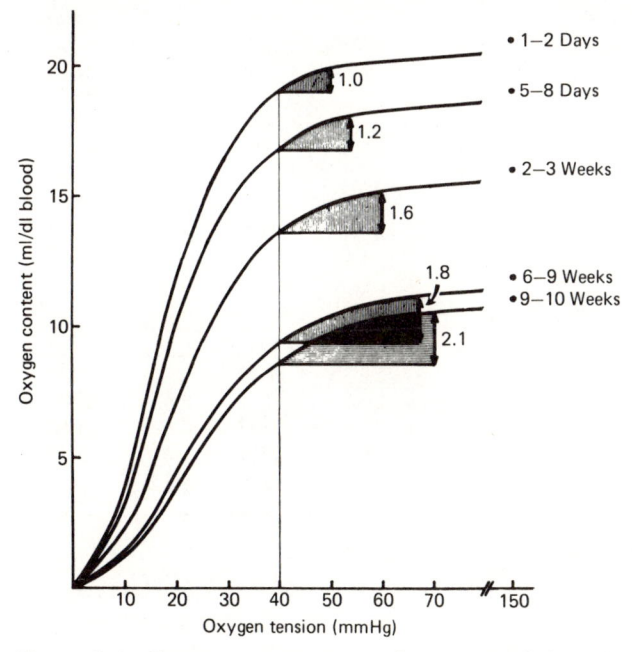

Figure 9.4 Oxygen content curves for preterm infants born weighing 1000–1500 g. The double arrows represent the oxygen-unloading capacity between a given 'arterial' and 'venous' P_{O_2}. (From Delivoria-Papadopoulos *et al.*[23], courtesy of the Editor and Publishers, *Pediatric Research*)

Table 9.3 Oxygen transport in preterm infants. (From Delivoria-Papadopoulos et al.[23], courtesy of the Editor and Publishers, *Pediatric Research*)

Age	Total Hb (g/dl)	PCV	MCHC (%)	O_2 capacity (ml/dl blood)	P_{50} at pH 7.40 (mmHg)	2,3-DPG nmol/ml blood	Fetal Hb (% of total)	FFDPG* (nmol/ml RBC)
Group I (<1000 g)†								
2 weeks	17.2	0.47	36.6	23.9	18.0	6255	83.0	1002
4 weeks	8.5	0.26	32.7	11.8	15.0	3923	81.0	761
9 weeks	7.2	0.22	32.7	10.0	15.0	4636	87.1	974
11 weeks	7.7	0.225	34.2	10.7	17.0	5867	78.0	1290
Group II (1001–1500 g)								
1–2 days	15.1	0.457	33.0	21.0	18.0	4124	86.6	580
	±1.3*§	±0.037	±0.7	±1.8	±1.7	±1562	±3.1	±287
5–8 days	13.4	0.414	33.5	18.7	18.9	4501	84.4	903
	±1.1	±0.032	±2.9	±1.5	±3.0	±1919	±3.8	±689
2–3 weeks	12.6	0.366	34.2	15.9	21.2	5721	83.3	1119
	±3.1	±0.06	±1.1	±3.1	±1.9	±1375	±5.1	±557
4–5 weeks	8.8	0.253	34.9	12.3	20.5	6095	85.2	931
	±0.9	±0.018	±1.7	±1.3	±1.7	±2081	±2.3	±456
6–9 weeks	9.1	0.245	35.1	11.8	23.4	8734	77.2	1995
	±1.7	±0.058	±2.2	±2.4	±1.1	±1854	±1.9	±480
9–10 weeks**	8.2	0.24	34.0	11.1	24.0	9000	77.0	2070
Group III (1501–2000 g)								
1–2 days	16.1	0.478	33.7	22.4	19.3	4475	87.2	703
	±0.9	±0.019	±1.9	±1.2	±0.9	±1174	±3.6	±331
5–8 days	16.8	0.485	34.7	25.3	19.8	5489	79.4	1056
	±3.3	±0.100	±0.5	±4.7	±1.3	±1428	±5.0	±590
2–3 weeks	13.6	0.404	34.4	18.8	21.3	6002	80.6	1184
	±3.0	±0.098	±1.5	±4.0	±1.8	±998	±5.8	±329
4–5 weeks	11.2	0.319	35.5	15.5	20.8	5841	75.8	1569
	±2.8	±0.099	±2.2	±3.8	±1.6	±839	±7.8	±577
6–9 weeks	8.0	0.221	35.9	11.1	24.0	7290	67.5	2457
	±0.7	±0.017	±0.7	±1.0	±0.9	±634	±6.2	±575
Group IV (2001–2500 g)								
1–2 days	15.9	0.462	35.8	21.9	20.2	5306	76.8	1258
	±0.9	±0.058	±1.9	±1.5	±1.6	±1075	±5.4	±392
5–8 days	15.6	0.47	34.2	21.5	21.3	6417	77.7	1457
	±1.7	±0.05	±1.1	±2.4	±3.3	±1527	±6.3	±603
2–3 weeks	12.3	0.351	34.9	17.1	22.0	7145	76.9	1666
	±1.1	±0.032	±0.5	±1.5	±1.3	±1737	±4.7	±472
6–9 weeks**	14.0	0.44	34.0	19.5	25.5	7100	43.0	3212

* Functioning fraction of 2,3-diphosphoglycerate.
† Only one patient.
§ Values are given as mean ± s.d.
** Less than five infants.

Table 9.4 Oxygen transport in term infants. (From Deliveria-Papadopoulos et al.[23], courtesy of the Editor and Publishers, *Pediatric Research*)

Number of infants	Age	Total Hb (g/dl)	PCV	MCHC (%)	O_2 capacity (ml/dl blood)	P_{50} at pH 7.40 (mmHg)	2,3-DPG (nmol/ml blood)	Fetal Hb (% of total)	FFDPG* (nmol/ml RBC)	Reticulocyte count (%)
19	1 day	17.8 ±2.0†	0.527 ±0.071	34.2 ±1.9	24.7 ±2.8	19.4 ±1.8	5433 ±1041	77.0 ±7.3	1246 ±570	4.7 ±1.74
18	5 days	16.2 ±1.2	0.469 ±0.060	34.1 ±0.8	22.6 ±2.2	20.6 ±1.7	6580 ±996	76.8 ±5.8	1516 ±495	2.15 ±1.64
14	3 weeks	12.0 ±1.3	0.335 ±0.043	35.9 ±1.2	16.7 ±1.9	22.7 ±1.0	5378 ±732	70.0 ±7.33	1614 ±252	0.88 ±0.71
10	6–9 weeks	10.5 ±1.2	0.302 ±0.039	34.9 ±0.6	14.7 ±1.6	24.4 ±1.4	5560 ±747	52.1 ±11.0	2670 ±550	1.63 ±0.65
14	3–4 months	10.2 ±0.8	0.303 ±0.024	33.8 ±1.7	14.3 ±1.2	26.5 ±2.0	5819 ±1240	23.2 ±16.0	4470 ±1380	1.36 ±0.45
8	6 months	11.3 ±0.9	0.340 ±0.036	33.4 ±0.7	14.7 ±0.6	27.8 ±1.0	5086 ±1570	4.7 ±2.2	4840 ±1500	1.42 ±1.15
8	8–11 months	11.4 ±0.6	0.348 ±0.019	32.8 ±0.9	15.9 ±0.8	30.3 ±0.7	7381 ±485	1.6 ±1.0	7260 ±544	0.82 ±0.27

* Functioning fraction of 2, 3-diphosphoglycerate.
† All values are given as mean ± 1 s.d.

of the blood is actually decreasing. The oxygen carrying capacity represents the product of the hemoglobin and the arterial oxygen saturation × 1.36 ml oxygen per gram of hemoglobin. This decline in oxygen carrying capacity is therefore independent of any change in oxygen affinity and merely represents the decline in hemoglobin. If all other factors remain equal, the fall in hemoglobin is more than compensated for by the rightward shift in the hemoglobin–oxygen dissociation curve so that the actual amount of oxygen capable of being delivered to tissues is continuously improving over the first several weeks of life. For example, a newborn weighing 1000 g with a hemoglobin of 15 g/dl, a P_{50} of 19 and a central venous oxygen tension of 40 mmHg (40 Torr) will unload 1.0 ml of oxygen to the tissues for every 100 ml of blood which passes through the capillary bed. This same infant, even though the hemoglobin has declined to 8 g/dl, will deliver 2.1 m' of oxygen per 100 ml of blood by 2–3 months of age because of the shift in P_{50} to 24 mmHg (24 Torr)[23] (*Figure 9.4*).

The changes which would be expected in preterm and term infants with respect to hemoglobin, oxygen carrying capacity, P_{50}, red cell 2, 3-DPG and fetal hemoglobin may be seen in *Tables 9.3* and *9.4*. It should be remembered that these serial changes were observed in a group of otherwise healthy infants. These same values might not be expected in ill infants. Red cell 2, 3-DPG levels are profoundly decreased in infants with severe respiratory distress[24]. This decrease with its associated lowering of the P_{50} value is most marked in infants with profound acidosis and is independent of the Bohr effect on the P_{50}.

CLINICAL CONSEQUENCES OF CHANGES IN OXYGEN TRANSPORT AND DELIVERY IN THE NEWBORN

There are relatively few studies which have emphasized the importance of changes in the clinical status of newborns caused by changes in oxygen transport and/or oxygen delivery. Those areas which seem to indicate that some cause and effect relationship does exist will be reviewed below. Much work has also been performed in other animal species and this will be briefly discussed.

Intrauterine transfusion

If adult red blood cells are transfused into the fetus or newborn, these cells will retain their characteristics as if they were still in the donor. The hemoglobin–oxygen equilibrium will be that of adult blood. Mathers *et al.*[40] and Novy *et al.*[45,46] found that adult red blood cells maintained their normal oxygen unloading properties for more than 2 months when given as an intrauterine transfusion. Fetuses born following such a procedure, if they have received sufficient quantities of blood, have P_{50} values characteristic of adult blood. Despite the decrease in oxygen affinity accompanied by intrauterine transfusion, no deleterious effects of this procedure with respect to placental uptake of oxygen by the fetus have been documented. The corollary of this is that infants born to mothers with 'high affinity' hemoglobinopathies have not demonstrated any ill effects as a consequence of decreased maternal oxygen release. Only in the lamb model has intrauterine transfusion produced any evidence of fetal hypoxia, and even here the effect was minimal[8].

The effect on the infant's oxygen delivery is largely a function of the storage characteristics of the type of blood used. For example, alterations of P_{50} produced by exchange transfusions performed with acid citrate dextrose (ACD) stored blood are related to the length of storage[22]. Blood stored as ACD rapidly looses its DPG content so that after just 4 to 5 days, exchange transfusion of such blood would actually be expected to transiently decrease the P_{50} of the newborn while the use of fresh heparinized blood or citrate phosphate dextrose blood stored up to one week produced a prompt rise in the P_{50} of newborns[22, 58].

The exact physiological significance of the manipulation of the oxygen affinity of infants *in utero* remains speculative. It is interesting to note the uncontrolled observation that the incidence of respiratory distress syndrome appears to be decreased in those infants receiving intrauterine transfusions of adult blood[67].

Extrauterine transfusions

Non-human studies

The physiological effects of left and right shifted curves have been studied on numerous occasions in newborn animals other than man[7, 38, 53]. Because of certain similarities of oxygen physiology, the lamb model has been most carefully investigated. The newborn lamb in the first 48 of life has a P_{50} of 18 to 20 mmHg, similar to newborn infants[7]. Manipulation of the hemoglobin–oxygen dissociation curve to the left in the newborn lamb can result in changes in both central venous P_{O_2} and cardiac output in order to maintain a constant oxygen consumption. Other data from newborn lambs show that mixed venous P_{O_2} does not remain constant but may drop as low as 20 mmHg[38]. Studies in rhesus monkeys in which an exchange transfusion was performed with stored DPG-depleted blood demonstrated that the major compensatory response to acute leftward shifts in the hemoglobin–oxygen dissociation curve was a marked decrease in mixed venous P_{O_2} with little or no effect on the cardiac output or oxygen consumption[53]. Lister *et al.* observed ameliorative effects of exhange transfusion with maternal blood (rise of P_{50} of 7 mmHg) on newborn lambs who were made to undergo a hypoxic stress[37]. Prior to the exhange transfusion, hypoxia caused an increase in cardiac output, a fall in arteriovenous oxygen difference and a decrease in oxygen consumption. Following exchange transfusion, under the same hypoxic stress, oxygen consumption returned to normal or above normal. This study suggests that exchange transfusion may be of benefit to hypoxic infants.

Human studies

Despite the similarities which exist between animal models and the human, physiological differences may well exist between these animal species and the human newborn. This has led to a great controversy over the real signficance of changes related to alterations of oxygen affinity in the postnatal period. Unfortunately there are not enough data available to settle this controversy. The reason for this is based on the fact that careful definition of the exact responses to manipulation of the oxygen affinity of the blood of newborn infants would require determination of such factors as oxygen consumption, cardiac output, arterial and central venous oxygen tensions, and alterations of regional blood flow effected by such manipulations. Because of the invasive nature of certain of the procedures required to make these determinations, we are left with only inferential data which, however, do suggest that manipulation of oxygen affinity can result in observable differences in the newborn. These data are now reviewed.

In 1973, DeLemos et al.[19] reported that exchange transfusions increased the survival rate of infants with the respiratory distress syndrome. The success of this procedure was attributed to the fact that the exchange transfusion corrected the coagulation abnormalities that were commonly present in such infants and reduced the incidence of fatal pulmonary and cerebral hemorrhages. In the same year, Delivoria-Papadopoulos et al.[20] reported that the use of early exchange transfusions increased the survival rate of infants who weighed less than 1000 g at birth and who did not have severe respiratory distress, and of infants who weighed 1000 to 1500 g and who had severe respiratory distress. It was speculated that the effect was due to the improvement in oxygen delivery associated with the shift to the right in the hemoglobin–oxygen dissociation curve, as Abrahamov and Smith had first shown in 1959 following exchange transfusion[1]. Theoretically, the exchange transfusion with fresh adult blood reduces the oxygen affinity of circulating blood, which in turn improves tissue oxygen tension and therefore the clinical state. A second study, reported by the same group of investigators in 1976, found that infants of birth weight less than 1250 g without severe respiratory distress who received exchange transfusion had a survival of 86 percent whereas in a non-exchanged group the survival was 57 percent[21]. In exchange-transfused infants with severe respiratory disease, survival was 59 percent compared with a 37 percent survival for the control group. In an associated study these investigators dismissed correction of coagulation abnormalities as the cause of the improvement in survival since the administration of fresh plasma alone did not reduce the mortality of the disease[30]. It was also observed that arterial oxygen tension improved following exchange transfusion. Since this response cannot be attributed to improved oxygen unloading as a result of a rightward shift in the hemoglobin-oxygen dissociation curve, the exact reason for improvement in survival was unclear. It should be noted that the procedure of exchange transfusion for facilitating oxygen delivery in infants with pulmonary disease remains highly controversial since other studies have not reproduced the same results[15].

One suggested clinical effect of manipulation of hemoglobin–oxygen affinity was thought to be a greater risk of retrolental fibroplasia. This was first mentioned by Aranda et al. in 1975[5]. It was felt that since tissue oxygenation was improved at any given partial pressure of oxygen, infants who were exchange transfused were unusually susceptible to the development of retrolental fibroplasia. Subsequent reports have demonstrated retrolental fibroplasia following exchange transfusion in infants who had never received supplementary oxygen. It must be said that these observations may not be significant since retrolental fibroplasia has now been reported in infants who received no supplementary oxygen and who were never given exchange transfusions[54].

A clearer indication of a clinical response to manipulation of the oxygen affinity of the blood of newborns may be noted by observing the reticulocyte and erythropoietin responses of infants who are given exchange or multiple transfusions. *Figure 9.5* depicts the reticulocyte index as a function of hemoglobin in two groups of infants weighing less than 1500 g[51]. In infants who were exchange transfused (an immediate rightward shift in the hemoglobin–oxygen dissociation curve from a P_{50} of 19 to 27) the reticulocyte index is lower at any given hemoglobin than in non-transfused controls. The exchange transfusions resulted in a greater fall in hemoglobin in the first 1 to 3 months of life before resumption of active erythropoiesis because of the improved oxygen delivery associated with replacement of fetal hemoglobin with adult hemoglobin.

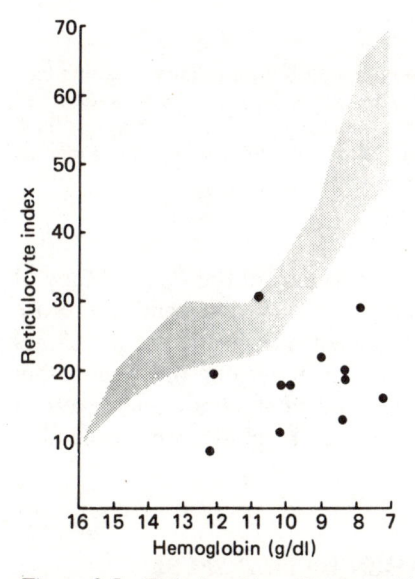

Figure 9.5 Relationship of hemoglobin value to reticulocyte index. The reticulocyte index is the hemoglobin multiplied by the percent reticulocytes. The shaded area represents the reticulocyte index for 60 infants weighing between 800 and 1500 g at birth who were studied for a 12 week period. Black dots represent observed values in 12 infants of similar birthweight who received exchange transfusions for non-hemolytic anemia at birth and were observed for 6–12 weeks. (From Oski and Stockman[51], courtesy of the Editor and Publishers, *British Journal of Haematology*)

In a study of a large number of infants at our institution, the erythropoietin responses of premature infants to varying levels of hemoglobin appeared to support this earlier observation. Although a significant inverse correlation was observed between hemoglobin level and plasma erythropoietin, a more striking correlation was observed between the plasma erythropoietin response and the inverse of the

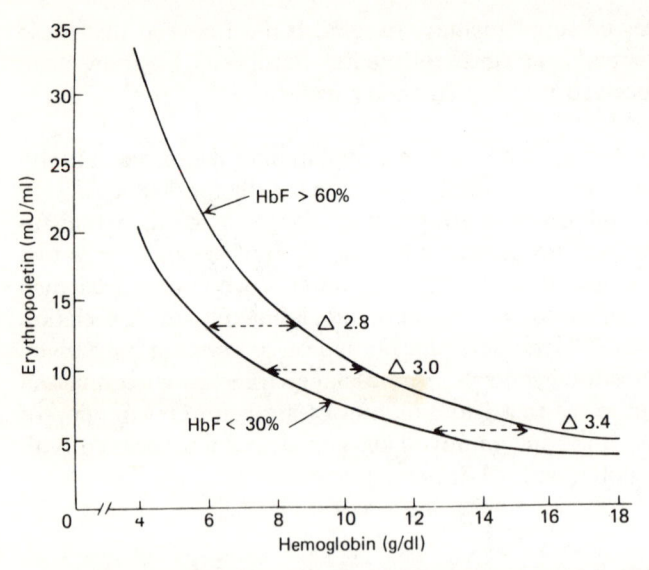

Figure 9.6 The relation of plasma erythropoietin and hemoglobin for infants weighing less than 1500 g at birth. The curve to the left represents the values for infants who had either been exchange-transfused or multiple-transfused so that the HbF concentration was less than 30 percent. (From Stockman *et al.*[63], courtesy of the Editor and Publishers, *New England Journal of Medicine*)

infant's oxygen unloading capacity (a function in great part of the P_{50})[63]. Many of these infants had received exchange or multiple transfusions and therefore demonstrated widely varying fetal hemoglobin concentrations. *Figure 9.6* shows that in infants with fetal hemoglobin values of less than 30 percent, the hemoglobin concentration fell 2 to 3 g/dl lower than in infants with fetal hemoglobin levels of more that 60 percent before comparable erythropoietin responses were noted.

FACTORS INFLUENCING THE DECISION WHEN TO TRANSFUSE

The most important reason for gaining insight into those factors which modify oxygen transport and delivery is to use this information to facilitate decisions concerning the need for transfusion. If all of these factors were known, such decisions would be relatively simple. As previously discussed, a truly informed decision would be based upon a knowledge of any given infant's ambient oxygen tension, arterial oxygen tension, hemoglobin level, arterial oxygen saturation, cardiac output, the position of the hemoglobin–oxygen equilibrium curve, the central venous oxygen tension and the oxygen requirements of the infant (basal metabolic rate or oxygen consumption). In the real world, it is not practical to make all of these determinations each time a decision is to be made concerning the need for transfusion. Most often, the guiding factors will be the hemoglobin and blood gases, a logical guess with respect to the other parameters, and good clinical judgement concerning the appearance of the infant. The latter consideration above all others is the basis upon which most decisions are made.

The clinical approach

Even though 'anemia' is common in the early weeks of life, its significance has remained controversial, especially in the preterm neonate. Although the anemia is usually regarded as 'physiological' because of its self-limiting nature, some infants do appear to benefit from transfusion. Commonly regarded as signs and symptoms of anemia at this age are the following: dyspnea, feeding difficulties, diminished activity, apnea, poor weight gain, tachypnea and tachycardia.

Wardrop et al.[66] have attempted to correlate these types of clinical signs and symptoms with alterations in the infant's hemoglobin levels and ability to deliver oxygen with respect to the position of the hemoglobin–oxygen dissociation curve.

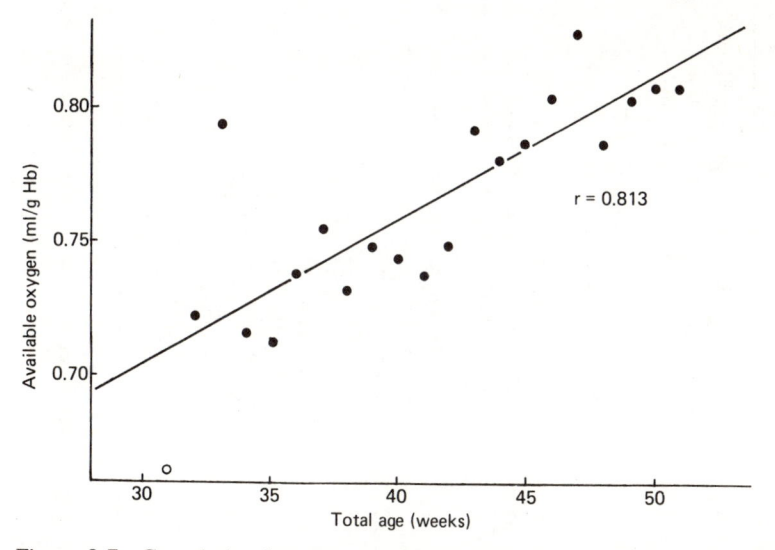

Figure 9.7 Correlation between 'available' oxygen/g hemoglobin and gestational age plus postnatal age (total age) in weeks. (From Wardrop et al.[66], courtesy of the Editor and Publishers, *Archives of Disease in Childhood*)

In infants who were not transfused, these investigators noted that the change in position of the hemoglobin–oxygen dissociation curve was quite predictable, obviating the need for an actual measurement in most cases. A linear correlation was found between the 'available' oxygen/g hemoglobin and gestational age at birth plus the postnatal age of preterm infants (*Figure 9.7*). This appears to be a reasonable assessment since one of the major determinants of oxygen affinity (changes in fetal hemoglobin concentration) is dependent on the time from conception rather than on the time from birth. 'Available' oxygen is the amount of oxygen capable of being released to tissues/g hemoglobin for every 100 ml of blood

Table 9.5 Clinical and hematological data of infants judged by medical staff to be anemic and to need blood transfusion on standard clinical grounds. (From Wardrop et al[66], courtesy of the Editor and Publishers, *Archives of Diseases in Childhood*)

Case	Gestational age at birth (weeks)	Age at Tx (days)	Hb (g/dl)	Available O_2 (ml/dl)	Indication for transfusion	Heart rate Before Tx	Heart rate After Tx	Respiration rate Before Tx	Respiration rate After Tx
1	28	29	10.3	6.5	↑ HR ↑ RR; poor weight gain; systolic murmur. ECG, chest X-ray normal	180	160	70	40
2	32	40	10.3	6.8	↑ HR ↑ RR, ECG, chest X-ray normal	170	140	58	40
3	30	44	9.6	6.5	↑ HR ↑ RR; lethargic, ECG, chest X-ray normal	162	140	56	40
4	31	31	9.7	5.1	↑ HR ↑ RR	172	150	50	48
5	32	39	8.0	5.6	Slow with feeds	158	150	50	48
6	31	46	8.0	6.5	Slow with feeds due to dyspnea	160	160	40	40
7	32	37	8.6	5.8	Systolic murmur; ECG, chest X-ray normal	172	156	40	40
8	30	27	9.5	7.2	Persistent apnea requiring O_2	160	150	70	54
9	31	30	8.5	6.1	Poor weight gain; lethargic	158	155	48	40
10	28	41	9.4	6.2	Dyspnea with feeds; lethargic	158	155	48	40
11	30	37	9.3	6.1	Dyspnea with feeds	150	140	50	40
12	32	46	8.6	6.8	Dyspnea with feeds	160	150	50	40
13	32	39	7.7	3.9	Dyspnea with feeds	160	150	52	40
14	33	24	8.1	5.8	Slow with feeds	170	160	50	48
15	34	21	8.1	5.9	Persistant severe apnea	160	158	48	48
16	34	34	9.1	7.5	↑ RR; systolic murmur, hepatosplenomegaly	164	158	60	40
17	34	27	9.3	6.8	↑ RR; pale; lethargic	160	160	60	40
18	36	35	9.8	6.9	↑ RR ↑ HR systolic murmur	170	140	60	40

HR = heart rate; RR = respiratory rate; Tx = transfusion.
Heart and respiration rates are means of 3-hourly observations during 24-hour periods before and 2 days after transfusion.

which passes through the capillary bed. Assuming a P_{50} appropriate for the age of the infant, the 'available' oxygen may be estimated from the following formula[66]:

'available' oxygen = (0.54 + 0.005 total age in weeks) × Hb concentration (g/dl)

In the Wardrop study, in infants born at less than 32 weeks gestation, clinical signs of anemia were present when the average available oxygen was about 6 ml/dl blood or less. More importantly, these clinical signs demonstrated improvement following blood transfusion. The hematological and clinical data in this group of infants may be seen in *Table 9.5*. It was apparent that anemia could have been the cause of signs and symptoms in the preterm infant if the hemoglobin level fell below 10.5 g/dl. This study is remarkable in that it is the first to suggest that clinical indications of anemia might be present at such high levels of hemoglobin.

The formula noted above is based on collective observations of many infants and may not be applicable in any given infant. It assumes that these infants have normal arterial oxygen saturations and that oxygen unloading can progress until a central venous oxygen tension of 20 mmHg (20 Torr) is reached. As noted, it is also based on a predicted P_{50} and therefore may not be useful in infants who have been transfused, who are acidotic or who have signficantly altered body temperatures. The formula of course makes no allowance for differing oxygen requirements among infants.

Failure to gain weight may also be a sign that a true anemia is present. In a study of a small group of infants, Stockman *et al.*[60] noted that some neonates who were not growing at an expected rate rapidly increased their growth velocity following transfusion. This increase in weight was most pronounced when the hemoglobin levels were less than 7.5 g/dl. In most cases, the transfusion was associated with a decline in oxygen requirements of about 15 percent and an increase in caloric intake. In a corollary study, these investigators also examined the utility of monitoring resting heart rate as an indicator of true anemia in preterm infants. No significant correlations could be obtained between the heart rate and changes in hemoglobin concentration[62]. The heart rate also did not correlate with the arterial oxygen tension or the P_{50}. A correlation did seem to exist, however, between the heart rate, the oxygen consumption of the infant and the required fall in central venous oxygen tension to achieve adequate oxygen delivery. These data indicate that an infant's resting heart rate is dependent on his or her metabolic needs. It is apparent that compensatory changes in heart rate do not simply reflect the level of hemoglobin, but rather the combined effects on oxygen delivery of the hemoglobin, the P_{50}, the arterial oxygen tension and the cardiac output as reflected in alterations of the central venous oxygen tension.

It appears that the most significant stimulus to erythropoietin production in these infants is not the decline in hemoglobin alone but rather the magnitude of the fall in central venous oxygen tension[61]. If all other modulators of oxygen delivery fail to provide adequate amounts of oxygen to tissues, the final 'safety valve' to permit adequate oxygenation is a lowering of the central venous oxygenation. In a sense then, this value represents the final adjustment caused by all the other variables which are important in oxygen transport and delivery. Once the central venous oxygen tension falls to less than 25 mmHg (25 Torr), it may be assumed that full compensatory mechanisms in the presence of anemia are operative, and depending on the clinical situation transfusion may be required. Some infants will not be doing well at even higher central venous oxygen tensions.

A practical approach to transfusion

Infants who manifest the clinical signs and symptoms of anemia noted previously may indeed be anemic and potentially may benefit from a transfusion. Assuming that there are no abnormalities in the ability to oxygenate arterial blood and that cardiac function is normal, it would be most unusual to observe such signs and symptoms in infants whose hemoglobin concentration is greater than 10 g/dl. Indeed, unless there are unusual oxygen requirements, even lower levels of hemoglobin than this should provide adequate oxygen to tissues.

A simple means to increase the probability that one's clinical impression is correct with respect to anemia in both term and preterm infants is to integrate all of the variables which influence the quantity of oxygen which is capable of being delivered. In the final analysis, the delivery of oxygen is the result of complex interactions among the pulmonary, cardiovascular and hematological systems of the body. As previously discussed, the major variables include cardiac output ($\dot{Q}$), oxygen consumption ($\dot{V}o_2$), hemoglobin (Hb), the partial pressure at which hemoglobin is 50 percent saturated (P_{50}), the arterial oxygen saturation (% Sao_2) and the central venous oxygen tension ($P\bar{v}o_2$). A simple means has been described which unifies these variables to assist in making clinical decisions[55]. This involves a description, in a single equation, of the interrelationships between these six variables (Hb, Sao_2, P_{50}, $\dot{Q}$ $\dot{V}o_2$, and $P\bar{v}o_2$). This equation may be expressed as follows:

$$Hb = \left(\frac{1000 \dot{V}o_2}{1.39 \dot{Q}} \times Sao_2\right) - \frac{100 P\bar{v}o_2}{P_{50}^{2.65} + P\bar{v}o_2^{2.65}}$$

The equation itself was derived by combining four relatively simple equations, each with only three variables. When these separate equations are suitably linked in terms of scale alignment, a single nomogram can be constructed which permits the functional interlocking of all the separate variables (*Figure 9.8*).

This nomogram can be used to assess whether oxygen delivery is adequate. The variable which provides the best indication of the adequacy of oxygen delivery is the value of the central venous oxygen tension. If this is very low (less than 25–30 mmHg) a truly anemic state is probably present.

It is obvious that not all the variables important in making these determinations will necessarily be known. The more variables which are known, the more accurate is the assessment. Certain assumptions, however, can be made. It is quite simple to measure the hemoglobin and arterial oxygen saturation, and if the equipment is available also the P_{50}. Determining the oxygen consumption and cardiac output is not so simple. Nonetheless, an average oxygen consumption of 7 ml · kg^{-1} · min^{-1} and an average cardiac output of 200 ml blood · kg^{-1} · min^{-1} can be used as a rough

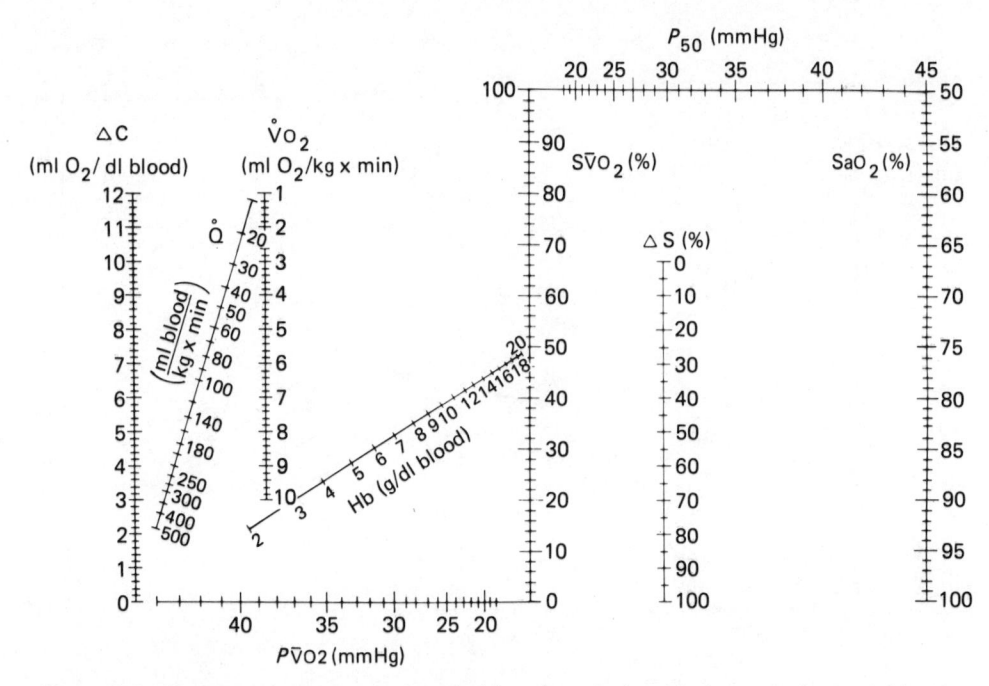

Figure 9.8 Composite nomogram interlocking the relationship between hemoglobin oxygen consumption, cardiac output, arterial oxygen saturation, P_{50}, and central venous oxygen tension. (From Schneider *et al.*[55], courtesy of the Editor and Publishers, *Critical Care Medicine*)

estimate of these values for most term and preterm infants. If the P_{50} cannot be directly measured, it should be recalled that the average P_{50} in a newborn is about 19 mmHg while in the adult it is about 27 mmHg. The expected changes after birth may be estimated from the values given in *Tables 9.3* and *9.4*.

Figure 9.9 illustrates the use of the nomogram. In this case, a term infant who had been exchange-transfused had unexplained tachycardia and tachypnea. The following laboratory values were obtained: Hb (12 g/dl), $\dot{Q}$ (170 ml · kg^{-1} · min^{-1}) and Sao$_2$ (96 percent). Since the child had been exchanged with adult blood the P_{50} was 27. The oxygen consumption ($\dot{V}o_2$) was estimated at 7 ml · kg^{-1} · min^{-1}. The question was whether reducing this infant's pre-exchange hemoglobin from 18 g/dl to 12 g/dl had caused him any significant compromise in oxygen delivery. The value that would answer this question best is the central oxygen tension. From the nomogram it can be seen that the central venous oxygen tension, despite a 6 g/dl fall in hemoglobin, is still well within the normal range at 38 mmHg (38 Torr). This decline in hemoglobin therefore does not appear to explain the infant's symptoms.

Although the optimal hemoglobin is a function of both cardiac output and oxygen consumption, the absolute values of these variables are of less consequence than their ratios. The ratio of these variables directly determines the arteriovenous oxygen content difference. In the resting state this difference generally ranges between 2.5–4 ml/dl at all ages, with the higher values observed in adults. An

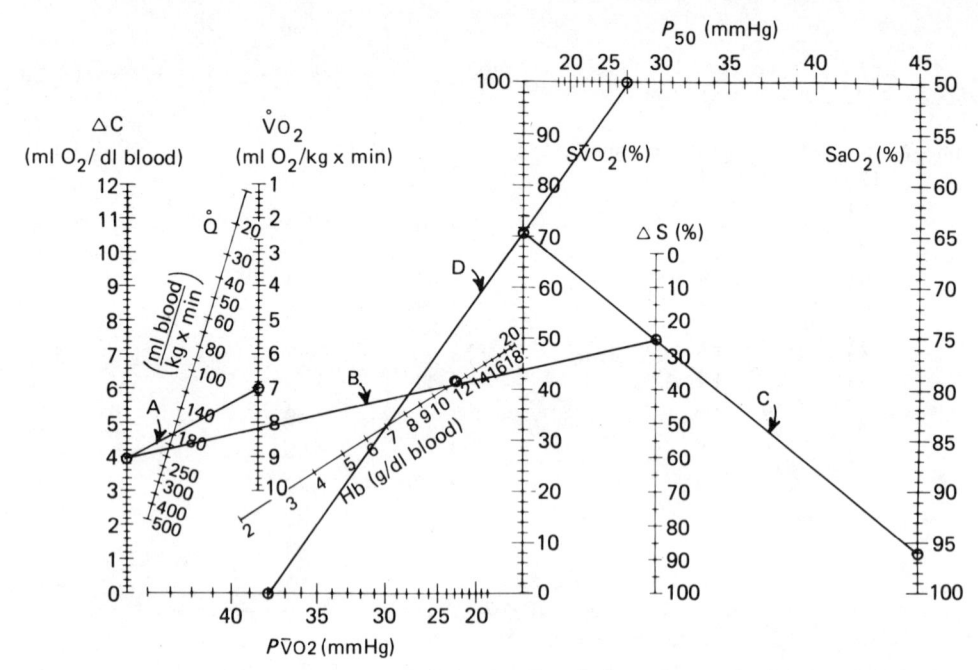

Figure 9.9 Use of the nomogram. *See* text for description of case then proceed with the following steps:
(1) Construct *line A* between the patient's $\dot{V}O_2$ of 7.0 ml/kg and the patient's $\dot{Q}$ of 170 ml · min^{-1} · kg^{-1} that intercepts ΔC. The change in oxygen content is 4.1 ml/dl blood.

(2) Construct *line B* from C that intercepts the line depicting a Hb of 12 g/dl and carry it to the line indicating ΔS (%). There is a 25 percent difference between the oxygen saturation of arterial and venous blood.

(3) Construct *line C* between the measured arterial oxygen saturation (SaO$_2$) of 96 percent and ΔS (%) of 25 percent and extend to the line depicting the $S\bar{v}O_2$ (central venous oxygen saturation). The value is 71 percent.

(4) Finally, construct *line D* from the P_{50} of 27 mmHg (27 Torr) through the $S\bar{v}O_2$ of 71 to intercept the line depicting the values for the central venous oxygen tension. The value is 38 mmHg (38 Torr) which is in the expected normal range.
(From Schneider et al.[55], courtesy of the Editor and Publishers, *Critical Care Medicine*)

approximate value of 3.4 ml/dl can be used for most clinical situations. With exercise this value may increase abruptly. In adults it may reach 5 ml/dl with modest exercise and 12 ml/dl with severe exercise.

Evident from the nomogram is the fact that whenever the central venous oxygen saturation exceeds 50 percent, the central venous tension must exceed the subject's P_{50}. Conversely, when the central venous oxygen saturation falls below 50 percent, the central venous oxygen tension will be less than the subject's P_{50}. In the neonate, as long as the central venous oxygen saturation exceeds 50 percent, the central venous oxygen tension will generally exceed 19–20 mmHg (19–20 Torr). Although no absolute lower limit of central venous oxygen tension that is compatible with life has been precisely defined, evidence suggests that a central venous oxygen tension in the range of 20–25 mmHg (20–25 Torr) may approach a critical limit below which oxygen transport to tissues is impaired. For example, in an infant with a hemoglobin of 5.2 g/dl, a P_{50} of 20, a typical arteriovenous oxygen content difference of 3.4 ml/dl and an arterial oxygen saturation of 96 percent, the central venous oxygen tension will be approximately 20 mmHg (20 Torr), a value which should be associated with clinical signs of a severe anemia.

The use of such 'armchair' calculations which integrate all of the factors important in oxygen delivery will never be a substitute for good clinical judgement. Such calculations can, however, simplify and clarify what otherwise appears as a complex situation.

SUMMARY

Although many years have now passed since it became apparent that multiple factors affect neonatal oxygen transport and oxygen delivery, the real significance of these in terms of human pathophysiology remains controversial. This controversy has permitted a lack of clarity in dealing with such basic questions as the indications for transfusing the newborn. This review has attempted to describe the expected or normal evolutionary changes which occur with respect to oxygen transport and delivery. Within this framework, guidelines in fact do exist which distinguish the aberrant from the normal. It is hoped that these, together with good clinical judgement, will assist those who care for ill newborns in answering many of these puzzling questions.

References

1 ABRAHAMOY, A. and SMITH, C. A. Oxygen capacity and affinity of blood from erythroblastic newborns. *American Journal of Disease of Children*, **97**, 15–19 (1959)

2 ALLEN, D. W. and JANDL, J. H. Factors influencing relative rates of synthesis of adult and fetal hemoglobin in vitro. *Journal of Clinical Investigation*, **39**, 1107–1113 (1960)

3 ALLEN, D. W., WYMAN, T. and SMITH, C. A. The oxygen equilibrium of fetal and adult hemoglobin. *Journal of Biological Chemistry*, **203**, 81–87 (1953)

4 ANSLEMINO, K. T. and HOFFMAN, F. The oxygen equilibrium of fetal and adult hemoglobin. *Archives of Gynecology*, **143**, 477–483 (1930)

5 ARANDA, J. V., CLARK, T. E., MANIELL, R. and PUTERBRIDGE, E. W. Blood transfusions: possible potentiating risk factor in retrolental fibroplasia. *Pediatric Research*, **9**, 362 (1975)

6 BARD, H. The postnatal decline of hemoglobin F synthesis in normal full-term infants. *Journal of Laboratory and Clinical Investigation*, **55**, 395–398 (1975)

7 BARD, H., FOURON, J. C., GROTHE, A. M., SOUKINI, M. A. and CORNET, A. The adaptation of the fetal red cells of newborn lambs to extrauterine life. *Pediatric Research*, **10**, 823 (1976)

8 BATTAGLIA, F. C., BOWES, W., McGAUGHEY, H. R., MAKOWSKI, F. C. and MESCHIA, G. The effect of fetal exchange transfusion with adult blood upon oxygenation. *Pediatric Research*, **3**, 60 (1969)

9 BENESCH, R. and BENESCH, R. E. The effect of organic phosphates from the human erythrocyte on the allosteric properties of hemoglobin. *Biochemistry and Biophysics Research Communications*, **26**, 162–167 (1967)

10 BRATTEBY, L. E., GARBY, L., GROTH, T., SCHNEIDER, W. and WADMAN, B. Studies on erythrokinetics in infancy. XIII. The mean life span and the life span frequency function of red blood cells formed during fetal life. *Acta Paediatrics Scandinavica*, **57**, 311–320 (1980)

11 BROCKHURST, G. and CHRISTI, J. Retrolental fibroplasia. *Archives Kinder Ophthalmoe*, **195**, 113 (1975)

12 BROMBERG, Y. M., ABRAHAMOV, A. and SALYBERGER, M. The effect of maternal anoxaemia on the foetal haemoglobin of the newborn. *Journal of Obstetrics, Gynaecology and Experimental Embryology*, **63**, 875–877 (1956)

13 BUNN, H. F. and BRIEHL, R. W. The interaction of 2, 3-diphosphoglycerate with various human hemoglobins. *Journal of Clinical Investigation*, **49**, 1088–1095 (1970)

14 BURMAN, D. and MORRIS, A. F. Cord hemoglobin in low birthweight infants. *Archives of Diseases of Childhood*, **49**, 382–385 (1974)

15 BUSTAMENTE, S. A. and SCOTT, K. E. Failure of exchange transfusion to alter course or outcome of RDS in very low birthweight infants. *Pediatric Reasearch*, **9**, 639 (1975)

16 CHANUTIN, A. and CURNISH, R. R. Effect of organic and inorganic phosphates on the oxygen equilibrium of human erythrocytes. *Archives of Biochemistry*, **121**, 196 (1967)

17 COLE, R. J. and PAUL, J. The effects of erythropoietin on haem synthesis in mouse yok sac and cultured fetal liver cells. *Journal of Embryology and Experimental Morphology*, **15**, 245–260 (1966)

19 deLEMOS, R. A., McLAUGHLIN, G. W., KOCH, H. F. and DISERENS, H. W. Abnormal partial thromboplastin time and survival in RDS: effect of exchange transfusion. *Pediatric Research*, **7**, 168 (1973)

20 deLIVORIA-PAPADOPOULOS, M., MILLER, L. D., BRANCA, K., FORSTER, R. E. and OSKI, F. A. Effects of exchange transfusion on altering mortality in: (1) infants weighing less than 1250 gm at birth and (2) infants with severe RDS. *Pediatric Research*, **7**, 63 (1973)

21 deLIVORIA-PAPADOLPOULOS, M., MILLER, L. D., FORSTER, R. E. and OSKI, F. A. The role of exchange transfusion in the management of low birthweight infants with and without severe respiratory distress syndrome. *Journal of Pediatrics*, **89**, 273–278 (1976)

22 deLIVORIA-PAPADOPOULOS, M., MORROW, G. and OSKI, F. Exchange transfusion in the newborn infant with fresh whole blood: the role of storage. *Journal of Pediatrics*, **79**, 898–903 (1971)

23 deLIVORIA-POPADOPOULOS, M., RONCEVIC, N. P. and OSKI, F. A. Postnatal changes in oxygen transport of term, premature, and sick infants: the role of adult hemoglobin and red cell 2, 3-diphosphoglycerate. *Pediatric Research*, **5**, 235–245 (1971)

24 DUC, G. and ENGEL, K. Hemoglobin-oxygen affinity and erythrocyte 2, 3-diphosphoglycerate content in hyaline membrane disease and cardiac malformations. *Proceedings of the Society for Pediatric Research*, **79**, 240 (1970)
25 FINNE, P. H. Erythropoietin levels in cord blood as an indicator of intrauterine hypoxia. *Acta Paediatrica Scandinavica*, **55**, 478–489 (1966)
26 FINNE, P. H. Erythropoietin levels in the amniotic fluid particularly in Rh-immunized pregnancies. *Acta Paediatrica Scandinavica*, **53**, 269–281 (1964)
27 FINNE, P. H. On pacental transfer of erythropoietin. *Acta Paediatrica Scandinavica*, **56**, 233–242 (1967)
28 FRESHNEY, R. I. and CONKIE, D. Effect of erythropoietin on haemoglobin synthesis and haem synthesizing enzymes of mouse foetal liver cells in culture. *Journal of Embryology and Experimental Morphology*, **27**, 525–532 (1972)
29 GARBY, L., SJOLIN, S. and VUILLE, J. C. Studies on erythrokinetics of synthesis of hemoglobin F and hemoglobin A during the first months of life. *Acta Paediatrica*, **51**, 245–254 (1962)
30 GOTTUSO, M. A., WILLIAMS, M. L. and OSKI, F. A. The role of exchange transfusion in the management of low birthweight infants with and without severe respiratory distress syndrome II. Further observations and studies of mechanisms of action. *Journal of Pediatrics*, **89**, 279–285 (1976)
31 HASSAN, M. W., LUTTON, J. D., LEVERE, R. D., RIEDER, R. F. and CEDERQUIST, L. L. In vitro culture of erythroid colonies from human fetal liver and umbilical cord blood. *British Journal of Haematology*, **41**, 477–484 (1979)
32 HUMBERT, J. R., ABELSON, H., HATHAWAY, W. E. and BATTAGLIA, F. C. Polycythemia in small-for-gestational-age infants. *Journal of Pediatrics*, **75**, 812–819 (1969)
33 INGRAM, V. M. Gene evolution and the hemoglobins. *Nature (London)*, **189**, 704 (1961)
34 JACOBSEN, L. O., GOLDWASSER, E., FRIED, W. and PFZAK, L. Role of the kidney in erythropoiesis. *Nature*, **179**, 633–634 (1957)
35 KAISER, I. H., CUMMINGS, J. N., REYNOLDS, S. R. M. and MARBARGER, J. P. Acclimatization response of the pregnant ewe and fetal lamb to diminished ambient pressure. *Journal of Applied Physiology*, **13**, 171–178 (1958)
36 KALPAKTSOGLOU, P. K. and EMERY, J. L. The effect of birth on the haemopoietic tissue of the human bone marrow. *British Journal of Haematology*, **11**, 453–460 (1965)
37 LISTER, G., FRICK, K. and TALNER, N. O_2 transport during hypoxia. *Pediatric Research*, **14**, 604 (1980)
38 LISTER, G., WALTER, T. K., VERSMOLD, H. T., DALLMAN, P. R. and RUDOLPH, A. M. Oxygen delivery in lambs: cardiovascular and hematologic development. *American Journal of Physiology*, **237**, H668–H675 (1979)
39 MacINTOSH, S. Erythropoietin excretion in premature infants. *Journal of Pediatrics*, **86**, 202–206 (1975)
40 MATHERS, N. P., JAMES, G. B. and WALKER, J. The oxygen affinity of blood of infants treated by intrauterine transfusion. *Journal of Obstetrics and Gynecology*, **77**, 648–654 (1970)
41 MATOTH, Y. and ZAIZOV, R. Absence of an inhibitor of erythropoiesis in postnatal plasma. *Israel Journal of Medical Science*, **3**, 477–479 (1967)
42 MATOTH, Y. and ZAIZOV, R. Regulation of erythropoiesis in the fetal rat. *Israel Journal Medical Science*, **7**, 839–843 (1971)

43 MATOTH, Y., ZAIZOV, R. and VARSANO, I. Postnatal changes in some red cell parameters. *Acta Paediatrica Scandanavica*, **60,** 317–320 (1971)

44 McCARTHY, E. F. The oxygen affinity of human maternal and foetal haemoglobin. *Journal of Physiology*, **102,** 55–61 (1943)

45 NOVY, M. J. Cord blood oxygen affinity following intrauterine transfusion for erythroblastoses program. *Society for Pediatric Research*, Abstract 141 (1969)

46 NOVY, M. J., FRIGOLETTO, F. D., EASTERLY, C. L., UMANSKY, I. and NELSON, N. M. Changes in cord blood oxygen affinity after intrauterine transfusions for erythrobastosis. *New England Journal of Medicine*, **285,** 589–595 (1971)

47 ORZALESI, M. M. and HAY, W. W. The regulation of oxygen affinity of fetal blood. In vitro experiments and results in normal infants. *Pediatrics* , **48,** 857–864 (1971)

48 OSKI, F. A. Fetal hemoglobin, the neonatal red cell, and 2, 3-diphosphoglycerate. *Pediatric Clinics of North America*, **19,** 907–917 (1972)

49 OSKI, F. A. and DELIVORIA-PAPADOPOULOS. The RBC, 2, 3-DPG and tissue O_2 release. *Journal of Pediatrics*, **77,** 941–956 (1970)

50 OSKI, F. A., GOTTLIEB, A. J., MILLER, W. and DELIVORIA-PAPADOPOULOS. M. The effects of deoxygenation of adult and fetal hemoglobin on the synthesis of red cell 2, 3-diphosphoglycerate and its in vivo consequences. *Journal of Clinical Investigation*, **49,** 400–407 (1970)

51 OSKI, F. A. and STOCKMAN, J. A. III. Anaemia in early infancy. *British Journal of Haematology*, **27,** 195 (1974)

52 REYNAFARJE, C., RAMOS, J., FAURA, J. and VILLAVICENCIO, D. Humoral control of erythropoietic activity in man during and after altitude exposure. *Proceedings of the Society for Experimental Biology and Medicine* , **116,** 649–650 (1964)

53 RIGGS, T. E., SHAFER, A. W. and GUENTER, C. A. Acute changes in oxyhemoglobin affinity. Effects on oxygen transport and utilization. *Journal of Clinical Investigation*, **52,** 2660–2663 (1973)

54 SACKS, L. M., SCHAFFER, D. B., PECKHAM, G. J., ANDAY, E. K. and DELIVORIA-PAPADOUPOULOS, M. Exchange transfusion and retrolental fibroplasia, lack of cause and effect. *Pediatric Research*, **12,** 533 (1978)

55 SCHNEIDER, A. J., STOCKMAN, J. A. III and OSKI, F. A. Transfusion nomogram: an application of physiology to clinical decisions regarding the use of blood. *Critical Care Medicine*, **9,** 469–473 (1981)

56 SCHOOLEY, J. C., GARCIA, J. F., CANTOR, L. N. and HAVENS, V. W. A summary of some studies on erythropoiesis using anti-EP immune serum. *Annals of the New York Academy of Sciences*, **149,** 266–280 (1968)

57 SEIP, M. The reticulocyte level, and the erythrocyte production judged from reticulocyte studies, in new born infants during the first week of life. *Acta Paediatrica*, **44,** 355–369 (1955)

58 SHAFER, A. W., TAGUE, L. L., WELCH, M. H. and GUENTER, C. A., et al. 2, 3-diphosphoglycerate in red cells stored in acid-citrate-dextrose and citrate-phosphate-dextrose: implications regarding delivery of oxygen. *Journal of Laboratory and Clinical Medicine*, **77,** 430–437 (1971)

59 SKJAELAAEN, P., HALVORSEN, S. and SEIP, M. Inhibition of erythropoiesis by plasma from newborn infants. In *proceedings of the Tel Aviv University Conference on Erythropoiesis,* (Petak Tikva), 35, New York, Academic Press (1970)

60 STOCKMAN, J. A. III, CLARK, D. and LEVIN, E. Weight gain, a response to transfusion in preterm infants. *Pediatric Research*, **14,** 612 (1980)
61 STOCKMAN, J. A., CLARK, D. A., KAVEY, R. E., McCLELLAN, K. and GARCIA, J. F. Anemia of prematurity, erythropoietin and central venous oxygen tension, indicators of adequate tissue oxygenation. *Pediatric Research*, **15,** 683 (1981)
62 STOCKMAN, J. A. III, CLARK, C. A., KAVEY, R. E. and McCLELLAN, K. Compensatory alterations in resting heart rate, and indicator of true anemia in preterm infants. *Pediatric Research*, **15,** 683 (1981)
63 STOCKMAN, J. A. III, GARCIA, J. F. and OSKI, F. A. The anemia of prematurity. Factors governing the erythropoietin response. *New England Journal of Medicine*, **296,** 647–650 (1977)
64 TCHERNIA, G., MIELOT, F., COULOMBEL, L. and MOHANDAS, M. Characterization of circulating erythroid progenitor cells in human newborn blood. *Journal of Laboratory and Clinical Medicine*, **97,** 322–331 (1981)
65 THOMAS, E. D., LOCHTE, H. L., GREENBOUGH, W. B. III and WALES, M. In vitro synthesis of foetal and adult haemoglobin by foetal haematopoietic tissues. *Nature (London)*, **185,** 396–398 (1960)
66 WARDROP, C. A. J., HOLLAND, B. M., VEALE, K. E. A., JONES, J. G. and GRAY, O. P. Non-physiological anaemia of prematurity. *Archives of Disease in Childhood*, **53,** 855–860 (1978)
67 WESTIN, B., NYBERG, R., MILLER, J. A. and WEDENBERG, E. Hypothermia with oxygenated blood in the treatment of asphyxia neonatorium. *Acta Paediatrica* (Suppl. 139), 51 (1962)
68 WILLIAMS, M. E., SHOTT, R. J., O'NEAL, P. L. and OSKI, F. A Role of dietary iron and fat on vitamin E deficiency anemia of infancy. *New England Journal of Medicine*, **292,** 887–890 (1975)
69 WOOD, W. G. Haemoglobin synthesis during human fetal development. *British Medical Bulletin*, **32,** 282–287 (1976)
70 ZIPURSKY, A., LARUE, T. and ISRAELS, L. G. The in vitro metabolism of erythrocytes from newborn infants. *Canadian Journal of Biochemistry and Physiology*, **38,** 727–738 (1960)

10
Thrombocytopenic purpura: current immunological and clinical aspects
Margaret Karpatkin

When thrombocytopenic purpura occurs in children the disease is generally of sudden onset and short duration with spontaneous recovery occurring within weeks or months. Adults more commonly have a chronic form of the disease in which spontaneous remission does not occur; fortunately this is rare in children. Thrombocytopenic purpura is an autoimmune disease in both its acute and chronic forms, with antibody-coated platelets being destroyed within the circulation. This autoimmune etiology, although well established in adults, has only relatively recently been confirmed in children.

In this review the evidence for the autoimmune nature of the disease will be reveiwed briefly. The clinical aspects of the disorder will then be discussed with particular emphasis on management.

Immune thrombocytopenia occurring in neonates due to transplacental passage of a maternal antibody will not be discussed and readers are referred to another review on this subject[28].

EVIDENCE FOR THE IMMUNE ETIOLOGY OF THROMBOCYTOPENIC PURPURA IN CHILDHOOD

In the adult, the immune nature of the disease known as idiopathic thrombocytopenic purpura (ITP) has been established for approximately 25 years. The observation that women with the disease frequently gave birth to children with transient thrombocytopenia suggested the presence of a humoral agent capable of crossing the placenta[11]. Harrington et al.[14,15] demonstrated this conclusively by taking plasma from patients with ITP and infusing it into normal volunteer recipients. A fall in the recipient's platelet count resulted, thus demonstrating the destruction of circulating platelets by an agent in the infused plasma. This observation was confirmed by Shulman et al.[48]. Attempts to demonstrate an antiplatelet antibody in sera of patients with ITP using *in vitro* techniques led to somewhat controversial results[16,20]. In 1969, Karpatkin and Siskind, using a platelet immuno-injury technique, demonstrated IgG antibody in the serum of

60–65 percent of patients with clinically diagnosed ITP[21]. Karpatkin et al.[25] subsequently identified this as belonging to the subclass IgG3. Karpatkin et al.[22] have suggested that with the autoimmune nature of the disease established it should more properly be called autoimmune thrombocytopenic purpura (ATP) rather than ITP.

None of the *in vivo* experiments described above were carried out in children, and antiplatelet antibody is rarely detected in sera of children with acute ITP[23, 26, 27]. Thus, the autoimmune nature of the disease in children remained in doubt. In 1975, Dixon et al.[9] described for the first time a method for detecting antibody on the surface of the platelet rather than in the serum. Using this technique, they demonstrated surface antibody on the platelets of all of 17 patients tested. Other laboratories have subsequently confirmed this finding using a variety of methods for detecting antibody on the platelet membrane[7, 17, 19, 36]. In 1977, Luiken et al.[36], using a Fab-anti-Fab assay system, demonstrated platelet-bound antibody in all of 37 patients studied, including six children with acute thrombocytopenia. Lightsey et al.[35] using the same technique, later demonstrated significantly increased platelet-associated IgG in 20 children with the disease. Seven of these had the acute form of the disease, and in those they were able to follow, the IgG fell to normal when remission occurred. Interestingly they found significantly greater amounts of IgG on the platelets of young patients with the acute variety of the disease than they did in children with chronic disease or in adults. They suggested that in the acute disease an immune complex is formed which binds to the platelet while in the chronic disease a specific immunoglobulin is directed against a platelet antigen.

As a result of the studies described above it seems that the immune nature of the childhood disease is now established and it should also be known as autoimmune rather than idiopathic thrombocytopenic purpura.

CLINICAL PRESENTATION

The disease may occur at any age but is most common between the ages of 2 and 6 years. It occurs with equal frequency in boys and girls. In adolescents, however, the relative number of girls affected begins to increase, resembling ATP in the adult, where the female to male ratio is 2–4:1. Also, a proportionately greater number of older children have the chronic form of the disease.

Onset of the disease is usually abrupt with a variety of hemorrhagic manifestations. Purpura is an almost invariable presenting sign, but bleeding from other sites, including epistaxis, conjunctival hemorrhage and menorrhagia, may also occur. There is a history of antecedent viral infection in 60 percent of cases and the disease occurs most commonly in the winter and spring, suggesting a viral etiology[38, 47]. Physical examination is unremarkable apart from signs of hemorrhage. Splenomegaly is not a feature of the disease and its presence should lead to the suspicion that another disease is causing the thrombocytopenia, such as mononucleosis, systemic lupus erythematous or leukemia.

Generally the only abnormal routine laboratory finding is a low platelet count, unless there has been sufficient hemorrhage to cause anemia. Platelets seen on a stained smear will appear larger than usual and electronic sizing will confirm that their volume is increased. This is an indication of rapid platelet turnover[13]. As mentioned earlier, serum antibodies against platelets are rarely demonstrable in childhood ATP but increased platelet-bound IgG is present.

Examination of the bone marrow most often shows an increase in the number of megakaryocytes. These may be small with only one or two nuclear lobes, and budding platelets are not usually seen. Such megakaryocytes are seen in conditions of rapid platelet destruction and are probably young megakaryoctes[4]. There is sometimes an increase in eosinophils in the marrow. Unless there has been sufficient hemorrhage to cause erythroid hyperplasia the other bone marrow elements appear normal. Examination of the bone marrow before instituting treatment is an absolute necessity in order to confirm the diagnosis and to rule out leukemia. In addition, a test for antinuclear antibodies should be done because systemic lupus erythematosis, although rare in childhood, may present with thrombocytopenia.

MANAGEMENT

The management of ATP may include administration of corticosteroids, splenectomy or use of chemotherapeutic agents. Each of these options will be discussed separately and then a general plan of management proposed.

Corticosteroids

The majority of children with ATP will show an increase in platelet count following the administration of corticosteroids. Shulman et al.[49] showed that the administration of steroids to a volunteer before administration of plasma from a patient with ATP prevented thrombocytopenia in the recipient (*Figure 10.1*). This implied that steroids do not act by lowering the antibody level but either by preventing antibody binding to the platelets or by preventing removal of antibody-coated platelets by the reticuloendothelial system. These authors also showed[49] that ATP plasma given to asplenic volunteers conferred a similar protection from thrombocytopenia (*Figure 10.2*), suggesting that the spleen is the major organ responsible for removal of antibody-coated platelets. It has been shown that phagocytosis of antibody-coated platelets can be inhibited by steroids[43], as can adhesion of platelets to granulocytes *in vitro*[53].

It is clear from the above remarks that steroids do not cure the disease. They simply maintain a hemostatic platelet count in the presence of antiplatelet antibody. In the majority of children the disease will remit spontaneously with disappearance of antibody in a relatively short period of time, and the steroids may then be discontinued. Because the drug does not actually cure the disease and has potentially harmful side-effects, such as growth impairment and immunosuppression, some pediatricians do not advocate the routine use of steroids in this disease but prefer to observe the patient and wait for spontaneous remission. The subject of steroid therapy in ATP has generated some controversy which will be reviewed below.

Lusher and Zuelzer[37], and Lusher and Iyer[38] reviewed data of 236 children with ATP followed at the Children's Hospital of Michigan. The mean time between onset of symptoms and return of the platelet count to normal in children who had received steroids was compared to that in children who had not received steroids.

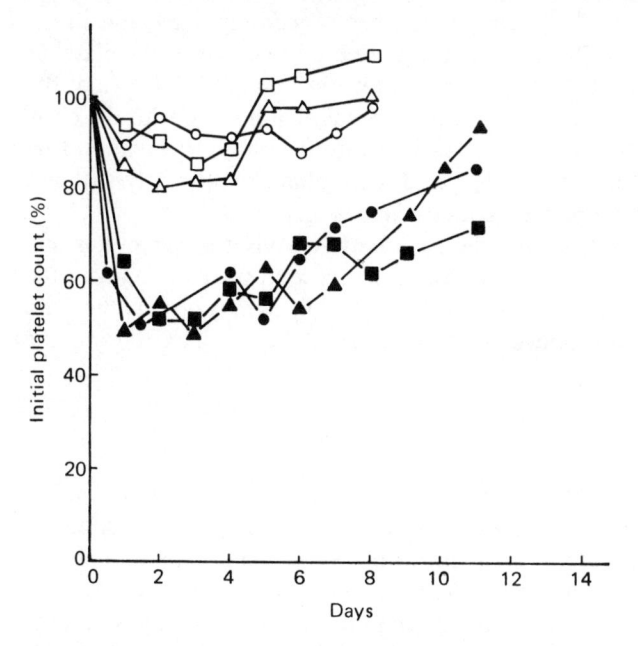

Figure 10.1 Effects of prednisone on the response to ITP plasma. Results of giving three normal individuals ITP plasma are shown by the solid symbols. The open symbols show results of giving the same dose of ITP plasma to the same individuals during administration of 60 to 80 mg of prednisone per day. In the different recipients, prednisone was started 3 h, 1 day and 3 days prior to infusing ITP plasma, and in each instance it was continued for a minimum of 7 days. The control infusions in two instances were given 1 and 2 months prior to the infusions with prednisone, and in one instance three weeks after the infusion with prednisone. (From Shulman et al.[49], courtesy of the Editor and Publishers, *Transactions of the Association of American Physicians*)

There was a significantly more rapid recovery in the untreated group. Choi and McClure[6] reviewed 161 patients and also found that recovery took longer in patients who had received steroids; however, no statistical analysis was undertaken. Lammie and Lovric[31] reviewed 152 patients under 13 years of age and concluded that steroids did not alter the duration of the disease or reduce the amount of bleeding. On the other hand, Simons et al.[50] showed that 14 children under 10 years of age who received steroids achieved significant increases in platelet counts far more rapidly than 19 children who did not. This comparison was made during the first 21 days of the illness. These workers did not find that use of steroids delayed spontaneous remission.

While many workers question the routine use of steroids in acute ATP, most advocate their use for a short period early in the illness in children with 'severe' disease[6, 37, 39, 40, 50, 54]. The classification of 'severe' is usually based upon clinical signs such as gastrointestinal bleeding, persistant epistaxis or very extensive purpura, although platelet counts of less than 10 000/mm³ have also been used as an indication of severity[7]. Use of a short course of steroids is advocated because intracerebral hemorrhage, a rare complication of ATP, occurs within a month of onset of symptoms[37, 38, 39, 41, 46, 54]. Only rarely has it been reported later in the course of the disease[3, 6, 34, 54]. Therefore steroids are used to maintain the platelets in a safe hemostatic range (50 000/mm³ or more) for the first critical weeks of the disease. The reason for the association of intracerebral hemorrhage with the early phase of the disease is not clear, but it is an interesting clinical observation that usually all hemorrhagic manifestations of the disease abate significantly within a few weeks of onset even if the platelet count is unchanged.

In summary, steroids do not shorten the time between onset of symptoms and drug-free remission; they do, however, cause an increase in platelet count in the majority of patients. Their use in the early weeks of the illness may protect the child from the potentially fatal complication of intracranial hemorrhage during the period of highest risk.

Splenectomy

The role of the spleen in ATP is twofold: (1) it removes antibody-coated platelets from the circulation and (2) it produces some antiplatelet antibody. Shulman et al.[49] showed that when plasma from a patient with ATP was infused into a person who had been splenectomized, the usual fall in platelet count did not occur (*Figure 10.2*), indicating that the spleen is of major importance in removing antibody-coated platelets. Najean et al.[44], using platelets labelled with chromium-51, demonstrated that in 61 percent of patients studied sequestration occurred predominately in the spleen, and this proportion was far greater in patients under the age of 15 years.

The role of the spleen in antibody production was first suggested by Karpatkin et al.[23], who showed that serum platelet antibody levels decreased in seven of eight patients with ATP following splenectomy. Luiken et al.[36] have reported a reduction in platelet-associated IgG after splenectomy. *In vivo* studies have demonstrated that spleens obtained surgically from patients with ATP synthesize significant amounts of IgG antiplatelet antibody when compared to control spleens[24, 42].

In the majority of children with ATP who remit within weeks or months of diagnosis the possibility of splenectomy does not have to be considered. In some of those who are not so fortunate, removal of the spleen may be indicated. Twenty years ago the accepted practice was to perform splenectomy if the disease persisted 6 months after diagnosis. At the present time a more conservative approach is advocated, as the literature now contains numerous examples of children who have achieved spontaneous remission after much longer periods. Walker et al.[54] in 1961 reported complete spontaneous recovery in four children more than a year after onset of disease, one child taking 2½ years to remit. Schulman[47] has also reported

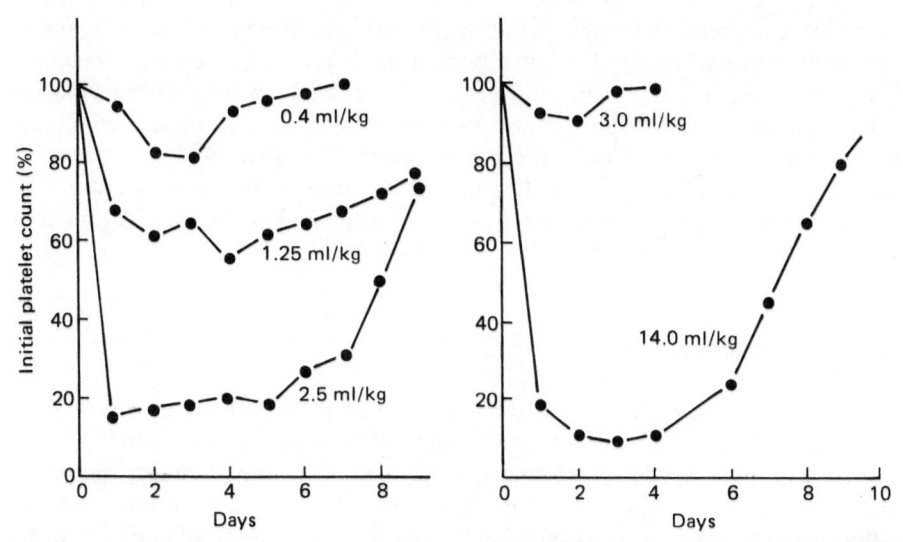

Figure 10.2 Comparison of response of normal and splenectomized persons to ITP factor. The graph on the left shows the effects of ITP plasma in a normal individual. The graph on the right shows the effects of the same ITP plasma in a splenectomized person. Note that the ITP plasma dose that did not produce thrombocytopenia in the splenectomized person was greater than the dose that produced marked thrombocytopenia in the normal invidual. (From Shulman et al.[49], courtesy of the Editor and Publishers, *Transactions of the Association of American Physicians*)

complete recovery after long periods of time and this observation has been confirmed by others[50]. Lusher and Iyer on the other hand, did not see complete recovery after 6 months in any child. However, a significant number of their chronic cases achieved platelet counts of more than 50 000/mm^3 and were virtually asymptomatic; they do not recommend splenectomy for these children[38]. Walker et al.[54] made the same observation when reviewing 31 cases of chronic purpura in children of whom 14 were not splenectomized. During an observation period of 3–12 years, the latter group had average platelet counts of 63 000/mm^3. These children were symptom-free and some girls achieved puberty without excessive menstrual bleeding. Most workers today would wait for at least 1 year in the hope of spontaneous remission before carrying out splenectomy and would not consider surgery in asymptomatic patients with platelet counts above 50 000/mm[31, 38, 47, 50, 54]. Rarely, patients will require splenectomy earlier in the course of the disease, sometimes within a few months of onset. These are patients who remain seriously symptomatic and unresponsive to steroids or only respond to large doses of steroids.

It has been reported that patients whose platelet counts do not increase in response to steroids are less likely to respond to splenectomy[5, 52]. This is presumably because these individuals sequester antibody-coated platelets in the liver rather than the spleen. However, others have reported successful outcome of splenectomy in such patients[10, 38], and some of the patients shown by Najean et al.[44] to sequester predominately in the liver did do well after splenectomy.

It has long been recognized that asplenic children under the age of 4 years are at risk for sudden overwhelming fatal infection. It has been recognized more recently that older children and adults who have been splenectomized are also at increased risk for overwhelming infection with the pneumococcus. For this reason all children who are splenectomized should receive a quadridecavalent antipneumococcal vaccine (Pneumovax, Merck). Not all strains of pneumococcus are included in this vaccine and some failures have been reported. Therefore, the additional prophylactic use of oral penicillin daily has been recommended[8].

Immunosuppressive agents

The first immunosuppressive agent to be employed in the treatment of ATP in children was azathioprine, which was used successfully in two small studies[18,30] but has not proved to be consistently effective[50]. In 1975, Laros and Penner[33] reported the successful use of cyclophosphamide in patients with ATP who were resistant to other forms of therapy, but no convincing success has been reported in children. In 1974, Ahn et al.[1] reported the successful use of vincristine in patients with refractory ATP. Of 21 patients treated, 16 responded with increased platelet counts. Two of the 21 patients were young boys, but the paper does not state their ages nor whether they were in the responsive group. Lanzkowsky[32] has given vincristine to seven children with refractory thrombocytopenia some of whom had been splenectomized. In each case there was a rapid significant rise in platelet count which then fell to the original pretreatment level within two weeks. In 1978, Ahn et al.[2] reported the successful treatment of ATP in adults by an infusion of vinblastine (velban)-loaded platelets. However other workers have not obtained the same good results[51].

Proposed plan of management

Children who have platelet counts of 40 000 or above and are relatively asymptomatic may be observed on an outpatient basis with restriction of physical activity. If the count is between 20 000 and 40 000/mm^3 and the patient displays only mild purpura he may also be observed as an outpatient, but with more stringent restriction of activity. A patient with significant symptoms of extensive purpura or other bleeding manifestations, or a platelet count of below 20 000/mm^3, should be treated with bedrest and prednisone 2 mg/kg per day. This will frequently result in an increase in platelet count into the normal range within a week. The prednisone may then be stopped, and in many instances the platelet count will remain in the normal range and no further treatment will be needed. In some patients the count will fall to pretreatment levels as soon as the prednisone is withdrawn. In this case the drug should be restarted and the patient maintained on sufficient prednisone to keep the platelet count at 50 000/mm^3. This is a safe count for hemostasis; it is not necessary to achieve counts in the normal range. At this level the child may be permitted to return to school and normal daily activities although vigorous contact sports such as football should be avoided. If at the end of one month spontaneous remission has not occurred, the prednisone is gradually decreased and then withdrawn. Usually the child will be relatively asymptomatic even if the platelet count falls to pretreatment levels. However, if significant symptoms recur steroids may be re-instituted with the lowest dose on which the patient can be maintained relatively asymptomatic regardless of platelet count. A small number of patients will not respond to the steroids with a rise in platelet count. These may nonetheless show symptomatic improvement, possibly due to a steroid effect on vascular integrity[12, 29, 45, 46], although this explanation has been questioned[38].

In patients who remain symptomatic and require large amounts of steroids to maintain hemostasis, splenectomy should be performed approximately 6 months after diagnosis, provided the child is more than 4 years of age. If bleeding manifestations are very severe, the operation may have to be done earlier. In patients who are asymptomatic or mildly symptomatic and in whom steroid requirement is little or none, a prolonged waiting period can be observed. Spontaneous remission to hemostatic platelet counts can occur years after diagnosis. Again, it should be emphasized that a platelet count of 50 000/mm^3 or above is generally adequate for hemostasis and return to the normal range is not necessary.

The management of patients who have undergone splenectomy and still remain thrombocytopenic and symptomatic is very difficult. Fortunately this clinical outcome occurs in only a very small number. Splenectomy may have made these patients more sensitive to steroids so that prednisone may be used intermittently to get them through hemorrhagic episodes such as surgery or menses. Menses may also be controlled by use of hormones. This author has had no experience with the use of immunosuppressive agents. It would seem that except for acute life-threatening emergencies they are not indicated, firstly because of their unpredictable long-term effects in young people and secondly because they do not meet with any consistent success. In an emergency, vincristine could be tried to obtain temporary improvement.

PROGNOSIS

The prognosis is generally excellent. Mortality has probably been between 1 and 2 percent and is almost entirely due to intracranial hemorrhage. Judicious use of steroids during the early weeks of the disease may reduce this mortality. The majority of children will recover spontaneously within 6 months of onset of disease. Lusher and Iyer[38], in reviewing 305 cases of children with ITP, found that such recovery occurs in 80–90 percent. Others have reported spontaneous recovery within six months in 65–70 percent[6, 31, 50, 54], although after the age of 10 spontaneous recovery becomes less frequent[50]. Of the 10–30 percent of children who do not recover rapidly a proportion will either recover completely over a longer period of time or achieve a 'safe' platelet count and become asymptomatic. A small percentage of children will remain significantly thrombocytopenic and will require splenectomy. Approximately 80 percent of these will benefit from the operation[38] with a rise in platelet count into the hemostatic range. The remaining 20 percent remain significantly thrombocytopenic and present a difficult clinical problem.

SUMMARY

Thrombocytopenic purpura in children is an autoimmune disease of unknown etiology. Platelets become coated by antibody or by immune complexes and are removed from the circulation by cells of the reticuloendothelial (RE) system. The spleen is the main RE organ which removes platelets. In 70–80 percent of patients spontaneous recovery occurs within 6 months, and a large number of the remainder will remit after longer periods. Steroids prevent removal of antibody-coated platelets by the spleen and can be used to maintain 'safe' platelet counts whilst awaiting spontaneous recovery. A small number of patients will remain significantly thrombocytopenic and symptomatic after long periods of time and will require splenectomy.

References

1 AHN, Y. S., HARRINGTON, W. J., SEELMAN, R. C. and EYTEL, C. S. Vincristine therapy of idiopathic and secondary thrombocytopenias. *New England Journal of Medicine*, **291**, 376 (1974)

2 AHN, Y. S., BYRNES, J. J., HARRINGTON, W. J., CAYER, M. L., SMITH, D. S., BRUNSKILL, D. E. and PALE, L. M. The treatment of idiopathic thrombocytopenia with vinblastine-loaded platelets. *New England Journal of Medicine*, **298**, 1101 (1978)

3 BENHAM, E. S. and TAFT, L. I. Idiopathic thrombocytopenic purpura in children: results of steroid therapy and splenectomy. *Australian Paediatric Journal*, **8**, 311 (1972)

4 BRANEHOG, I., KUTTI, J., RIDELL, B., SWOLIN, B. and WEINFELD. A. The relation of thrombokinetics to bone marrow megakaryocytes in idiopathic thrombocytopenic purpura. *Blood*, **45**, 551 (1975)

5 BRENNAN, M. F., RAPPAPORT, J. M., MOLONEY, W. C. and WILSON, R. E. Correlation between response to splenectomy for adult idiopathic thrombocytopenic purpura. *American Journal of Surgery*, **129**, 490 (1975)

6 CHOI, S. I. and McCLURE, P. D. Idiopathic thrombocytopenic purpura in childhood. *Canadian Medical Association Journal*, **97**, 562 (1967)

7 CINES, D. B. and SCHREIBER, A. D. Immune thrombocytopenia. Use in Coombs antiglobulin test to detect IgG and C_3 on platelets. *New England Journal of Medicine*, **300**, 106 (1979)

8 DICKERMAN, J. D. Splenectomy and sepsis: a warning. *Pediatrics*, **63**, 938 (1979)

9 DIXON, R., ROSSE, W. and EBBERT, L. Quantitative determination of antibody in idiopathic thrombocytopenic purpura. *New England Journal of Medicine*, **292**, 230 (1975)

10 DOAN, C. A., BOURONCLE, B. A. and WISEMAN, B. K. Idiopathic and secondary thrombocytopenic purpura. Clinical study and evaluation of 381 cases over a period of 28 years. *Annals of Internal Medicine*, **53**, 861 (1960)

11 EPSTEIN, R. D., LOZNER, E. L., COBBEY, T. S. and DAVIDSON, C. S. Congenital thrombocytopenic purpura. Purpura hemorrhagica in pregnancy and in the newborn. *American Journal of Medicine*, **9**, 44 (1950)

12 FALOON, W. W., GREENE, R. W. and LOZNER, E. L. The heomostatic defect in thrombocytopenia as studied by the use of ACTH and cortisone. *American Journal of Medicine*, **13**, 12 (1952)

13 GARG, S. K., AMOROSI, E. L. and KARPATKIN, S. Use of the megathrombocytes as an index of the megakaryocyte number. *New England Journal of Medicine*, **284**, 11 (1971)

14 HARRINGTON, W. J., MINNICH, V., HOLLINGSWORTH, J. W. and MOORE, C. V. Demonstration of a thrombocytopenic factor in the blood of patients with thrombocytopenic purpura. *Journal of Laboratory and Clinical Medicine*, **38**, 1 (1951)

15 HARRINGTON, W. J., MINNICH, V. and ARIMURA, G. The autoimmune thrombocytopenias. In *Hematology*, Vol. 1, 166 (1956) (in press)

16 HARRINGTON, W. J. and ARIMURA, G. Immune reactions of platelets. In *Henry Ford Hospital Symposium: Blood Platelets*, edited by S. A. Johnson, R. W. Monto, J. W. Rebuck and R. J. Horn, Jr. 659. Boston. Little, Brown (1961)

17 HEDGE, U. M., GORDON-SMITH, E. C. and WORLLEDGE, S. Platelet antibodies in thrombocytopenic patients. *British Journal of Haematology*, **35**, 113 (1977)

18 HILGARTNER, M. W., LANZKOWSKY, P. and SMITH, C. H. The use of azothioprine in refractory idiopathic thrombocytopenic purpura in children. *Acta Paediatrica Scandinavica*, **59**, 409 (1970)

19 HYMES, K., SHULMAN, S. and KARPATKIN, S. A solid phase radioimmune assay for bound antiplatelet antibody. *Journal of Laboratory and Clinical Medicine*, **94**, 639 (1979)

20 JACKSON, D. P., SCHMID, H. J., ZIEVE, P. O., LEVIN, J. and CONLEY, C. L. Nature of the platelet agglutinating factor in serum of patients with idiopathic thrombocytopenic purpura. *Journal of Clinical Investigation*, **42**, 383 (1963)

21 KARPATKIN, S. and SISKIND, G. W. In vitro detection of platelet antibody in patients with idiopathic thrombocytopenic purpura and systemic lupus erythematosis. *Blood*, **33**, 795 (1969)

22 KARPATKIN, S., GARG, S. K. and SISKIND, G. W. Autoimmune thrombocytopenic purpura and the compensated thrombocytolytic state. *American Journal of Medicine*, **51**, 1 (1971)

23 KARPATKIN, S., STRICK, N., KARPATKIN, M. and SISKIND, G. W. Cumulative experience with the detection of antiplatelet antibody in 234 patients with idiopathic thrombocytopenic purpura, systemic lupus erythematosus and other clinical disorders. *American Journal of Medicine*, **52**, 776 (1972)

24 KARPATKIN, S., STRICK, N. and SISKIND, G. W. Detection of splenic antiplatelet antibody synthesis in idiopathic autoimmune thrombocytopenic purpura (ATP). *British Journal of Haematology*, **23**, 167 (1972)

25 KARPATKIN, S., SCHUR, P. H., STRICK, N. and SISKIND, G. W. Heavy chain subclass of human antiplatelet antibodies. *Clinical Immunology and Immunopathology*, **2**, 1 (1973)

26 KARPATKIN, M., SISKIND, G. W. and KARPATKIN, S. The platelet factor 3 immuno-injury technique re-evaluated. *Journal of Laboratory and Clinical Medicine*, **89**, 410 (1977)

27 KARPATKIN, M. and KARPATKIN, S. Immune thrombocytopenia in children. *American Journal of Pediatric Hematology and Oncology*, **3**, 213–219 (1981)

28 KARPATKIN, M. and KARPATKIN, S. Immune neonatal thrombocytopenia. In *Acquired Bleeding Disorders in Children*, edited by J. Lusher and M. I. Barnhardt, 93–105 New York, Masson (1981)

29 KITCHENS, C. S. Amelioration of endothelial abnormalities by prednisone in experimental thrombocytopenia in the rabbit. *Journal of Clinical Investigation*, **60**, 1129 (1977)

30 KUZEMKO, J. A. and KEIDAN, S. E. Treatment of chronic idiopathic thrombocytopenic purpura with azathioprine and prednisone. A clinical trial with three children. *Clinical Pediatrics*, **7**, 216 (1968)

31 LAMMI, A. T. and LOVRIC, V. A. Idiopathic thrombocytopenic purpura; an epidemiologic study. *Journal of Pediatrics*, **83**, 31 (1973)

32 LANZKOWSKY, P. In *Pediatric Hematology and Oncology*, 257. New York, McGraw Hill (1980)

33 LAROS, R. J. and PENNER, J. A. Refractory thrombocytopenic purpura treated successfully with cyclophosphamide. *Journal of the American Medical Association*, **232**, 734 (1975)

34 LIGHTSEY, A. L., McMILLAN, R., KOENIG, H. M., SHANBERGER, J. G. and LANG, J. E. In vitro production of platelet binding IgG childhood idiopathic thrombocytopenic purpura. *Journal of Pediatrics*, **88**, 415 (1976)

35 LIGHTSEY, A. L., KOENIG, H. M., McMILLAN, R. and STONE, J. R. Platelet-associated immunoglobulin G in childhood idiopathic thrombocytopenic purpura. *Journal of Pediatrics*, **94**, 201 (1979)

36 LUIKEN, G. A., McMILLAN, R., LIGHTSEY, A. L., GORDON, P., ZEVELY, S., SCHULMAN, I., GRIBBLE, T. J. and LONGMIRE, R. L. Platelet-associated IgG in immune thrombocytopenic purpura. *Blood*, **50**, 317 (1977)

37 LUSHER, J. M. and ZUELZER, W. W. Idiopathic thrombocytopenic purpura in childhood. *Journal of Pediatrics*, **68**, 971 (1966)

38 LUSHER, J. M. and IYER, R. Idiopathic thrombocytopenic purpura in children. *Seminars in Thrombosis and Hemostasis*, **3**, 175 (1977)

39 McCLURE, P. D. Idiopathic thrombocytopenic purpura in children: diagnosis and management. *Pediatrics*, **55**, 68 (1975)

40 McCLURE, P. D. Idiopathic thrombocytopenic purpura in children. Should corticosteroids be given? *American Journal of Disease in Childhood*, **131**, 357 (1977)

41 McELFRESH, A. E. Idiopathic thrombocytopenic purpura – to treat or not to treat. *Journal of Pediatrics*, **87**, 160 (1975)

42 McMILLAN, R., LONGMIRE, R. L., YELENOSKY, R., SMITH, R. S. and CRADDOCK, C. G. Immunoglobulin synthesis in vitro by splenic tissue in idiopathic thrombocytopenic purpura. *New England Journal of Medicine*, **286**, 681 (1972)

43 McMILLAN, R., LONGMIRE, R. L., TAVASSOLE, M., ARMSTRONG, S. and YELENOSKY, R. In vitro platelet phagocytosis by splenic leukocytes in idiopathic thrombocytopenic purpura. *New England Journal of Medicine*, **290**, 249 (1974)

44 NAJEAN, Y., ARDAILLOU, N., DRESCH, C. and BERNARD, J. The platelet destruction site in thrombocytopenic purpura. *British Journal of Haematology*, **13,** 409 (1967)

45 ROBSON, H. N. and DUTHIE, J. Capillary resistance and adreno-cortical activity. *British Journal of Medicine*, **2,** 971 (1950)

46 SCHULMAN, I. Diagnosis and treatment: management of idiopathic thrombocytopenic purpura. *Pediatrics*, **33,** 979 (1964)

47 SCHULMAN, I. In *Clinical Disorders of the Platelets in Hematology of Infancy and Childhood*, edited by D. G. Nathan and F. A. Oski. Philadelphia, W. B. Saunders (1974)

48 SHULMAN, N. R., MARDER, V. J. and WEINRACH, R. S. Similarities between known antiplatelet antibodies and the factor responsible for thrombocytopenia in idiopathic purpura. *Annals of the New York Academy of Sciences*, **124,** 499 (1965)

49 SHULMAN, N. R., WEINRACH, R. S., LIBRE, E. P. and ANDREWS, H. L. The role of the reticuloendothelial system in the pathogenesis of idiopathic thrombocytopenic purpura. *Transactions of the Association of American Physicians*, **78,** 374 (1965)

50 SIMONS, S. M., MAIN, C. A., YAISH, H. M. and RUTZKY, J. Idiopathic thrombocytopenic purpura in children. *Journal of Pediatrics*, **87,** 16 (1975)

51 SLICHTER, S. J. and SCHWARTZ, K. Mechanism of action of vinblastine-loaded platelets in the treatment of chronic idiopathic thrombocytopenic purpura (ITP). *Clinical Research*, **27,** 307A (1979)

52 THOMPSON, R. L., MOORE, R. A., HESS, C. E., WHELBY, M. S. and LEAVELL, B. S. Idiopathic thrombocytopenic purpura. Long term results of treatment and the prognostic significance of response to corticosteroids. *Archives of Internal Medicine*, **130,** 730 (1972)

53 VERP, M. and KARPATKIN, S. Effect of plasma, steroids or steroid products on the adhesion of human opsonised thrombocytes to human leukocytes. *Journal of Laboratory and Clinical Medicine*, **85,** 478 (1975)

54 WALKER, J. H. and WALKER, W. Idiopathic thrombocytopenic purpura in childhood. *Archives of Disease in Childhood*, **36,** 649 (1961)

11
Clinical consequences and management of chronic iron overload

Jorge A. Ortega

INTRODUCTION

Despite remarkable advances in our understanding of the pathophysiology of chronic iron overload there has been little progress in its clinical management. Significant effort has gone into devising methods of removing iron from the body in patients affected with transfusion dependent anemia since chronic iron overload constitutes the major cause of death for these patients. Of the many chelating agents so far tried, Desferrioxamine (DF) is the best. Although recent improvements in the methods and techniques of DF administration are encouraging, the present status of iron chelation therapy is still far from a breakthrough in the management of chronic iron overload. Furthermore, the high cost of the presently available iron chelation regimes adds the economic factor to the extensive search for more efficient iron chelators.

CLINICAL MANIFESTATIONS

The clinical manifestations are given in *Table 11.1*. The human body guards its iron stores carefully and has no effective way of eliminating iron once excessive stores have developed. In patients with congenital or acquired anemias who are blood transfusion dependent, transfusional iron slowly but steadily is deposited in different tissues and organs; primarily the liver, heart and pancreas. This leads to progressive damage and eventually to the death of the patient in early adult life. The most frequent and often fatal complications of transfusional iron overload are related to the heart[2,10]. Children with thalassemia major constitute the major group of such patients, however a significant second group is made up of children with refractory Blackfan–Diamond Syndrome, aplastic anemia, and severe sickle cell anemia.

The frequency and severity of the cardiac complications increase in proportion to the number of transfusions. Nienhuis et al.[31] described three progressive stages in

Table 11.1 Chronic iron overload

Organ affected	Clinical manifestations
Heart	Left ventricular wall thickening
	Decreased ejection fraction
	Pericardial effusion
	Palpitation, arrhythmia
	Congestive heart failure
Pituitary	Delayed or absent puberty
Liver	Fibrosis
	Cirrhosis
	Parenchymal and reticuloendothelial siderosis
Pancreas	Diabetes mellitus
Parathyroid	Hypoparathyroidism
Adrenal	Adrenocortical insufficiency

cardiac deterioration in patients with chronic iron overload in relation to their previous transfusion records. In the asymptomatic first stage, the only abnormality present is slight ventricular wall thickening. During the second stage patients may complain of fatiguability and a radionuclide cineangiogram can reveal abnormalities in ejection fraction with exercise. The final and more advanced stage is characterized by the presence of palpitations and congestive heart failure. By this time significant abnormalities are present in the echocardiogram and radionuclide cineangiogram. Pericardial effusion is also commonly present in these patients as the cardiac condition deteriorates. Cardiac evaluation of asymptomatic iron overload patients by non-invasive techniques is warranted, since abnormalities prior to overt cardiac dysfunction can often be detected. These abnormalities include left ventricular wall thickening and decreased ejection fraction.

Endocrine abnormalities are frequent observations in patients with chronic iron overload. Delayed or absent pubescence or secondary hypogonadism due to failure of the pituitary to release follicle-stimulating hormone (FSH) and luteinizing hormone (LH) have been documented[32].

Adrenocortical deficiency at times requiring replacement therapy is also known to occur among patients with iron overload, especially after the second decade of life.

Endocrine pancreatic insufficiency, as evidenced by the presence of either overt clinical diabetes mellitus or abnormal glucose tolerance tests[5] becomes frequent as the number of transfusions increases.

In patients on chronic transfusional therapy, iron rapidly accumulates in the liver leading to progressive hepatic fibrosis and eventually to cirrhosis. This hepatic dysfunction is often the earliest complication of transfusional hemosiderosis and can also result in abnormal metabolism of steroid hormones.

Even though thyroid dysfunction is extremely rare in chronic iron overload, the excessive FSH response to thyrothropin-releasing hormone observed in some patients with thalassemia major suggests a mild compensating hypothyroidism[32].

Iron chelation therapy

The goal of iron chelation therapy should be to achieve negative iron balance by inducing urine iron excretion equal to or greater than iron intake via transfusion. In this way parenchymal damage and organ dysfunction may be prevented.

The value of iron chelation therapy has been studied thoroughly during the past-decade. Few new iron chelating agents had been clinically investigated and evaluated as potential drugs and emphasis has been placed mainly on the efficacy of known iron chelators. To date, the most extensively studied of the iron-chelating agents is DF. Presently it is the most widely used and accepted in the USA and abroad. The last few years have witnessed a considerable increase in the information and experience with the use of DF for iron chelation therapy.

In this chapter an attempt will be made to review the present status of the art of iron chelation. Since DF remains the primary drug available for treatment of transfusional iron overload, use of this agent will be emphasized.

Desferrioxamine

DF is a naturally occurring hydroxamic acid produced by *Streptomyces pilosus*. The colorless drug when administrated parenterally combines with iron and the rust-colored iron complex is then excreted in the urine. DF appears to cause significant iron excretion only in patients with substantial iron overload[1,27] suggesting that the iron storage compounds are the major source of chelated iron.

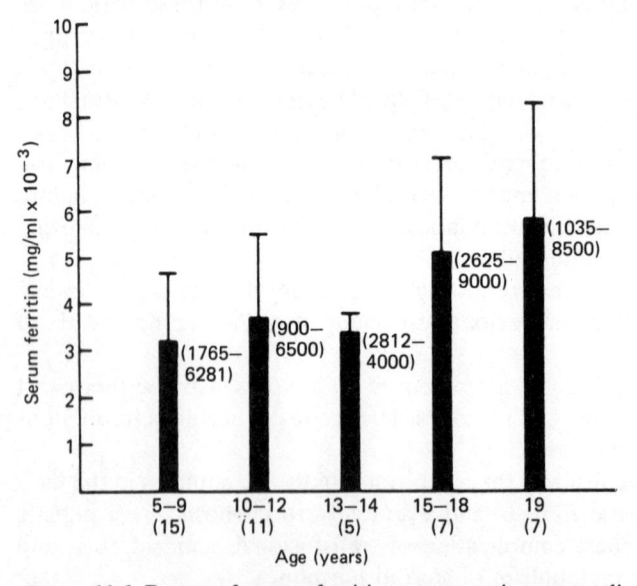

Figure 11.1 Range of serum ferritin concentrations according to age in transfusion dependent patients with thalassemia major. Number in parenthesis indicates number of patients for each age group. (From Nienhuis et al.[31], courtesy of the Editor and publishers, *Annals of the New York Academy of Sciences*)

Studies by Lipschitz et al.[24] seem to confirm that some compound on the pathway between the stores (ferritin and hemosiderin) and the plasma is probably the major source of iron chelation by DF. The serum ferritin concentration is generally accepted to be an index of body iron stores[32] and correlates well with the number of transfusions the patient has received (*Figure 11.1*). Evidence also exists that serum ferritin concentration reflects reticuloendothelial storage iron[42] and changes in reticuloendothelial iron are followed rapidly by changes in the serum concentration of ferritin[20]. Recently a decrease in serum ferritin concentration shortly after initiation of iron chelation therapy with DF has been observed[15] in patients with thalassemia major. Furthermore, a good correlation between serum ferritin and liver iron concentration has been documented[23]. The suggestion has been made that the observed drop in serum ferritin following initiation of DF therapy is due to a drop in nonglycosalated ferritin which reflects an improvement of liver function rather than a decrease in stores[21].

Results of controled studies have confirmed that prolonged administration of low dose DF to patients with thalassemia major significantly reduces liver iron and serum ferritin concentration[23] and retards hepatic fibrosis[1] as well as reversing of cardiac enlargement and electrocardiographic abnormalities.

Approximately two-thirds of iron bound by DF is excreted in the urine and one-third in the stools[7]. Fecal iron has been considered to be derived directly from the liver since experiments with ^{59}Fe ferrioxamine complex administered intravenously show that it does not appear in the stool[43]. However, recent studies by Pippard et al.[36] suggest that decreased iron absorption induced by DF may be partly responsible for the apparent increased fecal iron excretion. This decrease in iron absorption was observed in both ascorbate depleted and repleted animals.

Desferrioxamine and iron balance

Several factors influence iron balance in patients with transfusional hemosiderosis. Iron input is determined mainly by two major components: first, increased gastrointestinal absorption which, in anemic patients, can exceed 10 mg/day; and secondly, the iron received as blood which averages 1 mg/ml of sedimented red cells transfused. Since it is known that transfusion reduces iron absorption[11] this latter component does not play an essential role in the iron input of patients kept on a hypertransfusion program. In addition, the observation that DF decreases gastrointestinal iron excretion[36] further minimizes the importance of gastrointestinal absorption on iron input of patients receiving chelation therapy with DF. Spontaneous losses of iron in the urine and stool are minimal even when consideration is given to the higher than normal urine iron excretion which is observed in non-chelated patients with thalassemia[28].

These observations appear to justify the use of iron input as blood transfused and chelation induced urine iron excretion for monitoring iron balance in patients with transfusional hemosiderosis. Obviously the goal of any iron chelation therapy should be to attain negative iron balance, defined as urinary excretion of more iron than is received via blood transfusion.

Response to DF therapy has been shown to be proportional to body iron load[12] and significant effect is obtained only when the patient is already iron overloaded. This explains the poor response to DF therapy observed in transfusion dependent infants and young children where iron load is usually not established until three and four years of age[29,35]. Weiner et al.[46] have shown that in children with Cooley's anemia under three years of age, only 30 percent of the average daily transfused iron is excreted with daily administration of DF intramuscularly. It appears that the body iron load at which balance can be achieved is about 10 to 15 g[8,27], as opposed to the normal stores of 1 g; however, if such a large load remains toxic the treatment will achieve very little. Fortunately, the chronic administration of DF seems to protect to some extent the liver and the heart[27] from the damaging effects of iron and the initial results obtained with daily intramuscular administration of DF have recently been improved with the rapid evolution of different methods of administration of this chelating agent.

Desferrioxamine therapy dosage and administration techniques

The initial documentation by Sephton-Smith[40] in 1964 that administration of DF induces excretion of increased quantities of iron in thalassemic patients was followed by a rising interest on the field of iron chelation therapy.

Intramuscular desferrioxamine

Modell and Beck[28] have shown that a long-term therapeutic trial using DF, 500 mg, intramuscularly, six days a week, and 2 g/pint, in the blood at transfusion was able to achieve iron balance in some patients, However, they also found that a patient does not begin to respond to DF therapy until the body iron stores are about ten times normal. Studies of hepatic iron concentration and liver function suggested that a therapy program like the one used by Modell and Beck can slow the rate of liver iron accumulation and improve the serum transaminase level[1,41].

Results of subsequent trials[46] with intramuscular DF demonstrate that a program of daily intramuscular iron induces excretion of approximately 50 percent of the average daily transfused iron in children older than six years old. For these studies only urinary iron excretion was determined; losses in the stool were not determined.

Attempts to administer doses higher than 750 mg intramuscularly have resulted in significant pain and generally are not tolerated by patients.

Intravenous desferrioxamine

The evidences that the urinary iron excretion not only proportionally increases with the dose of intravenous administration[28] but also by prolonging the infusion time[18,38] (*Figure 11.2*) have encouraged different investigators to look for other

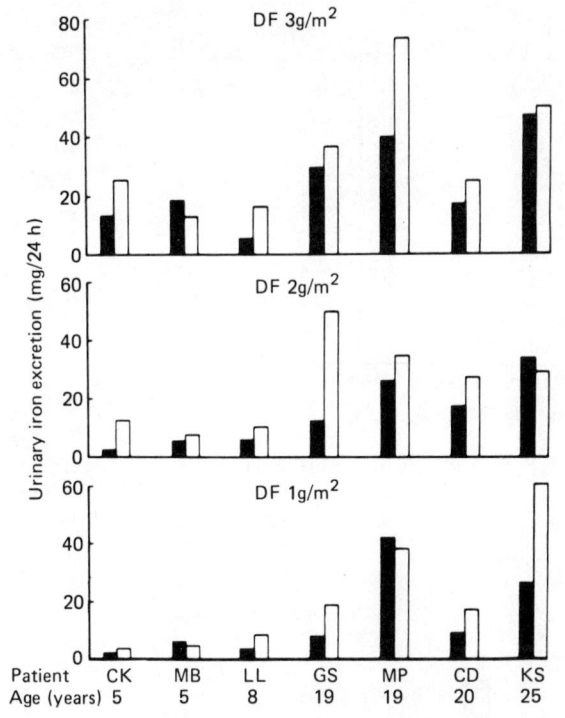

Figure 11.2 Relationship of desferrioxamine dose and infusion time of (■) 6 h i.v.; (□) 24 h i.v. to urinary iron excretion. (Reprinted from Hymam et al.[18], *Chelation Therapy in Chronic Iron Overload*, Symposia Specialists, Inc., PO Box. 610397, Miami, Florida 33161)

techniques of administration allowing use of larger doses. Furthermore, at equal doses both intravenous and subcutaneous infusions are much more effective inducing urinary iron excretion greater than intramuscular injections[17, 37, 38].

Subcutaneous desferrioxamine

Since daily intravenous infusion is not practical, the report by Propper et al.[39] in 1977 showing that administration of DF subcutaneously by portable infusion pump induces urinary iron excretion up to nearly twice that obtained with a single intramuscular injection of the same dose (*Figure 11.3*) and comparable to intravenous infusion (*Figure 11.4*) encouraged several groups to use this method of administration. Confirmation of Propper's results by other investigators[4, 15] has resulted in the acceptance of the subcutaneous administration via portable infusion pump as practical and effective, and the most compatible with a normal life style.

It seems that in children younger than 10 years old, little benefit is obtained with doses higher than 20 mg/kg, usually infused subcutaneously over a period of 8 to 10 h. In patients older than 10 years of age, at risk for cardiac and endocrine dysfunction and who responded significantly to higher doses of DF, it is justifiable to use doses up to 50 and 60 mg/kg.

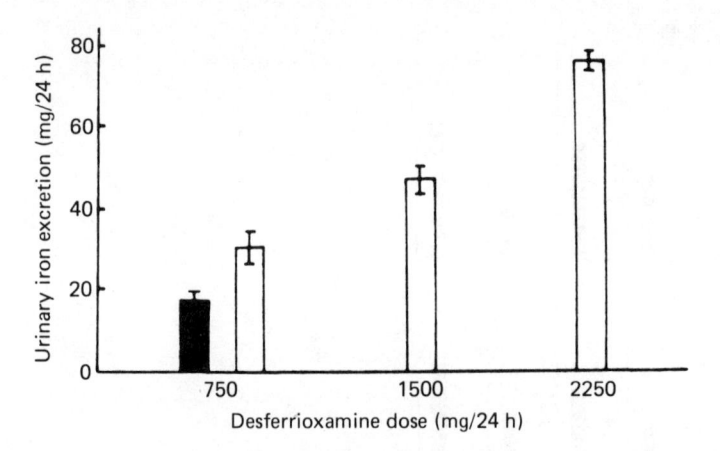

Figure 11.3 The effects of intramuscular (■) and subcutaneous (□) injections of desferrioxamine on iron excretion in thalassemia major patients. (From Propper, *Annals of the New York Academy of Science*, **344**, 375–383, 1980, by courtesy of the Editor and Publishers)

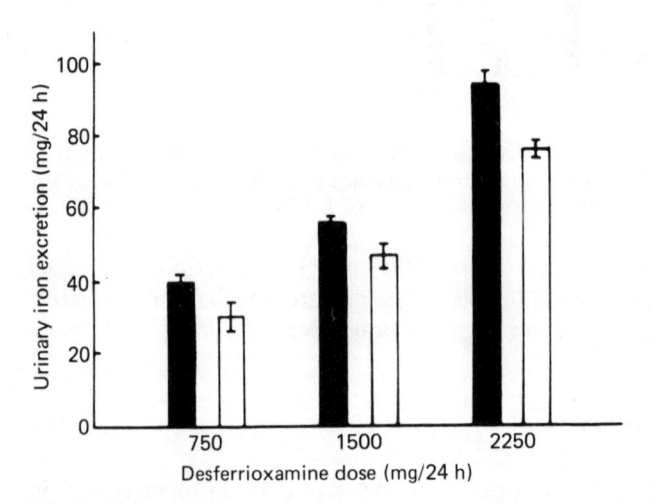

Figure 11.4 The effects of subcutaneous (□) and intravenous (■) administration of desferrioxamine at different doses on urinary iron excretion. (From Propper et al.[39] by permission of *The New England Journal of Medicine*, **297**, 420, 1977)

No serious toxicity have been noted with large doses of DF, except for occasional episodes of hypotension. In patients receiving the subcutaneous infusion, local pruritus and irritation can be observed, especially at the beginning of therapy. This can be avoided by adding 1 mg of hydrocortisone to the infused solution. Cataracts[26], a long-term side effect of DF, can be minimized by using the minimal effective dose of the drug. Most recently, Green[13] introduced a new method of administration using DF entrapped ghost red cells. Results of this study are preliminary and requiries further confirmation in a larger number of patients.

In general, the best method for iron chelation with DF has to be determined individually and tailored to each patient. Acceptability of the different routes of administration by the child and his family have to be considered, since serious attention should be given to patient compliance problems that may jeopardize results of the therapy.

Desferrioxamine and vitamin C

Depletion of ascorbic acid has been documented in a variety of conditions associated with iron overload, among them Cooley's anemia[44]. In this condition it has been shown that ascorbic acid can successfully increase the effectiveness of chelation therapy[45]. The mechanism of this effect is still uncertain. In animals, deficiency of ascorbic acid alters the iron distribution between the two storage compounds, ferritin and hemosiderin, with an increase in the insoluble form of hemosiderin[25] that is rapidly corrected by repletion of the vitamin. Futhermore, reducing agents such as ascorbic acid probably facilitate the release of iron from ferritin by its reduction to the ferrous state[6]. Since DF chelates ferric iron, it is reasonable to believe that the ferrous iron released is reconverted to the ferric state before chelation[45].

Ascorbic acid supplementation increases iron urinary excretion in response to DF in patients with thalassemia major[33], especially if they are ascorbate depleted. Doses in the range of 100 to 250 mg of ascorbic acid per day appear to be sufficient to maintain normal ascorbate white cell level[15] and to cause adequate augmentation of iron excretion in response to DF therapy. Caution should be taken in using higher doses that may cause excessive mobilization of iron resulting in catalysis of free radical reactions inducing lipid peroxidation and tissue damage[14]. Furthermore, concern has been expressed over the possibility that ascorbic acid, by promoting release of reticuloendothelial iron deposits, may lead to an increase in parenchymal iron with increased tissue damage[30].

In summary, an iron chelation therapy regimen consistent with the administration of DF subcutaneously via auto syringe at the dosage of 20–50 mg/kg body weight per day, over an 8 to 12 h period, supplemented by administration of ascorbic acid of 100–200 mg per day, can effectively prevent progressive iron deposition and apparently retard liver fibrosis.

These patients may also benefit from the administration of two to three days of continuous intravenous infusion of DF, repeated every four to six weeks.

Other iron chelators

Although long-term iron chelation therapy with DF, as currently used, significantly reduces liver iron accumulation and causes retardation in the progression of hepatic fibrosis, little difference has been documented in the severity of cardiac and endocrine complications [23], implying that improvement in iron chelation therapy is essential. A major international effort has been undertaken to improve not only the efficacy of iron chelation therapy, but also administration techniques resulting in a better quality of life.

Other iron chelates that have attracted attention in the past include:

2,3 Dihydrobenzoic acid (2,3-DHB)

This compound was found by Cerami et al.[3] to cause significant increase in urinary iron excretion in hypertransfused rats. Since the compound is also an effective free radical scavenger, it was thought that an additional benefical effect on lipid peroxidation and fibrotic changes of tissues might be obtained with its administration. Of further importance was also the fact that 2,3-DHB can be administered orally. However, results of a double blind clinical trial[34] over a one-year period failed to document an effect on liver iron accumulation. A significant variability in urinary iron excretion was also found from patient to patient. In some patients the amount of iron excreted was comparable to that observed with DF administration. Since the compound appears to be relatively free of toxicity and has the benefit of oral adminstration, it would be of interest to design an iron chelation regime combining subcutaneous DF with oral 2,3-DHB. At the present time, other 2,3-DHB derivative compounds[3] are under evaluation as iron chelators.

5-Hydroxypicolinzaldehyde thiosemicarbazone (5-HP)

5-HP was found to increase urinary iron excretion during a trial to evaluate its activity as a cancer chemotherapeutic agent. Results of a trial in seven patients[19] demonstrated that 5-HP at the dose of 6 to 12 mg/kg/day induced urinary iron excretion comparable to that of DF at a dose of 20 mg/kg given intravenously over a 15 minute period. The trial was subsequently abandoned due to the presence of mild to moderate symptoms of toxicity[19].

Rhodotorulic acid (RA)

Like DF, RA is a naturally occurring hydroxamic acid. It attracted attention as a potentially useful iron chelator in man because of its more economical production and use as a subcutaneous depot due to its relative insolubility in water[3]. However, pain and irritation at the injection site have limited its use and it appears that RA offers little advantage over DF in inducing urinary iron excretion.

It is noteworthy to mention that an intensive search for more effective iron chelators continues. The goal of this search must be to maintain a high quality of life with normal activities while removing the maximum amount of iron.

References

1 BARRY, M., FLYNN, D. M., LATSKY, E. A. and RISDON, R. A. Long-term chelation therapy in thalassemia major: effect on liver iron concentration, liver histology and clinical progress. *British Medical Journal*, **2,** 16–20 (1974)

2 BUJA, L. M. and ROBERTS, W. C. Iron in the heart: etiology and clinical significance. *American Journal of Medicine*, **51,** 209–221 (1971)

3 CERAMI, A., GRADY, R. W., PETERSON, C. M. and BHARGARA, K. K. The status of iron chelators. *Annals of the New York Academy of Sciences*, **344,** 425–435 (1980)

4 COHEN, A. and SCHWARTZ, E. Iron chelation therapy with desferrioxamine in Cooley's anemia. *Journal of Pediatrics*, **92,** 643–647 (1978)

5 COSTIN, G., KOGUT, M. D., HYMAN, C. and ORTEGA, J. A. Carbohydrate metabolism and pancreatic islet cell function in thalassemia major. *Diabetes*, **26,** 230–240 (1977)

6 CRICHTON, R. R. Structure and function of ferritin. *Angewandte Chemie*, **12,** 57–65 (1973)

7 CUMMING, R. L. C., MILLAR, J. A., SMITH, J. A. and GOLDBERG, A. Clinical and laboratory studies on the action of desferrioxamine. *British Journal of Haematology*, **17,** 257–263 (1969)

8 EDITORIAL. Desferrioxamine and transfusional iron overload. *Lancet*, **1,** 479–480 (1978)

9 EHLERS, K. H., LEVIN, A. R., MARKENSON, A. L., MARCUS, J. R., KLEIN, A. A., HILGARTNER, M. W. and ENGLE, M. A. Longitudinal study of cardiac functional in thalassemia major. *Annals of New York Academy of Sciences*, **344,** 397–404 (1980)

10 ENGLE, M. A. Cardiac involvement in Cooley's anemia. *Annals of New York Academy of Sciences*, **119,** 694–702 (1964)

11 ERLANDSON, M. E., WALDEN, B., STERN, G., HILGARTNER, M. W., WEHWAN, J. and SMITH, C. H. Studies on congenital haemolytic syndromes. IV. Gastrointestinal absorption of iron. *Blood*, **19,** 359–378 (1962)

12 FIELDING, J. Differential ferrioxamine test for measuring chelatable body iron. *Journal of Clinical Pathology*, **18,** 85–97 (1965)

13 GREEN, R., LAMON, J. and CURRAN, D. Clinical trial of desferrioxamine on trapped red cell ghosts. *Lancet*, **2,** 327–330 (1980)

14 GRAZIANO, J. H. Potential usefulness of free radical scavengers in iron overload. In *Iron Metabolism and Thalassemia*, edited by D. Bergsma., A. Cerami, C. M. Peterson and J. H. Graziano. New York, Alan R. Liss, Inc. (1976)

15 GRAZIANO, J. H., MARKINSON, A., MILLER, D. R., CHANG, H., BESTAK, M., MEYERS, P., PISCIOTTO, P. and RIJKIND A. Chelation therapy in B-thalassemia major. I. Intravenous and subcutaneous desferrioxamine. *Journal of Pediatrics*, **92,** 645–652 (1978)

16 HEINRICH, H. C., GABBE, E. E., OPPITZ, K. H. Absorption of inorganic and food iron in children with heterozygous and homozygous beta-thalassemia. *Zeitschrift für Kinderhuilkunde*, **115,** 1–22 (1973)

17 HUSSIAN, M. A. M., GREEN, N., FLYN, D. M., HUSSAIN, F. and HOFFBRAND, A. V. Subcutaneous infusion and intramuscular injection of desferrioxamine in patients with transfusion iron overload. *Lancet*, **2,** 1278–1280 (1976)

18 HYMAN, C. B., ORTEGA, J. A. and AFTERGOOD, L. Effects of different regimes of desferrioxamine and ascorbic acid administration and of serum or tocopherol level on urinary iron excretion. In *Chelation Therapy in Chronic Iron Overload*, edited by E. C. Zaino and R. H. Roberts, 109–144. Miami Symposia Specialists (1977)

19 HYMAN, C. B., ORTEGA, J. A., COSTIN, G., LANDING, B., LAZERSON, J. and LEIMBROCK, S. Management of thalassemia in Los Angeles. In *Iron Metabolism and Thalassemia*, edited by D. Bergsma, A. Cerami, C. M. Peterson and J. H. Graziano. 43–52. New York, Alan R. Liss, Inc. (1976)

20 JACOBS, A. Serum ferritin. In *Iron Metabolism and Thalassemia*, edited by D. Bergsma, A. Cerami, C. M. Peterson, J. H. Graziano, 97–103. New York, Alan R. Liss, Inc. (1976)

21 JACOBS, A. General discussion: clinical management. Sergio Riomelli, Moderator, *Annals of New York Academy of Sciences*, **344,** 418–424 (1980)

22 LETSKY, E. A., MILLER, F., WORWOOD, M. II. and FLYNN, D. M. Serum ferritin in children with thalassemia regularly transfused. *Journal of Clinical Pathology*, **27,** 652–655 (1974)

23 LETSKY, E. A. A controlled trial of long-term chelation therapy in homozygous B-thalassemia. In *Iron Metabolism and Thalassemia*, edited by D. Bergsma, A. Cerami, C. M. Peterson, J. H. Graziano, 31–41; New York, Alan R. Liss, Inc. (1977)

24 LIPSCHITZ, D. A., DUGARD, J., SIMON, M. O., BOTHWELL, T. H. and CHARLTON, R. W. The site of action of desferrioxamine. *British Journal of Haematology*, **20,** 395–404 (1971)

25 LIPSCHITZ, D. A., BOTHWELL, T. H., SEFTEL, H. C., WAPNICK, A. A. and CHARLTON, R. W. The role of ascorbic acid in the metabolism of storage iron. *British Journal of Haematology*, **20,** 155–163 (1971)

26 MALPAS, J. S. Current therapeutics – CCXII desferrioxamine. *Practitioner*, **195,** 369 (1965)

27 MODELL, C. B. and BECK, J. Long-term desferrioxamine therapy in thalassemia. *Annals of the New York Academy of Sciences*, **232,** 201–210 (1974)

28 MODELL, C. B. and BECK, J. Long-term desferrioxamine therapy in thalassemia. *Annals of the New York Academy of Sciences*, **232,** 201–210 (1974)

29 MODELL, B. Management of thalassemia major. *British Medical Bulletin*, **32,** 270–277 (1976)

30 NIENHUIS, A. W., DELEA, C., AZMODT, R., BARTTER, F. and ANDERSON, W. F. Evaluation of desferrioxamine and ascorbic acid for the treatment of chronic iron overload. In *Iron Metabolism and Thalassemia*, edited by D. Bergsma, A. Cerami, C. M. Peterson, J. H. Graziano, 177–185. New York, Alan R. Liss, Inc. (1976)

31 NIENHUIS, A. W., GRIFFITH, P., STRAWCZYNSKI, H., HENRY, W., BORER, J., LEON, M. and ANDERSON, W. F. Evaluation of cardiac function in patients with thalassemia major. *Annals of the New York Academy of Sciences*, **344,** 384–396 (1980)

32 NIENHUIS, A. W., PETERSON, D. T. and HENRY, W. Evaluation of endocrine and cardiac functions in patients with iron overload on chelation therapy. In *Chelation Therapy in Chronic Iron Overload*, edited by Edward C. Zaino and Richard H. Roberts, 1–15. Miami, Symposia Specialists (1977)

33 O'BRIEN, R. T. Ascorbic acid enhancement of desferrioxamine-induced urinary iron excretion in thalassemia major. *Annals of the New York Academy of Sciences*, **232**, 221–225 (1974)

34 PETERSON, C. M., GRAZIANO, J. H., GRADY, R. W., JONES, R. L., ULASSARA, H. V., CANALO, V. C., MILLER, D. R. and CERAMI, A. Chelation studies with 2-3 dihydrobenzoic acid in patients with thalassemia major. *British Journal of Haematology*, **33**, 477–485 (1976)

35 PIOMELLI, S., KARPATKIN, M. H., ARZANIAN, M., ZAMANI, M., BECKER, M. H., GENOISER, N., DANOFF, S. J. and KUHNS, W. J. Hypertransfusion regimen in patients with Cooley's anemia. *Annals of the New York Academy of Sciences*, **232**, 186–192 (1974)

36 PIPPARD, M. J., WARNER, G. T., CALLENDER, S. T. and WEATHERALL, D. J. Iron absorption in iron loading anemias: effect of subcutaneous desferrioxamine infusions. *Lancet*, **1**, 737–739 (1977)

37 PIPPARD, M. J., CALLENDER, S. T. and WEATHERALL, D. J. Intensive iron chelation therapy with desferrioxamine in iron-loading anaemia. *Clinical Sciences and Molecular Medicine*, **54**, 99–100 (1978)

38 PROPPER, R. D., SHURIN, S. B. and NATHAN, D. G. Reassessment of the use of desferrioxamine B in iron overload. *New England Journal of Medicine*, **294**, 1421–1423 (1976)

39 PROPPER, R. D., COOPER, B., RUJA, R., NIENHUIS, A. W., ANDERSON, W. F., PUNN, H. F., ROSENTHAL, A. and NATHAN, D. G. Continuous subcutaneous administration of desferrioxamine for iron overload. *New England Journal of Medicine*, **297**, 418–425 (1977)

40 SEPHTON-SMITH, R. Chelating agents in the diagnosis and treatment of iron overload in thalassemia. *Annals of the New York Academy of Sciences*, **119**, 776–787 (1964)

41 SESHADRI, R., CULBATCH, J. H. and FISHER, R. Urinary iron excretion in thalassemia after desferrioxamine administration. *Archives of Disease in Childhood*, **41**, 195–199 (1974)

42 SIIMES, M. A. and DALLMAN, P. R. New kinetic for serum ferritin in iron metabolism. *British Journal of Haematology*, **28**, 7–18 (1974)

43 WALSH, J. R., MASS, R. E., SMITH, F. W. and LANGE, V. Desferrioxamine's effect on iron excretion in hemochromatosis. *Archives of Internal Medicine*, **113**, 435–441 (1964)

44 WAPNICK, A. A., LYNCH, S. R., KRAWITZ, P., SEFTEL, H. C., CARLTON, R. W. and BOTHWELL, T. H. Effects of iron overload on ascorbic acid metabolism. *British Medical Journal*, **3**, 704–707 (1968)

45 WAPNICK, A. A., LYNCH, S. R., CHARLTON, R. W., SEFTEL, H. C. and BOTHWELL, T. H. The effect of ascorbic acid deficiency of desferrioxamine-induced urinary iron excretion. *British Journal of Haematology*, **17**, 563–568 (1969)

46 WEINER, M., KARPATKIN, M., HART, D., SEZMAN, C., SHOBHANA, K. V., HENRY, W. L. and PIOMELLI, S. Cooley's anemia: high transfusion regimen and chelation therapy results and perspective. *Journal of Pediatrics*, **92**, 654–658 (1978)

12
Home therapy in hemophilia and Christmas disease

Jack Lazerson

INTRODUCTION

During the past 15 years, dramatic changes have occurred in the care and treatment of patients suffering from hemophilia[1, 3, 12, 13, 18, 32]. Two major events have accounted for these changes. The first was the discovery by Dr Judith Graham Pool of a technically simple and rapid method for the concentration of factor VIII (cryoprecipitate) from plasma[38] and the second a commitment by those involved in the care of patients with hemophilia to a philosophy of maximal care and treatment for such patients[7, 10, 21, 23, 29, 31, 52]. The former allowed rapid administration of factor VIII to sufficient hemostatic levels to correct the defect, not only to abort hemorrhagic episodes but to assure adequate hemostasis under any circumstances. With the availability of this product the concept of prophylactic infusion therapy became a reality, although plasma infusions had been attempted in the past for such purposes[36, 54]. Unfortunately, the use of cryoprecipitate continued to be confined primarily to hospital care, except for a few hemophilia programs that began to train patients to use and administer this material at home[27, 29, 40, 47]. Because it had to be kept frozen until use, similar to plasma, it remained a cumbersome product for use at home. Fortunately, a number of pharmaceutical companies undertook the refinement of cryoprecipitate to produce a commercially available lyophilized material that could be stored at routine refrigerator temperatures (2–8°C), as well as at room temperature, for variable periods of time prior to its reconstitution and use[26]. Availability of this material allowed more patients to assume home storage and infusion in order to treat hemorrhagic episodes at the earliest suspicion of bleeding[14]. Parenthetically, although the concept of self-care by patients afflicted with a chronic disorder is not a new concept[53], until the availability of a therapeutic product that could alter the natural history of this disorder, little attention was paid to use of this self-care concept for patients with hemophilia.

As a result of early treatment regimens, dramatic improvement in health care for hemophilia patients began to be reported[28, 33, 35, 39, 41, 49], and it remained for the medical community to define treatment schedules, dosage requirements, criteria and standards for care.

The second major event that altered the course of treatment for hemophilia was in part a direct result of the availability of therapeutic products and their use. This was the concept that for the best possible patient care a comprehensive approach by a team of individuals with various areas of expertise was necessary in the treatment of this disorder[6,15]. Specifically, it became clear that prior to the institution of a home care infusion program for any given patient, an extensive evaluation by a team was necessary. Based on a variety of guidelines, a definitive plan of action could be provided that would then maximize care for any given patient. Although there were some hemophilia centers practising this type of philosophy, their geographical availability limited access to the majority of patients with hemophilia. In the early 1970s, the National Hemophilia Foundation in conjunction with a number of physicians and personnel from hemophilia treatment centers convinced the Federal Government that the natural course of this disorder could be dramatically altered for the 15–20 000 severely afflicted patients if sufficient seed federal monies could be provided to support the development and establishment of comprehensive care hemophilia centers throughout the United States[34]. By 1976, such funding had became available and approximately 20 centers were delineated on a regional basis to provide the expertise in the organization and treatment for patients with hemophilia.

The purpose of this review is to describe for the practitioner of medicine the present state of the art in the treatment of patients with hemophilia as well as to provide rational guidelines for the role of the physician[11] and patient in their interactions with comprehensive care centers. No attempt will be made to review all of the currently available data, as there are a number of excellent monographs[8,16] and reports[22,37,48] describing not only the history of this disorder but also therapy of specific problems. Rather, this review will deal with a philosophical and pragmatic approach that the physician should provide for patients with hemophilia.

CLASSIFICATION

The hemophilias are defined as a group of inherited hemorrhagic disorders characterized by either a deficiency or a defect of a specific procoagulant protein necessary to form a hemostatic fibrin clot. *Table 12.1* shows the three basic types of hemophilia, their pattern of inheritance and their incidence. Hemophilia C, or factor XI deficiency, does not in general lead to a major hemorrhagic diathesis unless the factor level is less than 5 percent. Even in such cases, there appears to be very little, if any, relationship between the factor level and the clinical bleeding diathesis. Fortunately, this disorder is fairly rare although the gene frequency appears to be high in families of Jewish descent. Patients affected by this disorder who require treatment can be treated with fresh frozen plasma. A number of reports[26] dealing with this disorder have been published and will not be further discussed.

Table 12.1 Classification of the types of hemophilia

Type	Plasma factor	Inheritance	Incidence
A	VIII	X-linked recessive	$5-10 \times 10^{-5}$ males
B	IX	X-linked recessive	$2-5 \times 10^{-5}$ males
C	XI	Autosomal recessive	1×10^{-6} (10×10^{-5})*

*In Jewish population.

Table 12.2 Classification of the severity

Procoagulant factor level	Class	Clinical problem
<1(<0.01 units/ml)	Severe	Spontaneous hemarthrosis
1–5% (0.01–0.05 units/ml)	Moderate	Hemorrhage after trauma
>5%(0.05 units/ml)	Mild	Hemorrhage at the time of surgery
50–150% (0.5–1.5 units/ml)	Normal	

Regardless of the specific procoagulant factor defect, the hemophilias are classified as to severity (Table 12.2) by the level of plasma procoagulant factor obtained from the patient's plasma. In general, the severity of the observed clinical problems relates to the decrease of the biological activity[43]. Specifically, a patient with severe (less than 1 percent) hemophilia A (factor VIII) will not only have an easy bruisability syndrome and recurrent hemorrhagic episodes with minor trauma, but also frequent spontaneous hemarthroses. In contrast, patients with the milder form of hemophilia (more than 5 to 10 percent procoagulant activity) have little if any systemic manifestations of hemorrhage except under surgical conditions, i.e. dental extractions, minor or major surgery, and infrequently require infusion therapy.

From the available data, it would appear that by increasing the patient's procoagulant factor level to 10 percent, sufficient hemostasis can be achieved to abort most hemorrhagic episodes[2, 9, 51]. However, to maintain adequate hemostasis for surgical procedures, levels of at least 30 percent must be achieved, and in many circumstances levels in excess of 50 percent are required. Details of treatment will be discussed below.

TREATMENT

To the causal observer, the treatment of hemophilia may simply seem to involve having the appropriate factor concentrate available for infusion to correct the hemostatic defect and thereby negate or abort any hemorrhagic episode[26, 55]. Although this may be true – and in fact is the single major medical advance that has altered the natural history of this disorder – from a practical point of view, a number of ancillary factors play a significant role in allowing patients to avail themselves of medical therapy. It has been said that hemophilia is a disorder

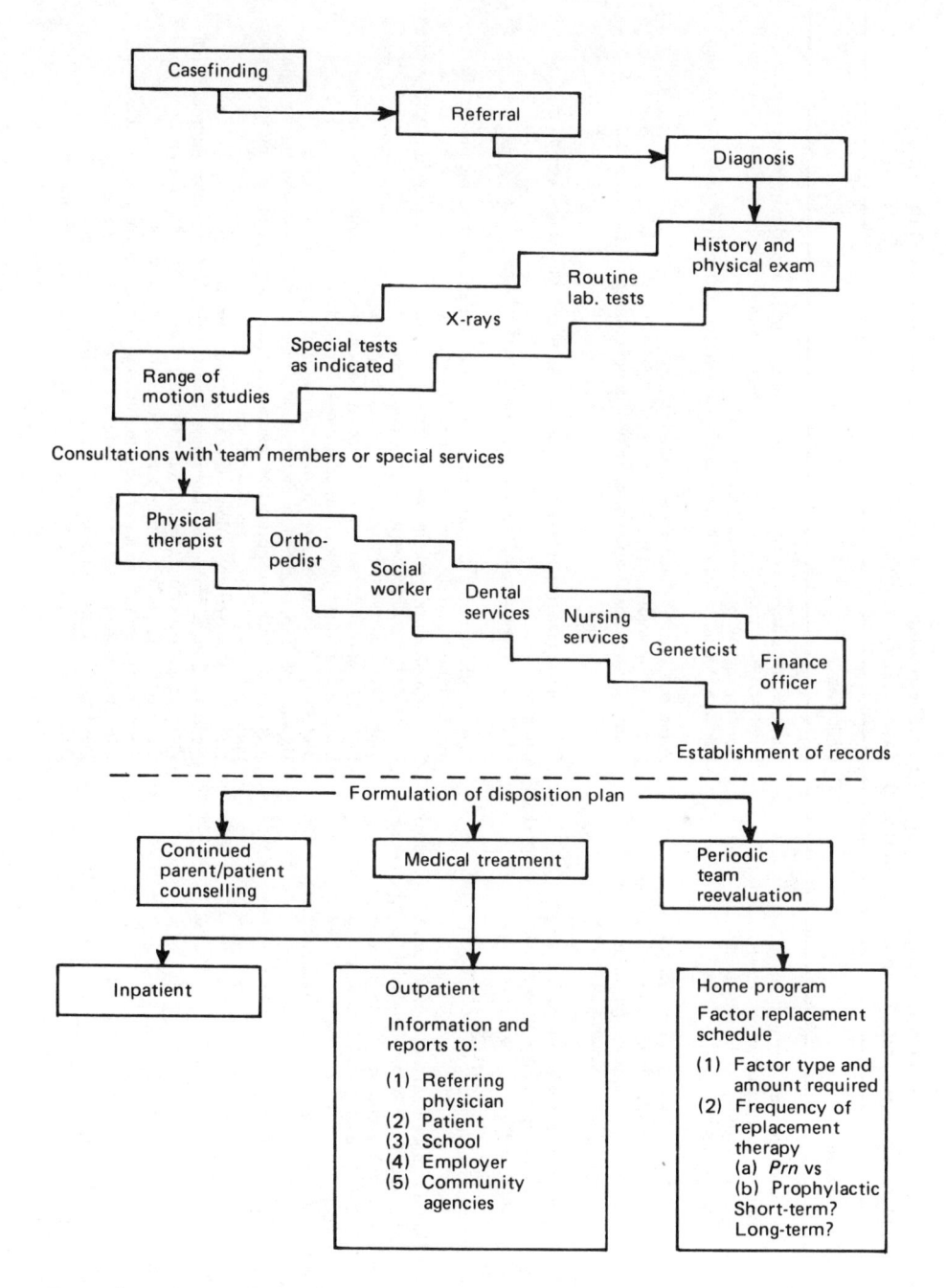

Figure 12.1 Comprehensive care approach to patients with hemophilia (Figure by A. Miller from Lazerson J: 'Prophylactic infusion therapy in hemophilia,' *Hospital Practice*, Vol. 14, No. 5, May 1979. Reproduced with permission)

Table 12.3 Basic information: living with hemophilia module (From *The Hemophilia Patient/Family Model*, courtesy of the Nursing Committee of the National Hemophilia Foundation and Baxter/Travenol Laboratories, 1982)

Topic	Explanation	Objectives
Definition	Normal coagulation versus defect in hemophilia (Optional: historical perspective of disorder; vasoconstriction, platelet plug formation, fibrin cascade system)	States what distinguishes person with hemophilia from one with normal coagulation Points out that hemophilia does NOT mean a person bleeds faster than normal but that bleeding may be prolonged if not treated Explains that apart from the coagulation defect, the patient is normal in most cases

Diagnosis	Method: blood test that measures clotting ability
	Meaning of results: diagnosis is permanent
	  type of disorder
	  severity of disorder
		Points out that this diagnosis is permanent
		States his type of hemophilia
		States his own classification of severity by his percentage of factor level

Manifestation	Implication of classification of severity Signs and complications of notable hemorrhages (see attached chart)	Explains the meaning of his severity classification as far as clinical symptoms are concerned Identifies signs and complications of notable hemorrhages
Treatment	No permanent cure Factor replacement therapy: definition, philosophy of early treatment, types of materials and their dosages and survival, method of administration, complications, record keeping, and supportive therapy Specific hemorrhages (see attached chart)	Shows understanding that no permanent cure is available at this time but that many manifestations and complications can be controlled States simple working definition of factor replacement, i.e. treating hemophilia with the factor that is defective in the patient's plasma States two reasons for early treatment of a hemorrhage Names type(s) of materials appropriate to patient for treatment of a hemorrhage States dosage that will be required for most hemorrhages States expected time of survival of factor material in his body Explains basic method of administering factor material, i.e. intravenous infusion Identifies at least two appropriate channels for receiving treatment (emergency room, parent) Lists at least two complications of factor replacement therapy Explains three advantages of keeping a record of bleeding episodes and treatments Patient regularly completes and submits a bleeding and treatment record Gives two examples of signs and treatments of notable bleeds Points out procedure necessary for treatment of minor superficial cuts and scrapes Gives two examples of comfort measures when treating a hemorrhage Has list of aspirin-containing and other contraindicated medications Patient consistently seeks early appropriate treatment for bleeding episodes

Genetics	Basic description of genetic patterns in hemophilia	Explains principle that carrier mother's son will have a 50% chance of having hemophilia and her daughter will have a 50% chance of being a carrier
States that all females born to a father with hemophilia will be carriers
Points out that a significant number of children born with hemophilia have no family history of the disorder, but once in the family it continues
States that factor classification remains the same in each family
General considerations	Financial
Comprehensive care
Defines the roles of participating treatment center team members
Inhibitor
Psychosocial
Dental
Exercise
Nutrition
Use of other medications
Preventive safety measures (i.e. approved car seats, sharp toys, gates on stairs)	Identifies methods of own financing coverage
Explains concept of comprehensive care in hemophilia
Evidences understanding of individual roles of treatment center team members
States definition and incidence of inhibitors
Lists advantages of wearing a medical identification tag/bracelet
Identifies at least one reason for contacting the hemophilia center prior to dental care
Explains three principles of good dental hygiene
Identifies three advantages of regular exercise
Explains need for good nutrition
Explains why aspirin and its compounds are contraindicated in the patient with hemophilia
Agrees to check with treatment center prior to using any medication not prescribed by them
Explains indication and side-effects of Amicar (aminocaproic acid)
Names three age-appropriate safety measures
Names person available to families who wish counseling

Goal: to provide the patient/learner with information which will allow for safe management of his disorder.
Note: this module should be the first covered with the learner.
Suggested instructors: physician, nurse, physician and nurse.

This test is to be used as a teaching tool only. You are not expected to know all the answers. You will not be graded on the results.

THE FOLLOWING QUESTIONS ARE ABOUT YOU OR YOUR FAMILY MEMBER WITH HEMOPHILIA. FILL IN THE BLANKS EITHER WITH A CHECK OR BY SUPPLYING THE CORRECT INFORMATION.

1. What type of hemophilia do you have?
   a. ___ Factor VIII defect (hemophilia A)
   b. ___ Factor IX defect (hemophilia B)
   c. ___ Other. Please specify _____

2. What is the level of severity of your hemophilia?
   a. ___ Mild (5–50%)
   b. ___ Moderate (1–5%)
   c. ___ Severe (less than 1%)

3. Do you have insurance coverage for factor replacement material?
   a. ___ Yes
   b. ___ No
   c. ___ Not sure

4. What type of factor material do you use? _____

5. What dosage of factor material do you use for most bleeding episodes? _____

THE REMAINING QUESTIONS WILL DEAL WITH HEMOPHILIA IN GENERAL. NOT ALL OF THEM WILL APPLY TO YOU DIRECTLY. PLEASE ANSWER THE QUESTIONS TO THE BEST OF YOUR ABILITY.

Multiple choice
In the following questions please place an X before each correct answer. There may be more than one correct answer for each question.
Example: Hemophilia is
   a. X genetic blood clotting disorder
   b. ___ a tropical plant
   c. X very rare in girls
   d. ___ I don't know

6. Symptoms of a joint bleed are the following
   a. ___ pain   d. ___ cold
   b. ___ nausea   e. ___ heat
   c. ___ stiffness f. ___ not sure

7. Factor concentrates
   a. ___ control or stop bleeding
   b. ___ contain clotting factor from normal blood
   c. ___ should only be used in extreme emergency
   d. ___ not sure

8. Use of factor concentrates can sometimes cause
   a. ___ hepatitis c. ___ allergic reactions
   b. ___ diabetes   d. ___ not sure

9. When a person thinks that he is beginning to bleed into a joint the *most important* thing to do is to
   a. ___ apply ice and ice bandages
   b. ___ wait and see if the bleeding will stop by itself
   c. ___ infuse with a factor replacement material
   d. ___ take pain medication
   e. ___ not sure

10. The reason(s) a patient with hemophilia should wear a medical identification tag or bracelet is/are to
    a. ___ alert his friends that he has a medical problem
    b. ___ alert medical personnel when the patient is unconscious
    c. ___ remind the patient he can't do things that other people do
    d. ___ not sure

11. A person with hemophilia should
    a. ___ eat a balanced diet
    b. ___ avoid all exercise
    c. ___ exercise regularly as directed by his doctor
    d. ___ take vitamin K supplements
    e. ___ not sure

12. A patient with hemophilia should keep a record of bleeding episodes and treatment for the following reason(s):
    a. ___ as an important part of his medical history
    b. ___ to remind him that he has a problem
    c. ___ so that the physician responsible for his care can supervise him properly
    d. ___ not sure

13. Factor replacement therapy is *usually* necessary in the following situations:
    a. ___ joint injury
    b. ___ bruising
    c. ___ head injuries
    d. ___ dental extractions
    e. ___ nose bleed
    f. ___ abrasions, such as a scraped knee
    g. ___ ileopsoas or retroperitonal bleed
    h. ___ not sure

True or false
Circle the true (T) false (F) answer appropriate to the following statements.
14. T F A person who has hemophilia bleeds faster than a normal person
15. T F When hemophilia is passed down from one generation to another the severity of the disorder usually varies individually
16. T F If carriers of hemophilia were prevented from giving birth to children the disorder would become extinct
17. T F All females born to fathers with hemophilia will be carriers of the disorder
18. T F Persons with hemophilia should be allowed to participate in most normal activites
19. T F Aspirin and factor replacement therapy are recommended for a painful joint hemorrhage
20. T F Regular tooth brushing and flossing are important for a person with hemophilia even if it causes some bleeding of his gums
21. T F Some patients outgrow hemophilia
22. T F If a patient with hemophilia has received a recent dose of factor material it is not necessary for him to wear a seat belt in the car.

Figure 12.2 Basic information: living with hemophilia; pre- and post-testing. (From *The Hemophilia Patient/Family Model*, courtesy of the Nursing Committee of the National Hemophilia Foundation and Baxter/Travenol Laboratories, 1982)

characterized by complex medical, psychosocial and financial problems. It therefore becomes necessary to discuss treatment as a complex modality that can best be approached and performed by a comprehensive care team. For all practical purposes, hemophilia centers have as one of their missions the availability of a multidisciplinary care team to evaluate and provide a treatment plan that will ultimately lead to a normalization of the patient's lifestyle[30]. As outlined in *Figure 12.1*, the elements of comprehensive care are listed not simply as an exercise but as a series of evaluations that must be performed in order to establish a data base from which a treatment plan can be derived. It is important to understand that 'normalization of lifestyle' is a relative term for hemophilia patients. What is meant, for the most part, is that patients 'are better off now than they were before' in regard to ease of treatment[20, 32, 42, 44, 45] and access to care with resultant avoidance of the consequences of untreated hemorrhagic episodes. Prior to outpatient and/or home therapy infusion programs, most hemophilia patients did not seek medical care unless life-threatening hemorrhage and/or pain from hemorrhage was significant enough to warrant it. As a result, the physical and psychosocial damage to most patients was great. Avoidance of medical care was the rule. The availability of rapid medical care to abort hemorrhage changed the relationship between patient and medical care community. It would appear that education of both the family and patient about the availability of appropriate treatment and a newer philosophy of care was the key to this change.

Emphasis on a comprehensive care team approach, educational programs for patients and families, and establishment of home care with self-infusion remain the basis for providing the maximum of care. For the pediatrician or physician who detects this disorder in a young patient, it is important to adopt a philosophy of early aggressive treatment. Therefore, it is important to start the educational program as soon as the diagnosis is established. In the United States, in conjunction with the National Hemophilia Foundation, the Hemophilia Educational Resource Project under the auspices of the Bureau of Maternal and Child Health has developed a highly effective didactic patient/family education module for training families and patients affected by this disorder. This module not only provides an excellent syllabus of material but follows the educational guidelines of using testing material to evaluate the learning process. In a more general sense, the module emphasizes the fact that the educational process requires a highly structured format to assure that the learner acquires information that can ultimately be used for the establishment of a successful home infusion program. *Table 12.3* and *Figure 12.2* are examples of the type of format and material being tested at a number of hemophilia centers in the United States.

Once the educational program has been instituted, the intravenous infusion program can be initiated with guidelines for successful completion as has been published[17]. Clearly, for most patients and their families, this latter step is what they are seeking and as such they may not realize that the former step is the critical and most important one. My experience would suggest that the I.V. training phase of the total care program is the easiest if a good foundation has been established by a strong educational program. The majority of problems that arise with home therapy are readily identifiable as to the infusionist and or patient not knowing the 'why's' of treatment rather than the technical 'how's'.

FACTOR CONCENTRATES

Table 12.4 lists the available therapeutic materials and some of their characteristics for treatment of hemophilia A and B patients. Regardless of which material is used, the biological effects are similar and dependent on achieving the same hemostatic level. The only differences between these materials, at the present time, relate to their ease of storage, reconstitutibility, and volumes administered. The biological half-life is similar to plasma or cryoprecipitate, i.e. 8 to 12 h. *In vivo* recovery of these materials varies from 60 to 100 percent and appears to be related to differences in the prepared lots. It should, however, be noted that there is a great

Table 12.4 Available therapeutic materials for treatment of hemophilia A and B

Product	Manufacturer	Storage requirements	Concentration of factors (units/ml)	Volume (ml)
Haemophilia A			*(VIII)*	
Fresh frozen plasma	Blood bank	Frozen at −20°C	0.5–1.5	225
Cryoprecipitate	Blood bank	Frozen at −20°C	4–8	10–15
Actif VIII	Merieux	RT or 2–8°C	5–20	50
Factorate	Armour	RT or 2–8°C	20–50	10–50
Hemophil	Hyland	RT or 2–8°C	25–35	10–30
Koate	Cutter	RT or 2–8°C	25–40	10–40
Profilate	Alpha	RT or 2–8°C	20–40	10–50
Hemophilia B			*(IX)*	
Fresh frozen plasma	Blood bank	Frozen at −20°C	0.6–1.3	225
Profilnine	Alpha	RT or 2–8°C	25–50	10–25
Konyne	Cutter	RT or 2–8°C	25–30	20
Proplex	Hyland	RT or 2–8°C	20–30	30

RT = Room temperature.

deal of difficulty in assaying factor VIII activity from commercially prepared materials, as the reference for this assay is based on normal plasma rather than concentrates 4b. In spite of this difficulty as well as the coefficient of variation of factor VIII assays, *in vivo* recovery appears reasonable for the product as labeled, although at least one report indicates major discrepancies of labeled assay and *in vivo* recovery[25]. A number of studies dealing with this problem are in progress and should within the next year provide reasonable guidelines as to the reliability and reproducibility of factor VIII unitage, as labeled on commercially available factor VIII material.

Dosage recommendations for treatment can be divided into three areas: prophylactic, as needed (p.r.n.) for early treatment, and surgical. *Table 12.5* lists treatment regimens used at present in a number of hemophilia centers. Although

Table 12.5 Dosage schedule

	Recommended dosage/infusion	
	Factor VIII	Factor IX
Prophylaxis	20–25 units/kg every other day	25–35 units/kg every third day
Early treatment	10–20 units/kg as needed (p.r.n.)	20–30 units/kg as needed
Surgical	50 units/kg preoperatively	100 units/kg preoperatively
	20–25 units/kg every 12 hours	40–50 units/kg every 24 hours
	100 units/kg preoperatively*	200 units/kg preoperatively*
	40–50 units/kg every 12 hours*	100 units/kg every 24 hours*

*Required for neurosurgical procedures.

very little scientific data are available as to the exact level of factor necessary to treat the various hemorrhagic manifestations of this disorder, the present guidelines suggest that early treatment of a suspected hemarthrosis requires approximately 10 units/kg per infusion. With such therapy, a second infusion may be required within 12 to 24 hours in 10 to 15 percent of cases, depending on the nature of the joint being treated[4a, 9]. Clearly, the current recommendation of 15–20 units/kg per infusion is more than adequate to abort the majority of suspected and/or early hemarthroses. Specific guidelines for soft tissue hemorrhage are more difficult to delineate, as many tend to be treated later in their course and may require repetitive doses during a 48–72 hour period. Once again, the clinical data suggest that single doses of 15–20 units/kg are more than adequate to abort and/or treat soft tissue hemorrhage, although it is suspected that much lower doses could be used if treatment were to occur earlier.

For patients undergoing surgical procedures, maintenance of relatively normal levels for 5 to 14 days is adequate, although duration of therapy relates to the type of surgical procedure, e.g. hernia repair or arthrodesis. Factor VIII replacement therapy during surgical procedures is primarily directed at maintaining adequate hemostasis, whereas the duration of therapy is directed at avoidance of hemorrhage during the patient's rehabilitative phase. Specifically, it would be prudent to provide adequate follow-up infusions until the patient returns to a relatively normal pattern of activity. As can be noted, neurosurgical procedures appear to require much higher factor levels to maintain hemostasis, for reasons that are not entirely clear. Caution should be used in treating hemophilia B patients with dosages in excess of 100 units/kg per 24 hours in view of the risk of thrombotic disease generated by infusion of factor IX concentrates. A number of reports have appeared relating thromboembolic disease to factor IX concentrate infusion and suggesting that an unknown factor (or a combination of factors) in this product induces intravascular coagulation predisposing the patient to clinical thrombosis. Anticoagulation with heparin in conjunction with high dosage factor IX replacement therapy has been recommended by some centers.

Prophylactic infusion therapy to completely prevent hemorrhage has been employed with varying degress of success depending on the dosage and frequency of administration[4, 19, 24, 30, 36, 46, 50]. It is the author's view that before any patient undertakes this form of treatment, specific guidelines as to need for treatment should be discussed. To date, although patients with this treatment regimen are known to do extremely well, no comparative data for early 'as needed' treatment regimens are available and/or indicate short-term (5 years) medical differences. The patient, family, physician and community must weigh the true costs, both financial and social, of complete prophylaxis with the currently available materials. Short periods of prophylaxis during times of high risk (sports activities, travel, etc.) combined with 'as needed' treatment may be preferable until data as to the long-term effects and consequences of these materials become available. Without these data, a great deal of concern remains as to induction of secondary disease as a result of chronic transfusion[56], i.e. chronic liver and/or renal disease.

SUMMARY

Improved therapy for hemophilia has clearly affected the lifestyle of patients suffering from the crippling effects of this disease. It has allowed patients to lead a physically and psychologically more 'normal' life, as the fears of major hemorrhages and their complications have been removed by the availability of replacement therapy. An air of optimism for young children affected with hemophilia now prevails. It would appear that newly diagnosed infants and children should have the opportunity to develop normally and to pursue lifestyles which do not differ greatly from those of their unaffected counterparts. Whether this can be achieved, and to what degree, remains to be seen. Clearly, the 15–20 year follow up of such patients will show whether the short-time gains of comprehensive care as presently dictated can be maintained.

References

1 ABILDGAARD, C. F. Current concepts in the management of hemophilia. *Seminars in Hematology*, **12**, 223–232 (1975)

2 ALLAIN, J. P. Dose requirement for replacement therapy in hemophilia A. *Thrombosis Hemostasis*, **42**, 825–831 (1979)

3 ALLAIN, J. P., ESTRABAUT, M. and TRAN, J. Traitement de l'hémophilie par l'autoperfusion. Etude clinique et psychologique. *Nouvelle Révue Française d'Hématologie*, **15**, 147–158 (1975)

4 ARONSTAM, A., ARBLASTER, P. G., RAINSFORD, S. G., TURK, P., SLATTERY, M., ALDERSON, M. R., HALL, D. E. and KIRK, P. J. Prophylaxis in hemophilia: a double-blind controlled trial. *British Journal of Haematology*, **33**, 81–90 (1976)

4a ARONSTAM, A., WASSEF, M., HAMAD, Z. and ASTON, D. L. The identification of high risk elbow hemorrhages in adolescents with severe hemophilia A. *Journal of Pediatrics*, **98**, 776–778 (1981)

4b BARROWCLIFFE, T. W. and THOMAS, D. P. Factor VIII standardisation. *Lancet*, **2**, 1342 (1981)

5 BIGGS, R. Recent advances in the management of hemophilia and Christmas disease. *Clinical Haemotology*, **8**, 95–114 (1979)

6 BOONE, D. C. (Editor) *Comprehensive Management of Hemophilia*, Philadelphia, F. A. Davis (1976)
7 BRECKENRIDGE, R. T. The therapy of classic hemophilia (factor VIII deficiency): past, present and future. *American Journal of the Medical Sciences*, **263**, 275–280 (1972)
8 BRINKHOUS, K. M. and HEMKER, H. C. (Editors) *Handbook of Hemophilia*, Part I and II. New York, American Elsevier Publishing Company (1975)
9 BRITTON, M., HARRISON, J. and ABILDGAARD, C. F. Early treatment of hemophilic hemarthroses with minimal dose of new factor VIII concentrate. *Journal of Pediatrics*, **85**, 245–247 (1974)
10 DIETRICH, S. L. Modern management of hemophilia and its implications for educational programs. *Journal of School Health*, **43**, 81–83 (1973)
11 EYSTER, M. E. Hemophilia: a guide for the primary care physician. *Postgraduate Medicine*, **64**, 75–82 (1978)
12 EYSTER, M. E., LEWIS, J. H., SHAPIRO, S. S., GILL, F., KAJANI, M., PRAGER, D., DJERASSI, I., RICE, S., LUSCH, C. and KELLER, A. The Pennsylvania hemophilia program 1973–1978. *American Journal of Hematology*, **9**, 277–286 (1980)
13 GILCHRIST, G. S. New advances in home treatment of hemophilia. *Medical Opinion*, March (1977)
14 GUENTHNER, E. E., HILGARTNER, M. W., MILLER, C. H. and VIENNE, G. Hemophilic arthropathy: effect of home care on treatment patterns and joint disease. *Journal of Pediatrics*, **97**, 378–382 (1980)
15 HILGARTNER, M. W. Comprehensive care of hemophilia. *Department of HEW Public Health Service Publication*, **(HSA) 79–5129** (1979)
16 HILGARTNER, M. W. (Editor) *Hemophilia in Children*. Publishing Sciences Group (1976)
17 HILGARTNER, M. W., AGLE, D. P., LAZERSON, J. and VAN EYS, J. *Home Therapy for Hemophilia: a Physician's Manual. The Treatment of Hemophilia*. National Hemophilia Foundation (1981)
18 HILGARTNER, M. W. Managing the child with hemophilia. *Pediatric Annuals*, **8**, 68–84 (1979)
19 HIRSCHMAN, R. J., ITSCOITZ, S. B. and SHULMAN, N. R. Prophylactic treatment of factor VIII deficiency. *Blood*, **35**, 189–194 (1970)
20 INGRAM, G. I. C., DYKES, S. R., CREESE, A. L., MELLOR, P., SWAN, A. V., KAUFERT, J., RIZZA, C. R., SPOONER, R. J. D. and BIGGS, R. Home treatment in haemophilia: clinical, social and economic advantages. *Clinical Laboratory Haematology*, **1**, 13–27 (1979)
21 JONES, P. Answering the needs of haemophilic children and their families. *Community Medicine*, July (1972)
22 JONES, P. Developments and problems in the management of hemophilia. *Seminars in Hematology*, **14**, 375–390 (1977)
23 KATZ, A. H. *Hemophilia: Study in Hope and Reality*, Springfield, Illinois, C. C. Thomas (1970)
24 KASPER, C. K., DIETRICH, S. L. and RAPAPORT, S. I. Hemophilia prophylaxis with factor VIII concentrate. *Archives of Internal Medicine*, **125**, 1004–1009 (1970)
25 KASPER, C. K. Problems with the potency of factor VIII concentrate. *New England Journal of Medicine*, **305**, 50–51 (1981)

26 LAZERSON, J. Clotting factor replacement. In *Enzymes As Drugs*, edited by J. S. Holcenberg and J. Roberts, 241–258. New York, Wiley and Sons (1981)

27 LAZERSON, J. Hemophilia home transfusion program: effect of cryoprecipitate utilization. *Journal of Pediatrics*, **82**, 857–859 (1973)

28 LAZERSON, J. Hemophilia home transfusion program: effect on school attendance. *Journal of Pediatrics*, **81**, 330–332 (1972)

29 LAZERSON, J. The prophylactic approach to hemophilia A. *Hospital Practice*, 99–109, February (1971)

30 LAZERSON, J. Prophylactic infusion therapy in hemophilia. *Hospital Practice*, 49–55, May (1979)

31 LEVINE, P. H. Effiacy of self-therapy in hemophilia. A study of 72 patients with hemophilia A and B. *New England Journal of Medicine*, **291**, 1381–1384 (1974)

32 LEVINE, P. H. Hemophilia and allied conditions. In *Current Therapy 1979*, 268–275. Philadelphia, W. B. Saunders (1979)

33 LEVINE, P. H. and BRITTEN, A. F. H. Supervised patient-management of hemophilia. *Annals of Internal Medicine*, **78**, 195–201 (1973)

34 National Heart and Lung Institute, National Blood Resource Program, Bethesda, Maryland. Summary report: NHLI's blood resource studies. June 30, *DHEW Publication*, (**HIH**) **73–416** (1972)

35 LE QUESNE, B., BRITTEN, M. I., MARAGAKI, C. and DORMANDY, K. M. Home treatment for patients with haemophilia. *Lancet*, **2**, 507–509 (1974)

36 NILSSON, I. M., BLOMBACK, M. and AHLBERG, A. Our experience in Sweden with prophylaxis on haemophilia. *Bibliotheca Haematologica*, **34**, 111–124 (1970)

37 PENNER, J. A. Therapeutic approaches to inhibitors: vitamin K-dependent factor concentrates. In *Haemophilia*, edited by V. Seligsohn, A. Rimon and H. Horoszowski, 97–106. New York, A. R. Liss (1981)

38 POOL, J. G. and ROBINSON, J. Observations on plasma banking and transfusion procedures for haemophilic patients using a quantitative assay for antihaemophiliac globulin (AHG). *British Journal of Haematology*, **5**, 17–23 (1959)

39 PROWSE, C. V. and CASH, J. D. The use of factor IX concentrates in man: a 9-year experience of Scottish concentrates in the south-east of Scotland. *British Journal of Haematology*, **47**, 91–104 (1981)

40 RABINER, S. F. and TELFER, M. C. Home transfusion for patients with hemophilia A. *New England Journal of Medicine*, **283**, 1011–1015 (1970)

41 RABINER, S. F., TELFER, M. C. and FAJARDO, R. Home transfusion of hemophiliacs. *Journal of the American Medical Association*, **221**, 885–887 (1972)

42 RABINER, S. F. and LAZERSON, J. Home management and prophylaxis of hemophilia. *Progress in Hematology*, **8**, 223–234 (1974)

43 RAINSFORD, S. G. and HALL, A. Clinical observations and their relationship to laboratory findings in the haemophilias. *Thrombosis et Diathesis Haemorrhagica*, **34**, 734–739 (1975)

44 RAINSFORD, S. G. and HALL, A. A three-year study of adolescent boys suffering from haemophilia and allied disorders. *British Journal of Haematology*, **24**, 539–551 (1973)

45 RAMSAY, D. M. and KHOO, K. K. A five-year study of a haemophilia reference centre. *Journal of Clinical Pathology*, **28**, 696–700 (1975)

46 RAMSAY, D. M. and PARKER, A. C. A trial of prophylactic replacement therapy in haemophilia and Christmas disease. *Journal of Clinical Pathology*, **26**, 243–247 (1973)

47 RIZZA, C. R. and SPOONER, J. D. R. Home treatment of haemophilia and Christmas disease: five years' experience. *British Journal of Haematology*, **37**, 53–66 (1977)

48 RIZZA, C. R. and MATTHEWS, J. M. Management of the haemophilic child. *Archives of Disease in Childhood*, **47**, 451–462 (1972)

49 SEELER, R. A., ASHENHURST, J. B. and LANGEHENNING, P. L. Behavioral benefits in hemophilia as noted at a special summer camp. *Clinical Pediatrics*, **16**, 525–529 (1977)

50 SHANBROM, E. and THELIN, G. M. Experimental prophylaxis of severe hemophilia with a factor VIII concentrate. *Journal of the American Medical Association*, **208**, 1853–1856 (1969)

51 STIRLING, M. L. and PRESCOTT, R. J. Minimum effective dose of intermediate factor VIII concentrate in hemophilia on home therapy. *Lancet*, **1**, 813–814 (1979)

52 STRAWCZYNSKI, H., STACHEWITSCH, A., MORGENSTERN, G. and SHAW, M. Delivery of care to hemophilic children: home care versus hospitalization. *Pediatrics*, **51**, 986–991 (1973)

53 TRAVIS, G. *Chronic Illness in Children. Its Impact on Child and Family*. California, Stanford University Press (1976)

54 VAN CREVELD, S. Prophylaxis of joint hemorrhages in hemophilia. *Acta Haematologica*, **45**, 120–127 (1971)

55 WHITE, G. C. II., LUNDBLAD, R. L. and KINGDON, H. S. Prothrombin complex concentrates: preparation, properties and clinical uses. *Current Topics in Hematology*, **2**, 204–244 (1979)

56 ZUCKERMAN, A. J. Viruses transmitted by blood clotting factors. In *Haemophilia*, edited by V. Seligsohn, A. Rimon, H. Horoszowski, 125–130. New York, A. R. Liss (1981)

13
Hemopoietic stem and progenitor cells: recent advances of physiopathologic relevance
C. Peschle

Hemopoietic tissues include both a lymphoid and a myeloid division. The latter comprises erythroid, granulocytic, eosinophilic, mast cell-basophilic, macrophage-monocytic and megakaryocytic lineages. This review is focused on the myeloid division, particularly on stem cells and progenitors of erythroid and granulomacrophage lineage.

DEVELOPMENT OF NEW TECHNOLOGY

Culture techniques

Hemopoiesis is a cell renewal system. A fraction of circulating blood cells is day-by-day replaced by newly produced elements, via homeostatic mechanisms modulating proliferation and differentiation of hemopoietic precursors.

Recent technology facilitates the investigation of the kinetics and control mechanisms of stem and progenitor cells. A crucial advance was represented by the development of an *in vivo* clonogenic assay for the stem element[185]. *In vitro* clonogenic assays for hemopoietic progenitors have been thereafter established[30, 119, 120, 143, 186]. In parallel, Dexter *et al.*[38] developed a culture technique allowing 'long-term' proliferation and differentiation of stem cells. An important experimental tool is also represented by hemopoietic lines, established from human or murine leukemias[12, 62, 96].

Clonogenic cultures in semi-solid medium

In these assays a progenitor cell, triggered by hemopoietic hormones, gives rise to a clonal colony (i.e. a progeny kept together in a network of agar, fibrin or methylcellulose). The number of colonies depends upon (1) the number of progenitors and (2) the hormonal activity(ies). The clonal origin of these colonies has been demonstrated by certified markers (glucose-6-phosphate dehydrogenase (G-6-PD) isoenzymes[156], sex chromosomes[178], etc.), as well as in unicellular cultures[92]. Strict clonality is insured in the presence of a low colony number, but not in overcrowded cultures[173].

The *in vitro* clonogenic techniques allowed identification of the progenitors of the various myeloid lineages, and further provided a large body of exceedingly useful information (*see* pp. 267–278). These assays, however, are subject to various limitations. Indeed, the culture medium includes elevated concentrations of fetal calf serum (FCS), which allows colony growth via obscure mechanisms, thus confusing both methodology and interpretation. It is emphasized however that, in murine[89] (*Figure 13.1*) and human[66] cultures, FCS may be effectively replaced by

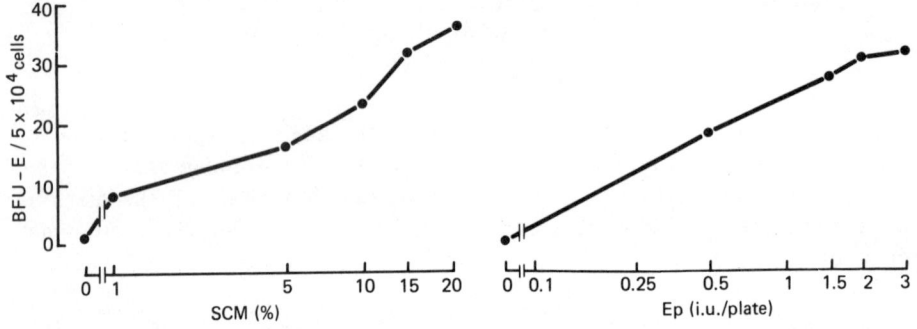

Figure 13.1 Growth of marrow BFU-E from CD1 mice in 'FCS-free' methylcellulose cultures: SCM (i.e., BPF) and Ep dose/response curves (number of bursts/hormonal activity), respectively in presence of plateau Ep or SCM levels. SCM = lectin-stimulated spleen conditioned medium from normal mice (containing 2 percent FCS, *see* [198]). Ep: Step III sheep hormone. FCS was replaced by deionized, delipidated bovine serum albumin (16 mg/dish), pure human transferrin (0.42 mg) and a lipid mixture (6 µl)[89]

its active constituents (albumin, selenium, iron-saturated transferrin, a lipid mixture, hemopoietic hormone(s)). Further confusion derives from impurity of the hemopoietic hormones plated routinely (erythropoietin (Ep), burst-promoting factor(s) (BPF)*, colony-stimulating factors (CSF)), and interactions between progenitors and other coseeded cells. Most important, culture experiments should always be corroborated by parallel *in vivo* observations, in order to exclude *in vitro* artefacts. All these aspects are dealt with in subsequent sections.

Long-term cultures in liquid-phase

These suspension cultures allow the proliferation and differentiation of normal splenic colony-forming units (CFU-S), which is dependent upon establishment of an underlayer of adherent cells[38]. In fact marrow murine cells[38, 39, 42, 47, 191],

---

* Also termed burst-promoting activity, burst-feeder activity, burst-enhancing factor or erythroid-potentiating activity.

cultured in a medium containing serum and hydrocortisone (10^{-7} mol/l)[71] at 33°C, rapidly form a foundation layer of adherent elements. These are a heterogenous population, which comprises large fat elements, macrophages, fibroblasts, endothelial cells, stem and progenitor cells, etc.[39]. Fat elements are hydrocortisone-dependent[71] and essential to maintain the system.

The intricate interplay between these adherent elements may reproduce in part the in vivo hemopoietic microenvironment[191]. Indeed, CFU-S and progenitors apparently proliferate in strict contact with the other adherent cells[191]. Stem and progenitor cells produced in the underlayer are shed in the overlayer medium[38], but only to a minor extent[111]. The underlayer may be in part substituted by a matrix of collagen gels[106].

In order to meet the metabolic requirement of these cultures, half of the supernatant is removed each week, and substituted by fresh medium[38]. This procedure entails depopulation of supernatant cells, which in turn provokes enhanced proliferation of stem cells in the underlayer[191] (see p. 271).

Long-term cultures for human and simian stem cells have been similarly developed[63, 80, 124, 126] (in the hamster species, however, adherent cells are not apparently required for prolonged stem cell proliferation[44]).

In these cultures, CFU-S differentiate prevailingly into the granulomacrophage pathway. In the murine system CFU-S and granulomacrophage CFU (CFU-GM) are maintained over a 3-month period or longer. Erythropoietic differentiation is expressed upon addition of crude Ep preparations (also containing BPF) or serum from irradiated, phenylhydrazine-treated anemic mice (containing presumably both BPF and Ep)[42, 47]. In human cultures CFU-GM are maintained for up to 2–3 months[80, 126] or 6 months[63], erythroid progenitors only for the initial 1–2 month period[63, 80, 124]. Lymphopoiesis is also present in both the murine[93] and human[80] system.

Deterioration of the cultures is characterized by a marked increase of the number of macrophages in supernatant and fibroblasts in the underlayer, as well as by the detachment of adherent cells[124].

Hemopoietic cell lines

Analysis of recent advances in this area[62, 96] is clearly beyond the scope of this review. It may be mentioned, however, that neoplastic T-lymphocyte or macrophage lines, grown in serum-free cultures, may soon provide a vast supply of various hemopoietic hormones (see p. 275). T lymphocytes, stimulated to release CSF and then fused with T lymphoma cells, were grown as a cell line producing CSF which was indistinguishable from the physiologic hormone[84].

Murine GM-progenitors derived from long-term cultures grow for at least several months in liquid phase, if CSF-rich medium is supplemented daily[40]. Similarly, sustained proliferation of GM-progenitors fractionated from normal human marrow is apparently observed in liquid cultures containing endogenous CSF, if supplemented with hydrocortisone and vitamin D (R. Gallo, personal communication). These studies clearly indicate that GM-progenitors are endowed with at least some self-renewal capacity.

Molecular aspects

In both ontogeny and cytogeny, cell differentiation is characterized by 'determination' and then 'maturation' of the differentiating elements. Stem cells are undetermined, i.e. endowed with the potential to feed into a wide spectrum of different cell lineages. Differentiation of stem cells is marked by gradual restriction of their pluripotent capacity, and an inverse rise of their determination or commitment to one or more lineages. Finally, differentiating cells enter irreversibly into a particular lineage, thereby initiating their specialization or maturation, i. e. expression of lineage-specific molecular markers.

The genetic programs underlying cell differentiation have not yet been unveiled[37]. In this regard, the hemopoietic system may provide a unique model to investigate these aspects. Indeed, recently developed genetic techniques, applied to hemopoietic cell populations, have already provided invaluable information. An example is the rearrangement of immunoglobin genes in the course of B lymphocyte maturation[85, 168]. Also of interest is the expression of the gene cluster coding for the non-α globin chains of Hb (5'-$^G\gamma$-$^A\gamma$-δ-β-3'): a transcriptional wave seems to progress along this gene sequence in both ontogenesis and adult erythroblastic maturation, as if cytogeny may recapitulate ontogeny[32, 153, 155a]. Most important, active globin genes in chicken embryos are apparently characterized by both an altered conformation and undermethylation[200]. Active globin genes in humans may also be undermethylated[193]. Last but not least, pioneer techniques for gene insertion have allowed successful transformation of cell lines[116], and more important of hemopoietic stem cells *in vivo*[31, 116, 117].

The genetic progam underlying hemopoietic differentiation is expressed by synthesis of multiple molecular markers, which characterize specific differentiation stages and/or cell lineages. In this regard, an area of particular interest is

Table 13.1 Expression of selected antigens on human hemopoietic stem and progenitor cells (After Fitchens et al.[57])

Antigen	Stem and progenitor cells		
	Stem cell	*BFU-E/CFU-E*	*CFU-GM*
HLA-A, B			
Allotypic	NR	NR	+
Common heavy-chain	NR	+*	+*
β_2-Microglobulin	NR	+	+
Ia-like (HLA-DR)	**	−/+	+*
T lymphocyte	−	−*	−*
Common ALL	−	−	−
Little i	NR	+	**
ABO	−	−	−

NR = Not reported.
*Confirmed with monoclonal antibody.
**Inconclusive results.

represented by cell surface markers[57, 160] (*Table 13.1*), and particularly by membrane receptors for hemopoietic hormones (*see* p. 273). Development of hybridoma technology[97] will greatly facilitate analysis of these surface markers. Furthermore, their recognition by fluoresceinated probes (monoclonal antibodies, lectins, etc.) should allow rapid cell sorting and improved cell purification[17, 128, 133]. This approach may in turn provide large numbers of homogeneous hemopoietic cells, which would be amenable to molecular analysis. Indeed, molecular studies on hemopoietic differentiation have been largely hampered so far by the heterogeneity of the analysed populations.

STEM AND PROGENITOR CELLS
The model of hemopoiesis

Stem cells are capable of extensive self-renewal, and also of differentiating into various progenitors. These are 'commited' to either myeloid (erythroid, granulocytic, eosinophilic, mast cell-basophilic, macrophage-monocytic, megakaryocytic) or lymphoid lineages[30, 119, 120, 143, 186]. Progenitors in turn give rise to the respective differentiated cell series. *In vivo*, hemopoietic elements are compartmentalized in specific sites (bone marrow, spleen, etc.), where they are intermixed with stromal cells. These are not the progeny of hemopoietic stem elements[55].

The *pluripotent stem cell* generates both myeloid and lymphoid progeny. Its existence has been demonstrated by means of radiation-induced chromosomal aberrations[11, 205]. In these studies marrow cells were irradiated and injected into stem cell deficient mice. Unique abnormalities of chromosomes were often demonstrated in both myeloid and lymphoid tissues[1].

The pluripotent stem cell may give rise to stem elements restricted to the myeloid lineages or the T lymphocytic one (*Figure 13.2*). This is suggested by occasional experiments whereby radiation-induced chromosomal aberrations were observed only in either myeloid lineages or T lymphocytes[1].

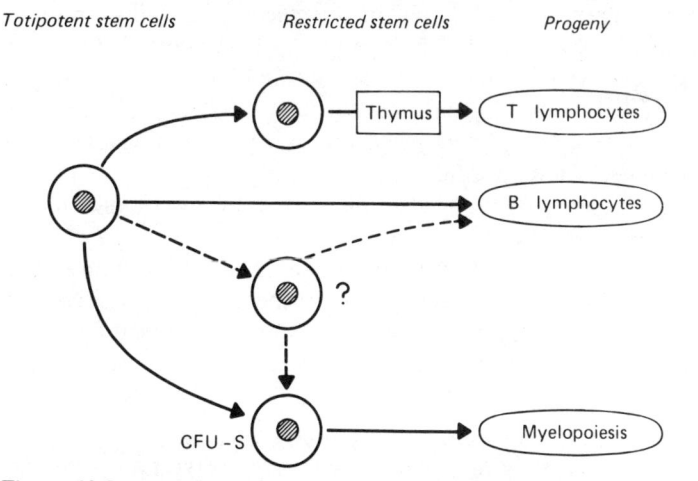

Figure 13.2 A model of hemopoietic stem cells. Interrupted lines indicate uncertain differentiation pathways. For further details, *see* text

Hemopoietic stem and progenitor cells

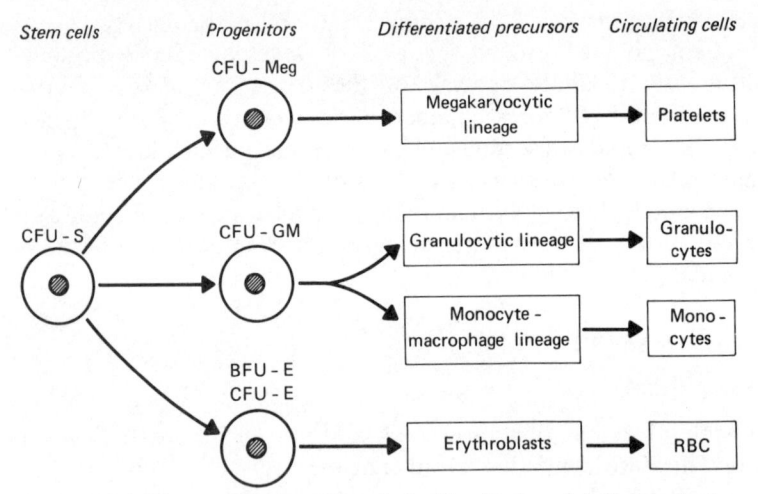

Figure 13.3 The model of myelopoiesis. For further details, see text

An important marker for stem cells is represented by G-6-PD isoenzymes[52,53] (A and B), which are coded by allelic genes in the X chromosome. Heterozygous females are functional mosaics, i.e. either one of the isoenzymes is expressed in individual cells. In polycythemia vera[2] (PV), chronic myelogenous leukemia[55] (CML) and essential thrombocythemia[54] heterozygous females show an homogeneous G-6-PD pattern in myeloid cells as compared with a heterogeneous one in fibroblasts. This indicates that these disorders derive from an abnormal myeloid stem cell, which gives rise to a clonal myeloid progeny. In the chronic phase of CML, the homogeneous 'myeloid' G-6-PD pattern is extended to B, but not T lymphocytes[52,53]. Accordingly, at least some myeloid stem cells might apparently function as B lymphocyte stem elements (*Figure 13.2*).

The *myeloid stem cell* (*Figure 13.3*) has been assayed in mice on the basis of its capacity to form macroscopic, mixed colonies in the spleen of lethally irradiated animals (CFU-S)[185]. These colonies are of clonal origin[14]. They contain all myeloid lineages, but not B and T lymphocytes (and perhaps not even lymphoid progenitors[105,138]) (cf. [186]). In semisolid cultures, murine[123] and human[51] stem cells generate mixed colonies, which contain erythroid, GM- and megakaryocytic lineages. In human colonies, T lymphocytes are occasionally present upon addition of their specific growth factor[51]. This suggests that these mixed colonies may in part derive from pluripotent stem cells.

Two erythroid *progenitors*, erythroid burst-forming unit(s) (BFU-E) and CFU-E, have been identified in mammals[7]. These give rise respectively to large colonies ('bursts') or small clusters of erythroblasts. Bursts are largely composed of CFU-E colonies*. BFU-E represent early erythroid progenitors, which differentiate into CFU-E. These precursors in turn feed into the erythroblastic pool.

*Very large, macroscopic murine bursts usually comprise granulocytic, erythroid and megakaryocytic series[85a]. Large ones often include both erythroid cells and megakaryocytes[197]. Small bursts, however, contain only erythroid elements[46]. Thus, murine CFU-S undergoing erythroid differentiation sequentially lose the potential to feed into the granulo- and then the megakaryopoietic lineage.

It is generally conceded that BFU-E are closely related to the CFU-S compartment[197]. Thus, BFU-E and CFU-S are characterized by identical cell size and buoyant density[197], although BFU-E show a slightly more elevated cycling activity[46, 86] than the slowly-proliferating CFU-S[104]*. BFU-E→CFU-E differentiation is characterized by a further increase of proliferative rate, as well as of pool amplification, cell size and buoyant density[46, 86, 197].

In both humans and mice, Eaves et al.[46] identified a third erythroid precursor, the 'mature' BFU-E (M-BFU-E), which is apparently intermediate between 'primitive' BFU-E (P-BFU-E or simply BFU-E) and CFU-E with respect to all the above parameters†.

The kinetics of CFU-E and proerythroblasts partially overlap, which suggests a close relationship between these elements[74].

A continuous spectrum of erythroid progenitors has been thus demonstrated. Their differentiation entails a gradual increase of their number, proliferative activity, cell size and density†. A further differential marker is progressive enhancement of Ep sensitivity, and decrease of response to BPF[45, 46, 87, 197] (*Figure 13.4*).

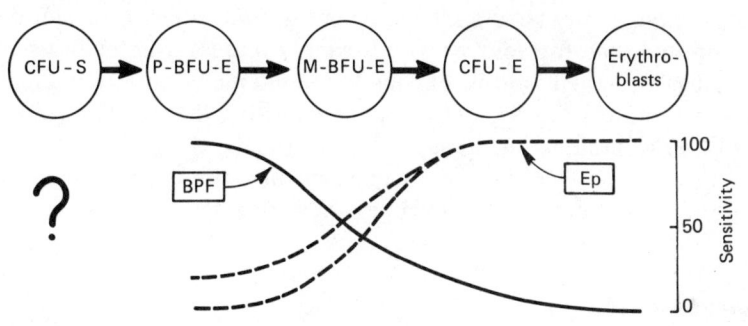

Figure 13.4 Sensitivity of erythroid progenitors to erythropoietic hormones (BPF, Ep), arbitrarily expressed as percentage of peak values. The Ep influence on early erythroid progenitors apparently differs among mammalian species and strains of mice (*see* text)

Similarly, a spectrum of *GM-progenitors* has been demonstrated[19, 20]. Their differentiation is also characterized by gradual increase of proliferative rate, cell size and density[19, 20]. Analysis of these aspects, however, is rendered difficult by the heterogeneity of GM-colonies (including G-, M- and GM-colonies) and CSF preparations (*see* [24] and p. 271). Murine CFU-GM are bipotential: they differentiate into unipotent CFU-G or CFU-M upon prolonged stimulus by pure GM-CSF or M-CSF respectively[121] (*see* p. 271). Here again, differentiation of progenitors entails a gradual restriction of their potential to feed into different cell lineages.

CFU-S, BFU-E and CFU-GM have been demonstrated in the *circulating blood* of humans[27, 136] and mice[159, 195]. These elements are apparently confined in the null lymphocyte blood fraction[131].

* It is apparent that some 'BFU-E' are in fact CFU-S. In the murine system, late-developing macroscopic 'bursts' are indeed mixed colonies (*see above*) which also contain CFU-S (i.e. derive from a stem cell undergoing both self-replication and differentiation)[85a].
† In mice, however, the M-BFU-E pool is not larger than that of P-BFU-E[86].

The number of circulating stem cells and CFU-GM is sharply increased by treatment with 'mobilizing' agents (endotoxin, lectins, dextran)[29, 204].

Stress erythropoiesis in humans and mice is associated with marked expansion of the pool of circulating CFU-S and BFU-E[77, 135, 155]. This suggests an increased traffic of these elements between different erythropoietic areas. Stress erythropoiesis in mice is associated with apparent migration of CFU-S and BFU-E from marrow to spleen via blood[77, 155]. This may contribute to the massive expansion of splenic erythropoiesis, observed under these conditions.

In conclusion, solid evidence has allowed an articulate model of hemopoiesis to be postulated (*Figures 13.2* and *13.3*). This model, although universally accepted, is still clouded by uncertainties. Stem or progenitor cells comprised within the same pool are fairly homogeneous when tested by 'cellular' criteria (clonogenic features, size and density, response to hemopoietic hormones, etc.). However, they may prove heterogeneous if subjected to molecular analysis. It is not possible to ascertain whether or not stem cells derive from an even less differentiated compartment[165], since an assay for this hypothetical population is not available. Other types of restricted stem cells, i.e. for both B and T or only B lymphocytic lineage may exist, although they have not been demonstrated so far. It cannot be excluded that pluripotent and myeloid stem cells simply represent an emergency reservoir, which plays a limited role in day-by-day hemopoietic differentiation: indeed, early GM-progenitors are apparently endowed with self-renewal capacity in the presence of CSF-containing medium[40] (cf. p. 265). The transition between different compartments is considered as strictly undirectional: this is not necessarily true for stem cell pools, and perhaps not even for those of early progenitors.

Hemopoietic hormones and inhibitors

Ep

The erythropoietic rate is largely or solely regulated by Ep[70, 99, 141], a glycoprotein hormone recently purified (molecular weight ~39 000 daltons[125]). Ep specifically induces differentiation of late erythroid progenitors to the recognizable erythroid compartment[56]. It also provokes an accelerated maturation of erythroblasts[176]. In stress erythropoiesis, enhanced Ep activity causes skipping of terminal divisions, and therefore macrocytosis[176].

The CFU-E compartment is amplified in face of elevated Ep levels, while depleted by suppressed Ep activity in transfusion-induced polycythemia[74, 86, 144, 145, 181, 192, 199]. The size of this pool is thus directly correlated with Ep activity. *In vitro*[88], and presumably *in vivo* as well[143], Ep allows survival of CFU-E. It is still debated whether or not Ep levels modulate BFU-E kinetics (pool size, cycling activity). In some murine strains, the Ep action on M-BFU-E is of minor significance, that on P-BFU-E is virtually absent (*Figure 13.4*)[7, 77, 86-88, 192, 196-199]. In other strains, however, the Ep influence on M-BFU-E is marked, and a transient action on P-BFU-E may be present (*Figure 13.4*)[144, 145, 181]. The Ep action on murine BFU-E is thus clearly strain-dependent, via a genetic mechanism[91]. In human marrow cultures, the Ep sensitivity of P-BFU-E is apparently very low, but low, but the hormonal response is gradually enhanced at the M-BFU-E and CFU-E level[45, 154].

The regulatory role of Ep is thus well-documented, both *in vivo* and *in vitro*[70, 99, 141]. Additionally, it has been confirmed by identification of polycythemic and anemic conditions mediated, at least in part, via excessive or defective Ep activity respectively[70, 99, 141].

BPF

Medium conditioned by T lymphocytes and/or macrophages contains glycoprotein factor(s) enhancing burst growth (BPF or BPA)[87, 88, 196, 197]. A murine BPF of ~24 000 daltons molecular weight has been purified to apparent homogeneity (G. Wagemaker, personal communication), via a 7-step chromatography procedure. In murine cultures, BPF allows survival of primitive BFU-E[87, 198]. It modulates the cycling activity of these early progenitors[198], as well as their differentiation to the M-BFU-E and perhaps the CFU-E stage[87, 198, 199] (*Figure 13.4*). In human[66] and perhaps murine[49] marrow cultures, it may also stimulate CFU-E growth in conjunction with Ep. The *in vivo* role of BPF is still under scrutiny (*see below*).

CSF

Survival, proliferation and differentiation of CFU-GM in culture is controlled by the level of CSF[24]. Two murine hormones have been purified: GM-CSF[23] triggers mainly G-colony formation, while M-CSF[175] induces M-colony growth. A G-CSF specific for G-colony growth has been recently identified, but not yet purified[132a]. GM-CSF forces resting CFU-GM into cycling and shortens the doubling time of GM-cells[24]. Although various murine GM-CSF show different molecular weight (m.w.) values, all had an homogeneous m.w. of ~23 000 daltons after neuraminidase or dodecyl sulfate treatment[132]. Purified M-CSF (m.w. ~70 000) is apparently composed of two subunits, each of m.w. 35 000[175].

Human CSFs have also been at least in part purified[24] (m.w. ~40 000–50 000 daltons). They stimulate proliferation of human (and occasionally murine) CFU-GM and also, in some instances, that of lymphocytes and endothelial cells[24].

The role of CSF *in vivo* is discussed below.

'CFU-S factor(s)'

In murine long-term cultures, regulation of CFU-S proliferation is apparently mediated by the balance between two opposing factors: the first one stimulates and the second one inhibits stem cell proliferation[191]. The former is elevated in culture medium during the initial phase after depopulation of the overlayer cells (cf. p. 265), which is associated with enhanced stem cell cycling[191]. The latter is elevated during the subsequent period, characterized by stem cell quiescence[191]. Moreover, an inhibitory or a stimulatory CFU-S factor can be purified respectively from the medium conditioned by normal or regenerating marrow[108, 109]. These factors exert their respective actions on CFU-S cycling when supplemented into long-term cultures[191].

Interestingly, Wagemaker[198] has apparently separated a glycoprotein of m.w. ~24 000 daltons, which modulates CFU-S cycling and is released by murine spleen T lymphocytes and/or macrophages (see below).

The role of BPF in vivo, and even more so, that of the putative 'CFU-S factor(s), is uncertain. Even the function of CSFs in vivo is not yet fully elucidated[24]. However, it is generally conceded that, in the hemopoietic microenvironment, these hormones exert regulatory roles similar to those documented in vitro. It is often suggested that small amounts of hemopoietins might be released by producer cells to act on closely-located target elements.

The role of these hormones in vivo has not yet been demonstrated by *direct* experimental evidence, i.e. injection in vivo of purified hormone or anti-hormone IgG. In the case of CSFs, these experiments have been repeatedly attempted, but failed to demonstrate the in vivo action of these hormones[119, 120], probably due to technical limitations[24]. Further observations are urgently needed to clarify these crucial aspects.

The role of CSF in vivo is *indirectly* but strongly supported by consensual fluctuations of CSF serum levels and granulopoietic activity[24, 119, 120]. A role for BPF in vivo may be suggested by its enhanced activity in cultures of splenic P-BFU-E from erythroleukemic mice infected by Friend virus (polycythemic or anemic strain)[146]. The BPA rise in vivo may underlie the erythropoietic type of these leukemias[146]. A role for a humoral 'CFU-S factor(s)' in vivo is suggested by observations on stem cell kinetics in diffusion chambers implanted in mice with subcutaneous inflammation and secondary myeloid hyperplasia[182].

Furthermore, no *human disease* documented so far can be related to excessive or defective production of these glycoproteins. An exception is apparently represented by cyclic neutropenia, whereby CSF serum levels fluctuate consensually with granulopoietic activity[75].

Confusion exists on the *identity* or not of BPF, GM-CSF and 'CFU-S factor(s)'. In unicellular cultures of fetal murine cells, massive amounts of pure GM-CSF stimulate CFU-S to proliferate, and in part differentiate into the erythroid lineage[122]. This may suggest either identity of these three factors or presence of a few CSF receptors on CFU-S. Alternatively, large amounts of plated GM-CSF might mimic the action of the other hormones (see below).

In human cultures, GM-CSF and BPF are seemingly distinct[1a, 66]. It has also been observed that a murine T lymphocyte cell line releases BPF, but virtually no CSF (*Figure 13.5*). Most important, Wagemaker[198] separated, via polyacrylamide gel electrophoresis, several glycoprotein hormones of ~24 000 daltons, which affect early hemopoiesis. Although in need of confirmatory evidence, these observations apparently identified: (1) a factor modulating CFU-S proliferation; (2) BPF; and (3) GM-CSF, which modulates growth of early CFU-GM. More distal progenitors of either granulocytic and macrophage or erythroid lineage would be mainly controlled by G- and M-CSF or Ep respectively[198].

The chemical similarity of different hormones affecting early hemopoiesis may in part explain the confusion of their possible identity. The similarity may underlie their capacity to mimic each other partially, particularly if plated in massive

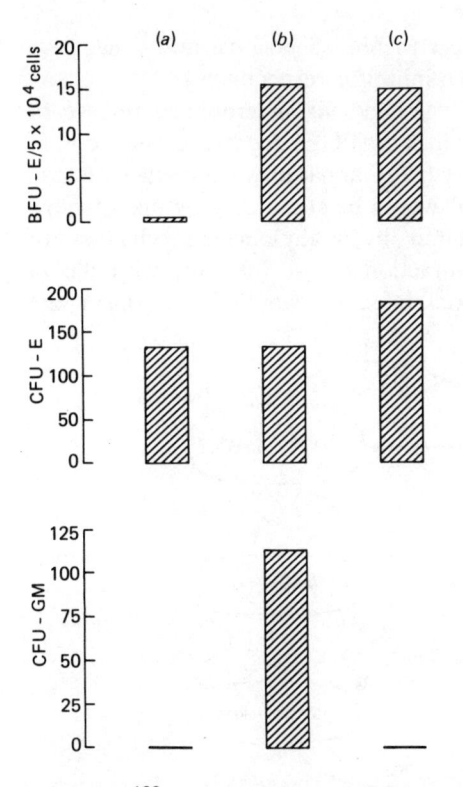

Figure 13.5 Growth of BFU-E, CFU-E and CFU-GM in FCS-free methylcellulose cultures (cf. *Figure 13.1*) upon addition of (a) Ep; (b) Ep + SCM (lectin-stimulated normal mouse spleen conditioned medium[198], containing both BPF and GM-CSF); and (c) Ep + medium conditioned by a T lymphocyte cell line (containing BPF but not GM-CSF). The line was kindly provided by Cudkowicz, G. (Buffalo, NY, USA)

amounts[122]. In phylogenetic development, these glycoproteins may derive from a single ancestor hormone, via gene duplication and subsequent mutations modifying different parts of the primitive molecule.

The *molecular mechanism of action* of hemopoietic hormones is still largely unknown. It is generally conceded that they may interact with surface receptors on hemopoietic target cells. This concept, however, is largely extrapolated from evidence on non-hemopoietic hormones. Some light has been shed on the mechanism of action of Ep[68, 69, 201]. This is apparently mediated via[68, 69]: (a) interaction of Ep with a putative membrane protein receptor; (b) activation of a protein cytoplasmic factor transferring the hormonal message to the genome; (c) transcription of specific RNA molecules. These results have been confirmed with pure Ep rigorously free of endotoxin[201]. Gangliosides in CFU-GM membranes may in part function as GM-CSF receptors[107], a mechanism suggested for other glycoprotein hormones.

Hemopoietic inhibitors

A balance between stimulatory and inhibitory factors might modulate the kinetics of stem and progenitor cells.

As mentioned above, CFU-S kinetics in long-term cultures is apparently regulated by this type of balance[191]. Axelrad[6a] recently suggested that the cycling activity of murine P-BFU-E is modulated by a protein inhibitor, controlled by the Fv-2 locus (determining susceptibility or resistance to Friend leukemia virus).

Thus, P-BFU-E proliferation may be subject to both a positive and a negative control mechanism (i.e. BPF and the protein inhibitor respectively).

CFU-M kinetics (*Figure 13.6*) may be controlled via macrophage release of either stimulatory (GM-CSF, M-CSF) or inhibitory (PGE) agents, respectively, in the face of low or high macrophage cellularity (PGE apparently exerts its effect via cAMP)[103, 140]. CFU-G kinetics (*Figure 13.6*) would be stimulated by macrophage release of GM- and G-CSF, and inhibited by granulocyte production of lactoferrin[21, 22, 103, 140], apparently via interaction of the inhibitor with the Ia antigen in CFU-G membrane[21, 22]. Bacterial infection would both trigger the

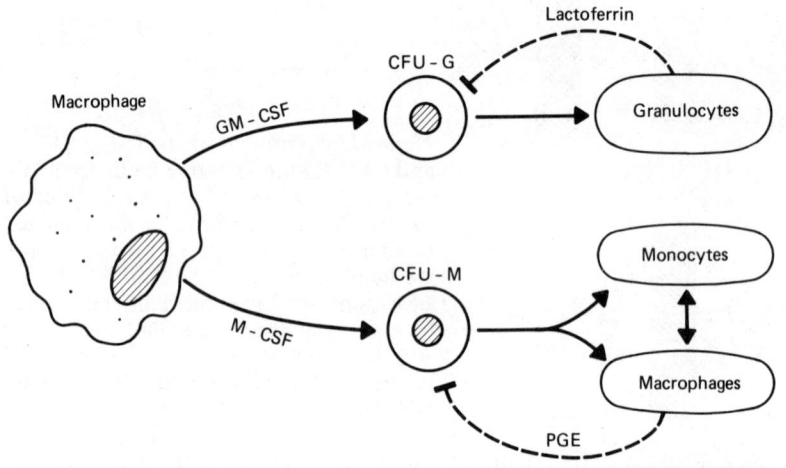

Figure 13.6 Kinetic regulation of CFU-G and CFU-M, according to Moore *et al.*[21, 103, 140]. Stimulatory (→) and inhibitory (---) influences are indicated. For further details, *see* text

former mechanism and dampen the latter one, thus leading to granulocytosis[140]. This attractive model is still under close scrutiny, particularly with regard to the lactoferrin component[24].

A possible role for the PGE–cAMP complex in the regulation of erythropoiesis is under analysis. These agents inhibit cloning of murine BFU-E, but stimulate that of human BFU-E (perhaps via interaction with macrophage and resulting BPF release)[162]. Recent experiments on murine BFU-E grown in 4 percent FCS cultures indicate that PGE exerts an inhibitory action at elevated dosages (10^{-6} mol/l) compared with a stimulatory effect at lower levels (10^{-8} mol/l) (C. Peschle, in preparation). The former phenomenon may be mediated via a direct action on BFU-E, the latter one via release of BPF by macrophages.

Studies on other inhibitors of erythropoiesis have unfortunately yielded a large number of uncertain results[70, 99, 141].

Production of hemopoietic hormones: the T lymphocyte–macrophage complex

In adult mammals, Ep is produced by the kidney[61, 90, 147] and liver[60, 151], which represent respectively its major and minor source. Thus, Ep control of adult erythropoiesis is largely or solely of long-range type. The liver is the main or exclusive Ep source in the mammalian fetus[151, 166, 206], thereby suggesting a short-range control of fetal erythropoiesis.

Fetal and adult Kupffer cells, and perhaps adult marrow macrophages, may play a role in Ep production[139, 152, 158] (see also below). In this regard, Bessis[15] postulated a functional erythropoietic unit in adult marrow, the 'erythroblastic island'. This structure is apparently characterized by a central macrophage surrounded by a crown of erythroblasts, which become gradually more differentiated from the center to the periphery. Erythroblastic islands have been also observed in long-term murine cultures (T. M. Dexter, personal communication).

Further insight into the biogenesis of Ep shall presumably derive by introduction of a recently-produced monoclonal antibody against Ep (E. Goldwasser, personal communication).

The T lymphocyte–macrophage complex is probably involved in production of BPF, GM- and M-CSF in the hemopoietic microenvironment*. Indeed, monocytic/ macrophage[4, 203] or T cell lines[66, 84] (see also [24] and *Figure 13.5*) produce these factors. More important, murine or human mononucleated cells from spleen, lymph node or peripheral blood, release these glycoproteins *in vitro*, particularly when either irradiated[196] or stimulated by lectins[6, 87, 123, 198] and allogeneic cell antigens[167]. Helper T cells and macrophages apparently cooperate in the process. In this regard, a helper T cell line of clonal origin and known antigenic specificity releases these glycoproteins upon both stimulation with specific antigen, and presence of accessory cells, apparently of macrophage type[167].

The T lymphocyte–macrophage complex may also release inhibitory factors, in physiological conditions[21, 22] as well as in aplastic anemia (cf. p. 280–281). T lymphocytes exerting either a stimulatory or an inhibitory action on erythroid progenitor growth coexist in murine thymus[98] and human peripheral blood[187a].

The mechanism(s) underlying release of hemopoietins and inhibitors by T lymphocytes and/or macrophages is totally unknown. Hypothetically, different clones of T lymphocytes might recognize different antigens on the membrane of early hemopoietic cells. The antigens would be selectively expressed in various stages of hemopoietic proliferation and/or differentiation. A specific antigen recognition may induce a particular clone of T lymphocytes to proliferate and release a specific hemopoietin or inhibitor, thus leading to modulation of stem and progenitor cells kinetics.

Physical interactions in the hemopoietic microenvironment

The role of physical interactions between hemopoietic cells, possibly via electrochemical or electrotonic influences at the level of cell membranes, is still unknown. Physical contact between stem and adherent cells in long-term cultures may modulate the cycling activity of the stem elements (see p. 265). It is

---

* Fibroblasts and endothelial cells are also capable of producing GM-CSF and/or M-CSF *in vitro*[24]. On the other hand, the T lymphocyte–macrophage system might release Ep, and perhaps other 'hemopoietins' (see above).

conceivable that physical interactions play a significant regulatory role in the hemopoietic microenvironment, which is characterized by a strikingly heterogeneous multitude of closely located cells.

Models for stem cell differentiation

The studies mentioned above give some insight into the regulation of stem and progenitor cells kinetics (*Figures 13.4* and *13.5*). However, the mechanism(s) underlying stem cell differentiation is still totally unknown.

A model of stem cell differentiation envisions 'hemopoiesis engendered randomly'[187]. Accordingly, stem cell proliferation, i.e. self-renewal and/or differentiation to the various hemopoietic lineages, occurs at random. Clone-to-clone variations occur stochastically. Instructive microenvironmental influences would modulate this process only in a *lax* way. This hypothesis is supported by marked variations of the number of stem and progenitor cells in different colonies generated by CFU-S in spleen[73] or in culture[85a].

An alternative model is based on the concept of a 'hemopoietic inductive microenvironment'[35]. According to this, stem cell differentiation is *strictly* controlled by the particular microenvironmental influences, represented by specific hormonal and/or cellular stimuli. In particular, the myeloid stem cell might be endowed with different receptors for various hemopoietic hormones[194]. If this were the case, competition between these hormones should take place. This competitive phenomenon has been observed at elevated (more than 10^5 cells/plate)[194], but not low (5×10^4 or less)[86], cell concentrations. Once again, purified stem cell populations, pure hemopoietic hormones and FCS-free cultures are required to probe effectively these intimate aspects.

An intriguing hypothesis has been suggested by Holtzer et al.[83], according to which asymmetric divisions ('quantal mitosis') may occur in early erythropoiesis: the two daughter cells would either become committed to terminal differentiation or remain uncommitted. Theoretically, stem cells might similarly undergo asymmetric divisions. Each asymmetric mitosis would generate a stem and a differentiating cell, thus explaining the capacity of stem elements for both self-renewal and hemopoietic differentiation. On the other hand, some stem cell divisions may be of a symmetric type, i.e. give rise only to either differentiating or uncommitted elements. Hypothetically, the mechanism(s) modulating the ratio between symmetric and asymmetric divisions may be of intrinsic and/or extrinsic type, thus leading again to the 'stochastic' and/or the 'microenvironment' model for stem cell differentiation.

A recent, interesting concept[161] postulates a linkage between stem cell proliferation and ontogenesis, whereby stem elements are capable only of a critical number of self-replicating divisions. After this number has been reached, the stem cell undergoes irreversible hemopoietic differentiation. Its part in blood formation is taken up by the next oldest stem cell, which is reaching the critical number of mitosis. The evidence supporting this 'generation-age' concept is still only indirect[161].

Ontogenic aspects

A detailed review of studies on fetal liver stem and progenitor cells is beyond the scope of this chapter. However, recent observations on fetal erythroid progenitors seem worthy of consideration.

Erythroid precursors generating colonies in semisolid cultures have been recently identified in human fetal liver[79, 163]. These reports included preliminary observations on their clonogenic properties. In recent studies[154], erythroid progenitors from 18 fetal livers in the 7–15-week gestational period were grown in methylcellulose cultures (additional experiments were carried out on 13 normal adult marrows, as well as 1 fetal, 15 neonatal and 26 adult blood specimens). Three classes of progenitors (P-BFU-E, M-BFU-E, CFU-E) have been thereby identified in fetal liver (and their presence confirmed in adult marrow[45]). Identification was based on their differential clonogenic characteristics, i.e. colony morphology and number, time/growth curve, differential Ep and BPF sensitivity, [^{3}H]thymidine suicide index *in vitro*. The multi-step differentiation of fetal erythroid progenitors is associated with: (1) gradual amplification of their pool size; (2) progressive decline of their BPF response; and (3) gradual enhancement of their Ep sensitivity. These findings are consistent with the concept[70, 99] that fetal erythropoietic activity is modulated by Ep. It is also apparent that BPF may play a similar regulatory role in both fetal and adult life.

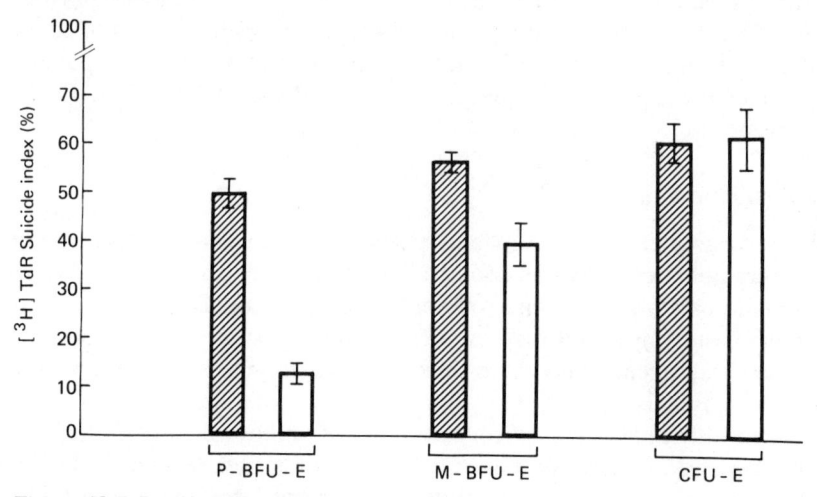

Figure 13.7 Proliferative rate (mean ± SEM values) of erythroid progenitors from human fetal liver (▨) and adult marrow (□), as evaluated on the basis of the percentage of cells in DNA synthesis (i.e., killed by [^{3}H-]TdR *in vitro*). (Reprinted by permission from C. Peschle *et al.*[154] courtesy of the Editor and Publishers, *Blood*)

Marked differences are observed, however, between the characteristics of corresponding fetal and adult erythroid progenitors[154]. Firstly, differentiation of adult precursors entails a gradual increase in their proliferative rate, while all fetal progenitors are characterized by maximal cycling activity (*Figure 13.7*). Interestingly, the doubling time of cells in fetal bursts (~19–21 h, mean value) is distinctly lower than in adult ones (~30–33 h), while intermediate values are observed in cord blood bursts (~25 h). These observations suggest that ontogenic maturation of the erythron is associated with a progressive decline in (1) proliferative activity of early and intermediate erythroid progenitors, and (2) cell doubling time in erythropoietic differentiation. Secondly, adherent cells apparently play a key role in BPF production in adult marrow cultures, but not in fetal liver ones. In the adult, the T lymphocyte–macrophage complex is apparently involved in hemopoietic hormone production (see p. 275). The placenta may release large amounts of the hormonal modulators of early hemopoiesis (cf. ref.[25], also our unpublished results). Finally, the sensitivity to added Ep on fetal CFU-E and M-BFU-E is apparently more elevated than that of corresponding adult progenitors.

APLASTIC ANEMIA

Congenital aplastic anemia (Fanconi's anemia)

This hereditary disorder is characterized by bone marrow hypoplasia leading to pancytopenia, multiple congenital malformations and increased spontaneous chromatin breakage[13,50].

Bone marrow cultures have uniformly shown a marked decrease of the number of both erythroid and GM-progenitors[58,110]. This is also observed in non-anemic patients[36]. Allogeneic bone marrow transplantation may induce complete normalization of the clinical condition, although most transplanted patients died of acute GVHD[65]. These findings strongly imply a functional defect of the stem cell pool of 'intrinsic' type (see below). This may be possibly related to a defect of the DNA repair mechanism[157,164].

Acquired aplastic anemia

This syndrome is characterized by peripheral pancytopenia, caused by fatty atrophy of bone marrow, and hence hypoplasia of all myeloid lineages. The syndrome should not include cases with: (1) marrow infiltration by neoplastic cells (myelophtisis) or fibroblasts (myelofibrosis), or (2) recent exposure to radiation and cytostatic drugs, i.e. agents known to induce constantly a transient marrow aplasia[142].

It is estimated that ~50 percent of cases are of unknown etiology[48]. The remainder have been exposed to either long-past radiation, chemical agents (benzene derivates, etc.), toxic drugs (choloramphenicol, etc.), infection (viral hepatitis), or else diagnosed for paroxymal nocturnal hemoglobinuria or antecedent autoimmune diseases[48]. Only a minority of these types of patients develop aplastic anemia; a genetic factor may therefore operate in its pathogenesis. In this regard, a small dose of choloramphenicol induced aplastic anemia in two pairs of identical twins[16,129].

On the basis of current concepts on hemopoiesis, aplastic anemia clearly derives from a functional defect of myeloid stem cells, leading to impaired differentiation into the myeloid lineages. Indeed, cultures of marrow or blood have constantly shown deficient cloning of stem cells[76], BFU-E[134] and CFU-GM[72] (see also below).

Latent and overt stem cell damage

A reduced number of stem and progenitor cells may still support an almost normal hemopoiesis. In chronically-irradiated mice, a 90–95 percent depleted CFU-S pool can sustain a near-normal erythropoietic rate[18]. Similarly, patients recovering from aplastic anemia show a decreased number of BFU-E[134] and CFU-GM[94] in marrow and blood, in spite of absence of erythroid and granulopoietic hypoplasia.

A depleted stem cell pool may thus sustain a near normal hemopoiesis via enhanced proliferation. This compensatory mechanism, however, cannot operate indefinitely, in that the proliferative potential of stem cells is limited. In this regard, mice chronically treated with busulfan show initially a decrease of the number of CFU-S and CFU-GM in marrow, which is not associated with granulopoietic hypoplasia[127]. After several months, further depletion of CFU-S and CFU-GM pools to less than 1 percent of the control value leads to frank marrow aplasia[127]. The limited proliferative potential of stem cells is also indicated by the progressive decline of their repopulating capacity after serial transplantations[34].

These findings suggest that in aplastic anemia a distinction may be established between *latent* and *overt* stem cell damage. The former condition would be characterized by depletion of the pools of stem and progenitor cells in the presence of near-normal hemopoiesis (as evaluated by standard hematological parameters in marrow and blood); and the latter one by a more marked and/or prolonged depletion of stem and progenitor cells, which causes hypoplasia and frank peripheral pancytopenia.

Intrinsic versus extrinsic mechanisms

On a theoretical basis, a stem cell defect may be attributed to either 'intrinsic' or 'extrinsic' mechanisms. An 'intrinsic' mechanism was thought to operate in the W/W^v mouse[115] (i.e., its CFU-S are unable to colonize sublethally irradiated normal recipients, whereas normal CFU-S generate efficiently mixed splenic colonies in W/W^v recipients). Recently, transplantation of normal T lymphocytes in W/W^v mice cured their anemia[202], thus suggesting that an immunological defect contributes to the disease (*see below*). A typical model for stem cell defect of 'extrinsic' type is provided by the Sl/Sl^d mouse[115]: its CFU-S show normal colony-forming capacity in normal recipients, but normal stem cells do not generate effectively spleen colonies in recipient Sl/Sl^d mice. Similarly, Dexter-type long-term cultures showed that a W/W^v adherent layer allows growth of Sl/Sl^d progenitors[41]. It is apparent, therefore, that a microenvironmental defect is responsible for this type of anemia.

A possible role for stromal factors in marrow hypoplasia has been suggested by studies involving local irradiation of bone marrow[33,95]. The irradiation induced a prompt aplasia, via death of stem cells. This was followed by restoration of hemopoiesis, mediated by stem cell migration from unirradiated areas into aplastic marrow. A second aplastic period was observed two months later: it was suggested that it results from progressive damage of the slowly proliferating sinusoidal cells.

In line with this concept, restoration of hemopoiesis was observed following curettage and local transplantation of syngeneic marrow. It cannot be excluded that, in some idiopathic or drug-induced aplastic anemia cases, extensive destruction of marrow sinusoids might be caused by an immune reaction (*see below*).

Autoimmune mechanisms in aplastic anemia

Several reports[169, 174, 184] indicated that in patients with aplastic anemia recovery may occasionally follow treatment with immunosuppressive agents (usually anti-lymphocyte globulin). In parallel, pioneer studies showed that coculture of aplastic anemia lymphocytes with normal marrow induced suppression of normal CFU-E growth[81]. Similarly, removal of lymphocytes from aplastic marrow enhanced its CFU-GM cloning capacity, while cocultures of both aplastic and normal marrow were characterized by defective growth of normal CFU-GM[5]. These findings led to the hypothesis that cellular autoimmune mechanisms may play a crucial role in some cases of aplastic anemia.

Both lines of evidence, however, were soon clouded by serious reservations. Spontaneous recovery is known to occur in aplastic anemia, thus casting doubt on the significance of the recovery observed after immunosuppressive therapy. Coculture studies were also subjected to sharp criticisms. In this regard, most patients are subjected to transfusion, which causes lymphocyte sensitization; in cocultures, aplastic anemia lymphocytes may exert a cytotoxic effect against normal progenitors. Indeed, blood lymphocytes from 12 of 34 transfused patients with aplastic anemia inhibited the growth of HLA-identical normal BFU-E, while those from 8 non-transfused cases did not[188]. A similar discrepancy was observed for CFU-GM[171]*. These aspects have been carefully analysed in a dog model. In DLA-identical dogs, a single transfusion from a littermate can induce T lymphocyte sensitization in the recipient[190]. The sensitization was shown to reduce erythroid colony formation when donor marrow is coincubated with recipient lymphocytes[190]. Furthermore it was predictive of graft rejection following transplantation of the recipient dog with donor marrow[189].

Recent studies suggest however that, in *some* aplastic anemia cases, a cellular autoimmune mechanism may indeed operate. Thus, mononuclear blood cells (of lymphocytic-macrophage type) from *untransfused* patients exert occasionally an inhibitory action on growth of cocultured normal BFU-E and/or CFU-GM[172, 179, 183]. As previously mentioned, this inhibition was not observed in another series of untransfused cases[188]; in these patients, however, autologous marrow cultures showed that T cell depletion usually provoked BFU-E proliferation, which was inhibited again upon T cell addition[188]. In patients in remission, mononuclear blood cells of macrophage type[134] or purified marrow T lymphocytes[8,9], suppressed growth of *autologous* BFU-E[134] or CFU-GM[8,9]. In the latter studies, T lymphocytes with IgG receptors (T_{G+}) were apparently responsible for the inhibitory action[9]. Most important, medium conditioned by either normal T_{G+} stimulated by

---

* In some studies even lymphocytes from transfused cases were not inhibitory[180].

lectin[8] or T_{G+} from aplastic anemia in the absence of lectin[9] exerted an inhibitory effect on cloning of *autologous* CFU-GM. It is possible, therefore, that CFU-GM proliferation is physiologically regulated by T_{G+} released inhibitor(s) (*see* p. 275), the production of which would be uncontrolled and hence severely inhibitory in aplastic anemia. Finally, a positive correlation was documented between clinical response to immunosuppressive therapy and tests for suppression of growth of *autologous* progenitors by T lymphocytes *in vitro*[10].

Recent results on marrow transplantation among identical twins strongly confirm that autoimmune mechanisms operate in some cases of aplastic anemia. In this regard, engraftment of HLA-compatible marrow occurs in a large majority of non-transfused patients[177]. However, this does not necessarily imply that an 'intrinsic' stem cell defect is cured by replacement with normal CFU-S; indeed, allogeneic transplantation is always associated with massive immunosuppressive therapy, which may abolish an 'extrinsic' inhibitory mechanism. This dilemma is bypassed in studies on identical twins. In two cases, transplantation of aplastic anemia with identical twin marrow allowed engraftment in the absence of immunosuppressive treatment[3]. This clearly indicates a stem cell defect of 'intrinsic' type. In two other observations, however, treatment with cyclophosphamide was necessary to allow the engraftment[3]. Furthermore, mononuclear blood cells from the recipient inhibited growth of donor BFU-E and CFU-GM[3]. This strongly suggests that extrinsic mechanism(s), possibly of autoimmune cellular type, contributed to the genesis of aplastic anemia in these two patients.

Conclusion

Although the pathogenesis of aplastic anemia is still under scrutiny, it may be suggested that, in some patients, the stem cell is intrinsically defective, as a result of exposure to physicochemical or viral agents. The damage, possibly favored by a genetic factor, may be first latent and then overt. In some cases, an 'extrinsic' mechanism may operate, via T lymphocyte- and/or macrophage-mediated inhibition. In this regard, the inhibitory role of T_{G+} under normal conditions and in aplastic anemia deserves further scrutiny. Finally, the possibility cannot be excluded that other mechanisms (stromal defects, immunocomplexes[26] etc.) may play a significant role in a small fraction of patients.

PURE RED CELL APLASIA (PRCA): CONGENITAL (BLACKFAN-DIAMOND SYNDROME) AND ACQUIRED TYPE

Congenital PRCA (*Blackfan–Diamond syndrome*) is a rare condition[43] of unknown pathogenesis. The presence of humoral inhibitors has been first suggested[137] then denied[64]. Peripheral lymphocytes from these patients, co-incubated with normal marrow, inhibit CFU-E colony formation[82]. However, the inhibitory phenomenon has not been observed in other cases[59]. As in aplastic anemia, results are obscured by the possibility of transfusion-induced sensitization in the examined patients (*see* p. 280). Interestingly, a transient erythroblastic crisis after anti-lymphocyte globulin therapy has been observed in one case[113]. Adequately controlled studies are clearly necessary to elucidate the pathogenesis of this disease.

Adult PRCA is a rare condition, characterized by near absence of erythroblasts in an otherwise normal marrow. A mild decrease of the number of platelets or leukocytes in peripheral blood is occasionally observed[102, 150]. PRCA is often coexistent with thymoma, various immunological abnormalities and/or autoimmune diseases (hemolytic anemia, myasthenia gravis, etc.). Thymectomy induces a remission in 25–30 percent of PRCA cases harboring a thymic tumor[102, 150]. PRCA may be successfully treated with immunosuppressive agents[102, 114, 150] or repeated plasmapheresis[118].

These clinical observations concur with the concept of a humoral autoimmune pathogenesis in PRCA, as indicated by frequent presence of a serum IgG inhibitor(s) to erythropoiesis[102, 150]. In this regard, the IgG fraction inhibits heme synthesis in both autologous and allogeneic marrow cultures, thus excluding the possibility of a transfusion-induced sensitization[100, 102, 114, 150]. The IgG inhibitor exerts a cytotoxic action on erythroblasts[101] but also inhibits CFU-E and BFU-E growth (CFU-GM are however unaffected) (PRCA *type I*)[118, 148]. In some cases, it may inhibit even murine erythroid progenitors[148]. In exceptional patients, the IgG inhibitor seems to interact with circulating Ep (PRCA *type II*), which is then nearly absent in spite of low hematocrit values[114, 149]. In occasional cases PRCA represents a preleukemic condition (PRCA *type III*), progressing to acute myeloid leukemia[150]; an IgG inhibitor has not been reported in these patients[150]. Finally, the rare cases of PRCA associated with chronic lymphocytic leukemia (PRCA *type IV*) may be mediated via a T lymphocyte autoimmune mechanism[112, 130].

Acknowledgements

Supported by Grants from Volkswagen Foundation, Hannover; EURATOM (No. BIO-C-353-I), Bruxelles; CNR, Rome (Progetto Finalizzato Controllo Crescita Neoplastica, No. 80.01615.96, 81.01437.96).

References

1 ABRAMSON, S., MILLER, R. G. and PHILLIPS, R. A. The identification in adult bone marrow of pluripotent and restricted stem cells of the myeloid and erythroid systems. *Journal of Experimental Medicine*, **145**, 1567–1579 (1977)

1a ABBOUD, C. N., BRENNAN, J. K., BARLOW, G. H. and LICHTMAN, M. A. Hydrophobic absorption chromatography of colony-stimulating activities and erythroid-enhancing activity from the human monocyte-like cell line, GCT. *Blood*, **58**, 1148–1154 (1981)

2 ADAMSON, J. W., FIALKOW, P. J., MURPHY, S., PRCHAL, J. F. and STEINMAN, L. Polycythemia vera: stem cell and probable clonal origin of the disease. *New England Journal of Medicine*, **295**, 913–916 (1976)

3 APPELBAUM, F. R., FEFER, A., CHEEVER, M. A., SANDERS, J. E., SINGER, J. W., ADAMSON, J. W., MICKELSON, E. M., HANSEN, J. A., GREENBERGER, P. D. and THOMAS, E. D. Treatment of aplastic anemia by bone marrow transplantation in identical twins. *Blood*, **55,** 1033–1039 (1980)

4 ASCENSAO, J. L., KAY, N. E., EARENFIGHT-ENGLER, T., KOREN, H. S. and ZANJANI, E. D. Production of erythroid potentiating factor(s) by a human monocytic cell line. *Blood*, **57,** 170–173 (1981)

5 ASCENSAO, J., KAGAN, W., MOORE, M., PAHWA, R., HANSEN, J. and GOOD, R. Aplastic anemia: evidence for an immunological mechanism. *Lancet*, **1,** 669–671 (1976)

6 AYE, M. T. Erythroid colony formation in cultures of human marrow; effect of leukocyte conditioned medium. *Journal of Cellular Physiology*, **91,** 69–78 (1977)

6a AXELRAD, A. A., CROIZAT, H. and ESKINAZI, D. A washable macromolecule from $Fv2^{rr}$ marrow negatively regulates DNA synthesis in erythropoietic progenitor cells BFU-E. *Cell*, **26,** 233–244 (1981)

7 AXELRAD, A. A., McLEOD, D. L., SHREEVE, M. M. and HEATH, D. S. Properties of cells that produce erythropoietic colonies *in vitro*. In *Hemopoiesis in Culture*, edited by W. A. Robinson, 226–234. Washington, GPO (1974)

8 BACIGALUPO, A., PODESTÀ, M., MINGARI, M. C., MORETTA, L., PIAGGIO, G., VAN LINT, M. T., DURANDO, A. and MARMONT, A. M. Generation of CFU-C/suppressor T cells *in vitro*: an experimental model for immune-mediated marrow failure. *Blood*, **57,** 491–496 (1981)

9 BACIGALUPO, A., PODESTÀ, M., MINGARI, M. C., MORETTA, L., VAN LINT, M. T. and MARMONT, A. M. Immune suppression of hematopoiesis in aplastic anemia: activity of T-gamma lymphocytes. *Journal of Immunology*, **125,** 1449–1543 (1980)

10 BACIGALUPO, A., PODESTÀ, M., VAN LINT, M. T., VIMERĆATI, R., CERRI, R., ROSSI, E., RISSO, M., CARELLA, A., SANTINI, G., DAMASIO, E., GIORDANO, D. and MARMONT, A. M. Severe aplastic anemia: correlation of *in vitro* tests with clinical response to immunosuppression in 20 patients. *British Journal of Haematology*, **47,** 423–433 (1981)

11 BARNES, D. W., FORD, C. E., GRAY, S. M. and LOUTIT, J. F. Spontaneous and induced changes in cell populations in heavily irradiated mice. *Progress in Nuclear Energy (Biol.)*, **2,** 1–10 (1959)

12 BARNES, D. and SATO, G. Serum-free cell culture: a unifying approach. *Cell*, **22,** 649–655 (1980)

13 BEARD, M. E. J. Fanconi anaemia. In *Congenital Disorders of Erythropoiesis: Ciba Foundation Symposium*, 103–114. Amsterdam, Elsevier (1976)

14 BECKER, A. J., McCULLOCH, F. A. and TILL, J. E. Cytological demonstration of the clonal nature of spleen colonies derived from transplanted mouse marrow cells. *Nature*, **197,** 452–454 (1963)

15 BESSIS, N. L'îlot erythroblastique, unité fonctionelle de la moëlle osseuse. *Nouvelle Revue Française d'Hématologie*, **13,** 8–13 (1958)

16 BEST, W. R. Chloramphenicol-associated blood dyscrasias. *Journal of American Medical Association*, **201,** 181–188 (1967)

17 BEVERLY, P. C. L., LINCH, D. and DELIA, D. Isolation of human hemopoietic progenitor cells using monoclonal antibodies. *Nature*, **287,** 332–333 (1981)

18 BLACKETT, N. M. Erythropoiesis in the rats under continuous γ-irradiation at 45 rads/day. *British Journal of Haematology*, **13,** 915–923 (1967)

19 BOL, S., VISSER, J. and VAN DEN ENGH, G. The physical separation of three subpopulations of granulocyte-macrophage progenitor cells from mouse bone marrow. *Experimental Hematology*, **7,** 541–553 (1979)

20 BOL, S. and WILLIAMS, N. The maturation state of three types of granulocyte/macrophage progenitor cells from mouse bone marrow. *Journal of Cellular Physiology*, **102,** 233–243 (1980)

21 BROXMEYER, H. E., SMITHYMAN, A., EGER, R. R., MYERS, P. A. and De SOUSA, M. Identification of lactoferrin as the granulocyte-derived inhibitor of colony stimulating activity production. *Journal of Experimental Medicine*, **148,** 1052–1067 (1978)

22 BROXMEYER, H. E., De SOUSA, M., SMITHYMAN, A., RALPH, P., HAMILTON, J., KURLAND, J. I. and BOGNACKI, J. Specificity and modulation of the action of lactoferrin, a negative feedback regulator of myelopoiesis. *Blood*, **55,** 324–333 (1980)

23 BURGESS, A. W., CAMAKARIS, J. and METCALF, D. Purification and properties of colony-stimulating factor from mouse lung-conditioned medium. *Journal of Biological Chemistry*, **252,** 1998–2003 (1977)

24 BURGESS, A. W. and METCALF, D. The nature and action of granulocyte macrophage colony stimulating factors. *Blood*, **56,** 947–958 (1980)

25 BURGESS, A. W., WILSON, E. M. A. and METCALF, D. Stimulation by human placental conditioned medium of hemopoietic colony formation by human marrow cells. *Blood*, **49,** 573–583 (1977)

26 CALLIGARIS CAPPIO, F., NOVARINO, A., CAMUSSI, G. and GAVOSTO, F. Immune complexes in aplastic anaemia. *British Journal of Haematology*, **45,** 81–87 (1980)

27 CHEVERNICK, P. A. and BOGGS, D. R. *In vitro* growth of granulocytic and mononuclear cell colonies from blood of normal individuals. *Blood*, **37,** 131–135 (1971)

28 CLINE, M. J. and GOLDE, D. W. Production of colony-stimulating activity by human lymphocytes. *Nature*, **248,** 703–704 (1974)

29 CLINE, M. J. and GOLDE, D. W. Mobilization of hemopoietic stem cells (CFU-C) into the peripheral blood of man by endotoxin. *Experimental Hematology*, **5,** 186–190 (1977)

30 CLINE, M. J. and GOLDE, D. W. Cellular interactions in hematopoiesis. *Nature*, **277,** 177–181 (1979)

31 CLINE, M. J., STANG, H. D., MERCOLA, K. E., MORSE, L., RUPRECHT, R., BROWNE, S. and SALSER, W. Gene transfer in intact animals. *Nature*, **284,** 422–425 (1980)

32 COMI, P., GIGLIONI, B., OTTOLENGHI, S., GIANNI, A. M., POLLI, E., BARBA, P., COVELLI, A., MIGLIACCIO, G., CONDORELLI, M. and PESCHLE, C. Globin chains synthesis in single erythroid bursts from cord blood: studies on γ–β and $^G\gamma$–$^A\gamma$ switches. *Proceedings of the National Academy of Sciences of USA*, **77,** 362–365 (1980)

33 CROSBY, W. J. Experience with infused and implanted bone marrow: relation of function to structure. In *Hemopoietic Cell Differentiation*, edited by F. Stohlman Jr., 87–96. New York, Grune and Stratton (1970)

34 CUDKOWICZ, G., UPTON, A. C., SHEARER, C. M. and HUGHES, W. L. Lymphocyte content and proliferative capacity of serially transplanted mouse bone marrow. *Nature*, **201,** 165–167 (1964)

35 CURRY, J. L. and TRENTIN, J. J. Hemopoietic spleen colonies studies. I: growth and differentiation. *Developmental Biology*, **15,** 395–413 (1967)

36 DANESHBOD-SKIBBA, G., MARTIN, J. and SHAHIDI, N. T. Myeloid and erythroid colony growth in non-anemic patients with Fanconi's anaemia. *British Journal of Haematology*, **44,** 33–38 (1980)

37 DAWID, I. B. and WAHLI, W. Application of recombinant DNA technology to questions of developmental biology: a review. *Developmental Biology*, **69,** 305–328 (1979)

38 DEXTER, T. M., ALLEN, T. D. and LAJTHA, L. G. Conditions controlling the proliferation of haemopoietic stem cells *in vitro*. *Journal of Cellular Physiology*, **91,** 335–344 (1977)

39 DEXTER, T. M., ALLEN, T. D., LAJTHA, L. G., KRIZSA, F., TESTA, N. G. and MOORE, M. A. S. *In vitro* analysis of self-renewal and commitment of hematopoietic stem cells. In *Differentiation of Normal and Neoplastic Cells*, edited by B. Clarkson, P. A. Marks, and J. E. Till, 63–80. New York, Cold Spring Harbor Laboratory (1978)

40 DEXTER, T. M., GARLAND, J., SCOTT, D., SCOLNICK, E. and METCALF, D. Growth of factor-dependent hemopoietic precursor cell lines. *Journal of Experimental Medicine*, **152,** 1036–1047 (1980)

41 DEXTER, T. M. and MOORE, M. A. S. *In vitro* duplication and 'cure' of hemopoietic defects in genetically anemic mice. *Nature*, **269,** 412–414 (1977)

42 DEXTER, T. M., TESTA, N. G., ALLEN, T. D., RUTHERFORD, T. and SCOLNICK, E. Molecular and cell biologic aspects of erythropoiesis in long term bone marrow cultures. *Blood*, **58,** 699–707 (1981)

43 DIAMOND, L. K. and BLACKFAN, K. D. Hypoplastic anemia. *American Journal of Diseases of Children*, **56,** 464–466 (1938)

44 EASTMENT, C., DENHOLM, F., KATSNELSON, I., ARNOLD, F. and TS'O, P. O. P. *In vitro* proliferation of hemopoietic stem cells in the absence of an adherent layer. *Blood*, (in press)

45 EAVES, C. J. and EAVES, A. C. Erythropoietin (Ep) dose-response curves for three classes of erythroid progenitors in normal human marrow and in patients with polycythemia vera. *Blood*, **52,** 1196–1210 (1978)

46 EAVES, C. J., HUMPHRIES, R. K. and EAVES, A. C. *In vitro* characterization of erythroid precursors cells and the erythropoietic differentiation process. In *Cellular and Molecular Regulation of Hemoglobin Switching*, edited by G. Stamatoyannopoulos and A. W. Nienhuis, 251–273. New York, Grune and Stratton (1979)

47 ELIASON, J. F., TESTA, N. G. and DEXTER, T. M. Erythropoietin-stimulated erythropoiesis in long-term bone marrow culture. *Nature*, **281,** 382–384 (1979)

48 ERSLEV, A. J. Aplastic anemia. In *Hematology*, edited by W. J. Williams, E. Beutler, A. J. Erslev and R. W. Rundles, 258–278. New York, McGraw-Hill (1977)

49 FAGG, B. Is erythropoietin the only factor which regulates late erythroid differentiation? *Nature*, **289,** 184–186 (1981)

50 FANCONI, G. Familiäre infantile perniziosaartige Anämie (FA) (pernizioses Blutbild und Konstitution). *Jahrbuch für Kinderheilkunde*, **117,** 257–280 (1927)

51 FAUSER, A. A. and MESSNER, H. A. Granulo-erythropoietic colonies in human bone marrow, peripheral blood and cord blood. *Blood*, **52,** 1243–1248 (1979)

52 FIALKOW, P. J. Clonal origin of human tumors. *Annual Review of Medicine*, **30**, 135–143 (1979)

53 FIALKOW, P. J. Clonal and stem cell origin of blood cell neoplasms. In *Contemporary Hematology/Oncology*, **1**, edited by R. Silber, J. LoBue and A. S. Gordon, 1–43. New York, Plenum (1980)

54 FIALKOW, P. J., FAGUET, G. B., JACOBSON, R. J., VAIDYA, K. and MURPHY, S. Evidence that essential thrombocythemia is a clonal disorder with origin in a multipotent stem cell. *Blood*, **58**, 916–919 (1981)

55 FIALKOW, P. J., JACOBSON, R. J. and PAPAYANNOPOULOU, T. Chronic myelocytic leukemia: clonal origin in a stem cell common to the granulocyte, erythrocyte, platelet and monocyte/macrophage. *American Journal of Medicine*, **63**, 125–130 (1977)

56 FILMANOWICZ, E. and GURNEY, C. W. Studies on erythropoiesis. XVI. Response to a single dose of erythropoietin in the polycythemic mouse. *Journal of Laboratory Clinical Medicine*, **75**, 65–72 (1961)

57 FITCHENS, J. H., FOON, K. A. and CLINE, M. J. The antigenic characteristics of hematopoietic stem cells. *New England Journal of Medicine*, **305**, 17–25 (1981)

58 FREEDMAN, M. H. and SAUNDERS, E. F. Deficient erythroid colony growth (CFU-E) in constitutional (congenital) aplastic anemia. *Blood*, **46**, 1023 (Abst.) (1975)

59 FREEDMAN, M. H. and SAUNDERS, E. F. Diamond-Blackfan syndrome: evidence against cell-mediated erythropoietic suppression. *Blood*, **51**, 1125–1128 (1978)

60 FRIED, W. The liver as a source of extrarenal erythropoietin production. *Blood*, **40**, 671–677 (1972)

61 FRIED, W., BÀRONE-VARELAS, J., BARONE, T. and HELFGOTT, M. Extraction of erythropoietin from kidneys. *Experimental Hematology*, **8**, (Supp. no. 8), 41–51 (1980)

62 FRIEND, C., SCHER, W., HOLLAND, J. G. and SATO, T. Hemoglobin synthesis in murine virus-induced leukemic cells *in vitro*: stimulation of erythroid differentiation by dimethyl sulfoxide. *Proceedings of the National Academy of Sciences of USA*, **68**, 378–382 (1971)

63 GARTNER, S. and KAPLAN, H. S. Long-term culture of human bone marrow cells. *Proceedings of the National Academy of Sciences of USA*, **77**, 4756–4759 (1980)

64 GELLER, G., KRIVIT, W., ZALUSKY, R. and ZANJANI, E. D. Lack of erythropoietic inhibitory effect of serum from patients with congenital pure red cell aplasia. *Journal of Pediatrics*, **2**, 198–201 (1975)

65 GLUCKMAN, E., DAVERGIC, A., SCHAISON, G., BUSSEL, A., BERGER, R., SOHIER, J. and BERNARD, J. Bone marrow transplantation in Fanconi anaemia. *British Journal of Haematology*, **45**, 557–564 (1980)

66 GOLDE, D. W., BERSCH, N., QUAN, S. G. and LUSIS, A. J. Production of erythroid-potentiating activity by a human T-lymphoblast cell line. *Proceedings of the National Academy of Sciences of USA*, **77**, 593–596 (1980)

67 GOLDE, D. W. and CLINE, M. J. Identification of the colony-stimulating cell in human peripheral blood. *Journal of Clinical Investigation*, **51**, 2981–2983 (1972)

68 GOLDWASSER, E. Some molecular aspects of red cell differentiation. In *Regulation of Erythropoiesis*, edited by A. S. Gordon, M. Condorelli and C. Peschle, 227–233. Milano, Il Ponte (1971)

69 GOLDWASSER, E. and INANA, G. Molecular aspects of the initiation of erythropoiesis. In *Hematopoietic Cell Differentiation*, edited by D. W. Golde, M. J. Cline, D. Metcalf and C. F. Fox, 15–24. New York, Academic (1978)

70 GORDON, A. S. Erythropoietin. *Vitamins and Hormones*, **31**, 105–174 (1973)

71 GREENBERGER, J. S. Sensitivity of corticosteroid-dependent insulin-resistant lipogenesis in marrow preadipocytes of obese diabetic (db/db) mice. *Nature*, **275**, 752–754 (1978)

72 GREENBERG, P. L. and SCHRIER, S. L. Granulopoiesis in neutropenic disorders. *Blood*, **41**, 753–769 (1973)

73 GREGORY, C. J. and HENKELMAN, R. M. Relationship between early hemopoietic progenitor cells determined by correlation analysis of their numbers in individual spleen colonies. In *Experimental Hematology Today*, edited by S. J. Baum and G. D. Ledney, New York, Springer, 93–101 (1977)

74 GREGORY, C. J., TEPPERMAN, A. D., McCULLOCH, E. A. and TILL, J. E. Erythropoietic progenitors capable of colony formation in culture: response of normal and genetically anemic W/W^v mice to manipulations of the erythron. *Journal of Cellular Physiology*, **84**, 1–12 (1974)

75 GUERRY, D., ADAMSON, J. W., DALE, D. C. and WOLFF, S. M. Human cyclic neutropenia. Urinary colony stimulating factor and erythropoietin levels. *Blood*, **44**, 257–262 (1974)

76 HARA, H., KAI, S., FUSHIMI, M., TANIWAKI, S., OKAMOTO, T., OHE, Y., FUJITA, S., NOGUCHI, K., SENBA, M., HAMANO, T., KANAMARU, A. and NAGAI, K. Pluripotential hemopoietic precursors *in vitro* (CFU mix) in aplastic anemia. *Experimental Hematology*, **8**, 1165–1171 (1980)

77 HARA, H. and OGAWA, M. Erythropoietic precursors in mice under stimulation and suppression. *Experimental Hematology*, **5**, 141–148 (1977)

78 HARA, H. and OGAWA, M. Erythropoietic precursors in murine blood. *Experimental Hematology*, **5**, 159–163 (1977)

79 HASSAN, M. W., LUTTON, J. D., LEVERE, R. D., RIEDER, R. F. and CEDERQUIST, L. *In vitro* culture of erythroid colonies in human fetal liver and umbilical cord blood. *British Journal of Haematology*, **41**, 477–484 (1979)

80 HOCKING, W. G. and GOLDE, D. W. Long-term human bone marrow cultures. *Blood*, **56**, 118–124 (1980)

81 HOFFMAN, R., ZANJANI, E. D., LUTTON, J. D., ZALUSKY, R. and WASSERMAN, L. R. Suppression of erythroid-colony formation by lymphocytes from patient with aplastic anemia. *New England Journal of Medicine*, **296**, 10–13 (1977)

82 HOFFMAN, R., ZANJANI, E. D., ZALUSKY, R., LUTTON, J. D. and WASSERMAN, L. R. Diamond-Blackfan syndrome. Lymphocyte-mediated suppression of erythropoiesis. *Science*, **193**, 899–900 (1976)

83 HOLTZER, H., WEINTRAUB, H., MAYNE, R. and MOCHAN, B. The cell cycle, cell lineages, and cell differentiation. *Current Topics in Developmental Biology*, **7**, 229–256 (1972)

84 HOWARD, M., BURGESS, A. W., PcPHEE, D. and METCALF, D. T-cell hybridoma secreting hemopoietic regulatory molecules: granulocyte-macrophage and eosinophil colony-stimulating factors. *Cell*, **18**, 993–999 (1979)

85 HOZUMI, N. and TONEGAWA, S. Evidence for somatic rearrangement of immunoglobin genes coding for variable and constant regions. *Proceedings of the National Academy of Sciences of USA*, **73**, 3628–3632 (1976)

85a HUMPHRIES, R. K., EAVES, A. C. and EAVES, C. J. Self-renewal of the hemopoietic stem cells during mixed colony formation *in vitro*. *Proceedings of the National Academy of Sciences of the USA*, **78**, 3629–3633 (1981)

86 ISCOVE, N. N. The role of erythropoietin in regulation of population size and cell cycling of early and late erythroid precursors in mouse bone marrow. *Cell and Tissue Kinetics*, **10**, 323–334 (1977)

87 ISCOVE, N. N. Erythropoietin-independent stimulation of early erythropoiesis in adult bone marrow cultures by conditioned media from lectin-stimulated mouse spleen cells. In *Hemopoietic Cell Differentiation*, edited by D. W. Golde, M. J. Cline, D. Metcalf and C. F. Fox, 37–52. New York, Academic (1978)

88 ISCOVE, N. N. and GUILBERT, L. J. Erythropoietin-independence of early erthropoiesis and a two-regulator model of proliferative control in the hemopoietic system. In *In Vitro Aspects of Erythropoiesis*, edited by M. J. Murphy Jr., C. Peschle, A. S. Gordon, and E. A. Mirand, 3–7. New York, Springer (1978)

89 ISCOVE, N. N., GUILBERT, C. J. and WEYMAN, C. Complete replacement of serum in primary cultures of erythropoietin-dependent red cell precursors (CFU-E) by albumin, transferrin, iron, unsaturated fatty acid, lecithin, and cholesterol. *Experimental Cell Research*, **126**, 121–126 (1980)

90 JACOBSON, L. D., GOLDWASSER, E., FRIED, W. and PLAK, L. F. Role of the kidney in erythropoiesis. *Nature*, **179**, 633–634 (1957)

91 JOHNSON, G. R. Control of erythropoiesis: genetic and regulatory interactions. *Experimental Hematology*, **9**, (Suppl. no. 9), 176 (Abst.) (1981)

92 JOHNSON, G. R. and METCALF, D. Pure and mixed erythroid colony formation *in vitro* stimulated by spleen conditioned medium with no detectable erythropoietin. *Proceedings of the National Academy of Sciences of USA*, **74**, 3879–3882 (1977)

93 JONES-VILLENEUVE, E. V., RUSTHOVEN, J. J., MILLER, R. G. and PHILLIPS, R. A. Differentiation of thyl-bearing cells from progenitors in long-term bone marrow cultures. *Journal of Immunology*, **124**, 597–601 (1980)

94 KERN, P., HEIMPEL, H., HEIT, W. and KUBANEK, B. Wachstum peripherer Blutzellen in der Agarkultur bei Gesunden und bei Patienten mit Panmyelopathie. *Blut*, **28**, 213 (Abst.) (1974)

95 KNOSPE, W. H., BLOM, J. and CROSBY, N. H. Regeneration of locally irradiated bone marrow. I Dose dependent long-term changes in the rat, with particular emphasis upon vascular and stromal reaction. *Blood*, **28**, 398–415 (1966)

96 KOEFFLER, H. P. and GOLDE, D. W. Human myeloid leukemia cell lines: a review. *Blood*, **56**, 344–350 (1980)

97 KOHLER, G. and MILSTEIN, C. Continuous cultures of fused cells FL secreting antibody of predefined specificity. *Nature*, **256**, 495–497 (1975)

98 KRAMMER, P. H., KEES, U., HÜLTNER, L., STABER, F. G., KIRCHNER, H. and MARCUCCI, F. Frequency, activity, and clonal analysis of immune interferon, T-cell growth factor and colony stimulating factor producing murine T-cells. *Experimental Hematology*, **9**, (Suppl. no. 9), 4 (Abst.) (1981)

99 KRANTZ, S. B. and JACOBSON, L. O. (Eds.). Erythropoietin and Regulation of Erythropoiesis, 329 pp. Chicago, Ill., University of Chicago (1970)

100 KRANTZ, S. B. and KAO, V. Studies on red cell aplasia. I. Demonstration of a plasma inhibitor to heme synthesis and an antibody to erythroblast nuclei. *Proceedings of the National Academy of Sciences of USA*, **58**, 493–500 (1967)

101 KRANTZ, S. B., MOORE, W. H. and ZAENTZ, S. D. Studies on red cell aplasia. V. Presence of erythroblast cytoxicity in γ-globulin fraction of plasma. *Journal of Clinical Investigation*, **52**, 324–336 (1973)

102 KRANTZ, S. B. and ZAENT, S. D. Pure red cell aplasia. In *The Year in Hematology*, edited by A. S. Gordon, R. Silber, and J. LoBue, 153–190. New York, Plenum (1977)

103 KURLAND, J. I., BROXMEYER, H. E., PELUS, L. M., BOCKMAN, R. S. and MOORE, M. A. S. Role of monocyte-macrophage derived colony-stimulating factor and prostaglandins E in the positive and negative feedback control of myeloid stem cell proliferation. *Blood*, **52**, 388–407 (1978)

104 LAJTHA, L. G., POZZI, L. V., SCHOFIELD, R. and FOX, M. Kinetic properties of hemopoietic stem cells. *Cell and Tissue Kinetics*, **2**, 39–49 (1969)

105 LALA, P. K. and JOHNSON, G. R. Monoclonal origin of B-lymphocyte colony forming cells in spleen colonies formed by multipotential hemopoietic stem cells. *Journal of Experimental Medicine*, **148**, 1468–1477 (1978)

106 LANOTTE, M., SCHOR, S. and DEXTER, T. M. Collagen gels as a matrix for haemopoiesis. *Journal of Cellular Physiology*, **106**, 269–277 (1981)

107 LENZ, R. and PLUZNICK, D. H. Membranal gangliosides present on committed hemopoietic stem cells (CFU-C): possible receptors for colony-stimulating factor (CSF). In *Experimental Hematology Today*, edited by S. J. Baum, G. D. Ledney, and D. W. Van Bekkum, 13–18. New York, Karger (1980)

108 LORD, B. I., MORI, K. J. and WRIGHT, E. G. A stimulator of stem cell proliferation in regenerating bone marrow. *Biomedicine*, **27**, 223–226 (1977)

109 LORD, B. I., MORI, K. J., WRIGHT, E. G. and LAJTHA, L. G. An inhibitor of stem cell proliferation in normal bone marrow. *British Journal of Haematology*, **34**, 441–445 (1976)

110 LUI, V. C., RAYAB, A. M., FINDLEY, H. S. and FRAUEN, B. J. Bone marrow cultures in children with Fanconi's anaemia and TAR syndrome. *Journal of Pediatrics*, **91**, 925–954 (1977)

111 MANCH, P., GREENBERGER, J. S., BOTNICK, L., HANNON, E. and HELLMAN, S. Evidence for structured variation in self-renewal capacity within long-term bone marrow cultures. *Proceedings of the National Academy of Sciences of USA*, **77**, 2927–2930 (1980)

112 MANGAN, K. F., CHIKKAPPA, G. and SCHARFAMN, W. B. Modulation of erythropoietic peripheral blood burst forming unit (BFU-E) proliferation by T-lymphocytes bearing Fc receptors for IgM and IgG: possible pathogenic role in the pure red cell aplasia of chronic lymphocytic leukemia. *Experimental Hematology*, **8**, (Suppl. no. 7), 45 (Abst.) (1980)

113 MARMONT, A. M. Congenital hypoplastic anemia refractory to corticosteroids but responding to cyclophosphamide and antilymphocyte globulin. *Acta Haematologica*, **60**, 90–99 (1978)

114 MARMONT, A., PESCHLE, C., SANGUINETI, M. and CONDORELLI, M. Pure red cell aplasia (PRCA): Response of three patients to cyclophosphamide and/or antilymphocyte globulin (ALG) and demonstration of two types of serum IgG inhibitors to erythropoiesis. *Blood*, **45**, 247–261 (1975)

115 McCULLOCH, E. A., SIMINOVITCH, L., TILL, J. E., RUSSEL, E. S. and BERNSTEIN, S. E. The cellular basis of the genetically determined hemopoietic defect in anemic mice of phenotype Sl/Sl^d. *Blood*, **26**, 399–410 (1965)

116 MERCOLA, K. E. and CLINE, M. J. The potentials of inserting new genetic information. *The New England Journal of Medicine*, **303**, 1297–1300 (1980)

117 MERCOLA, K. E., STANG, H. D., BROWNE, J., SALSER, W. and CLINE, M. J. Insertion of a new gene of viral origin into bone marrow cells of mice. *Science*, **208**, 1033–1035 (1980)

118 MESSNER, H. A., FAUSER, A. A., CURTIS, J. E. and DOTTEN, D. Control of antibody-mediated pure red-cell aplasia by plasmapheresis. *New England Journal of Medicine*, **304**, 1334–1338 (1981)

119 METCALF, D. Hemopoietic colonies. *In vitro* cloning of normal and leukemic cells. In *Recent Results in Cancer Research*. 227 pp. Berlin, Springer (1977)

120 METCALF, D. Hemopoietic colony stimulating factors. In *Tissue Growth Factors*, edited by R. Baserga. New York, Springer (1980)

121 METCALF, D. Commitment of bipotential GM progenitor cells to granulocyte or macrophage formation by GM-CSF or M-CSF. *Experimental Hematology*, **9**, (Suppl. no. 9), 3 (Abst.) (1981)

122 METCALF, D., BURGESS, A. W. and JOHNSON, G. R. Stimulation of multipotential and erythroid precursor cells by GM-CSF. In *Experimental Hematology Today*, edited by S. J. Baum, G. D. Ledney and D. W. Van Bekkum, 3–12. New York, Karger (1980)

123 METCALF, D., JOHNSON, G. R. and MANDEL, T. E. Colony formation in agar by multipotential hemopoietic cell. *Journal of Cellular Physiology*, **98**, 401–420 (1979)

124 MIGLIACCIO, G., GABUTTI, V., MIGLIACCIO, A. R., QUATTRIN, S., MASTROBERARDINO, G. and PESCHLE, C. Proliferation and differentiation of stem and progenitor cells in long-term cultures: studies in normal and β-thalassemic subjects. In *Hemolymphopoiesis: Normal and Pathological Cell Differentiation*, edited by F. Gavosto, G. P. Bagnara, M. A. Brunelli and C. Castaldini, 23–27. Bologna, Esculapio (1981)

125 MIJAKE, T., KUNG, C. K. H. and GOLDWASSER, E. Purification of human erythropoietin. *Journal of Biological Chemistry*, **252**, 5558–5564 (1977)

126 MOORE, M. A. S. and SHERIDAN, A. P. Pluripotential stem cell replication in continuous human, prosimian, and murine bone marrow culture. *Blood Cells*, **5**, 279–311 (1979)

127 MORLEY, A. and BLAKE, J. An animal model for chronic aplastic marrow failure. Late marrow failure after busulfan. *Blood*, **44**, 49–56 (1974)

128 MORSTYN, G., NICOLA, N. A. and METCALF, D. Purification of hemopoietic progenitor cells from human marrow using a fucose-binding lectin and cell sorting. *Blood*, **56**, 798–805 (1980)

129 NAGAO, T. and MAUER, A. M. Concordance for drug-induced aplastic anemia in identical twins. *New England Journal of Medicine*, **281,** 7–11 (1969)
130 NAGASAWA, T., ABE, T. and NAKAGAWA, T. Pure red cell aplasia and hypogammaglobulinemia associated with Tr-cell chronic lymphocytic leukemia. *Blood*, **57,** 1025–1031 (1981)
131 NATHAN, D. G., CHESS, L., HILLMAN, D. G., CLARKE, B., BREARD, J., MERLER, E. and HOUSMAN, D. E. Human erythroid burst-forming unit: T-cell requirement for proliferation *in vitro*. *Journal of Experimental Medicine*, **147,** 324–339 (1978)
132 NICOLA, N. A., BURGESS, A. W. and METCALF, D. Similar molecular properties of granulocyte-macrophage colony stimulating factors produced by different mouse organs *in vitro* and *in vivo*. *Journal of Biological Chemistry*, **254,** 5290–5299 (1979)
132a NICOLA, N. A. and METCALF, D. Biochemical properties of differentiation factors for murine myelomonocytic leukemic cells in organ-conditioned media. – Separation from colony-stimulating factors. *Journal of Cellular Physiology*, **109,** 253–264 (1981)
133 NICOLA, N. A., METCALF, D., VON MELCHNER, H. and BURGESS, A. W. Isolation of murine fetal hemopoietic progenitor cells and selective fractionation of various erythroid precursors. *Blood*, **58,** 376–386 (1981)
134 NISSEN, C, CORNU, P., GRATWOHL, A. and SPECK, B. Peripheral blood cells from patients with aplastic anaemia in partial remission suppress growth of their own bone marrow precursors in culture. *British Journal of Haematology*, **45,** 233–243 (1980)
135 OGAWA, M., GRUSH, O. C., O'DELL, R. F., HARA, H. and Mac EACHERN, M. D. Circulating erythropoietic precursors assessed in culture: characterization in normal men and patients with hemoglobinopathies. *Blood*, **50,** 1081–1092 (1977)
136 OGAWA, M. and SEXTON, J. Circulating erythropoietic precursors in human blood. *Clinical Research*, **24,** 316a (Abst.) (1976)
137 ORTEGA, J. E., SHORE, M. A., DUKES, P. P. and HAMMOND, D. Congenital hypoplastic anemia. Inhibition of erythropoiesis by sera from patients with congenital hypoplastic anemia. *Blood*, **45,** 83–89 (1975)
138 PAIGE, C. W., KINCADE, P. W., MOORE, M. A. S. and LEE, G. The fate of fetal and adult B-cell progenitors grafted into immunodeficient CBA/N mice. *Journal of Experimental Medicine*, **150,** 548–563 (1979)
139 PAUL, P., ROTHMANN, S. A., NAUGHTON, B. A. and GORDON, A. S. Presence of erythropoietin (Ep) in Kupffer cell conditioned medium. *Experimental Hematology*, **9,** (Suppl. no. 9), 57 (Abst.) (1981)
140 PELUS, I. M., BROXMEYER, H. E., KURLAND, J. and MOORE, M. A. S. Regulation of macrophage and granulocyte proliferation: specificities of prostaglandin E and lactoferrin. *Journal of Experimental Medicine*, **150,** 277–292 (1979)
141 PESCHLE, C. Regulation of erythropoiesis and its defects. *British Journal of Haematology*, **31,** (Suppl.), 69–81 (1975)
142 PESCHLE, C. Bone marrow hypoplasia. In *Kidney Hormones*, **2,** *Erythropoietin*, edited by J. W. Fisher, 495–530. London, Academic (1977)
143 PESCHLE, C. Erythropoiesis. *Annual Review of Medicine*, **31,** 303–314 (1980)

144 PESCHLE, C., CILLO, C., MIGLIACCIO, G. and LETTIERI, F. Fluctuations of BFU-E and CFU-E cycling after erythroid perturbations: correlations with variations of pool size. *Experimental Hematology*, **8**, 96–102 (1980)

145 PESCHLE, C., CILLO, C., RAPPAPORT, I. A., MAGLI, M. C., MIGLIACCIO, G., PIZZELLA, F. and MASTROBERARDINO, G. Early fluctuations of BFU-E pool size after transfusion or erythropoietin treatment. *Experimental Hematology*, **7**, 87–93 (1979)

146 PESCHLE, C., COLLETTA, G., COVELLI, A., CICCARIELLO, R., MIGLIACCIO, G. and ROSSI, G. B. The erythropoietic component of Friend virus erythroleukemias: role of erythropoietic hormone(s) and SFFV genome. In *Expression of Differentiated Functions in Cancer Cells*, edited by R. Revoltella, G. Pontieri, G. Rovera, C. Basilico, R. Gallo and J. Subake-Sharp. New York, Raven (in press)

147 PESCHLE, C. and CONDORELLI, M. Biogenesis of erythropoietin: evidence for pro-erythropoietin in a subcellular fraction of kidney. *Science*, **190**, 910–911 (1975)

148 PESCHLE, C., MAGLI, M. C., CILLO, C., LETTIERI, F., PIZZELLA, F., MIGLIACCIO, G. and MASTROBERARDINO, G. Erythroid stem cell kinetics. Experimental and clinical aspects. *Blood Cells*, **4**, 233–252 (1978)

149 PESCHLE, C., MARMONT, A. M., MARONE, G., GENOVESE, A., SASSO, G. F. and CONDORELLI, M. Pure red cell aplasia: studies on an IgG serum inhibitor neutralizing erythropoietin. *British Journal of Haematology*, **30**, 411–417 (1975)

150 PESCHLE, C., MARMONT, A., PERUGINI, S., BERNASCONI, C., BRUNETTI, P., FONTANA, G., GHIO, R., RESEGOTTI, L., RIZZO, S. C. and CONDORELLI, M. Physiopathology and therapy of adult pure red cell aplasia (PRCA): a cooperative study. In *Aplastic Anemia*, edited by S. Hibino, F. Takaku and N. T. Shahidi, 285–303. Tokyo, University of Tokyo (1976)

151 PESCHLE, C., MARONE, G., GENOVESE, A., MAGLI, M. C. and CONDORELLI, M. Erythropoietin production in the rat: additive role of kidney and liver. *American Journal of Physiology*, **230**, 845–848 (1976)

152 PESCHLE, C., MARONE, G., GENOVESE, A., RAPPAPORT, I. A. and CONDORELLI, M. Increased erythropoietin production in anephric rats with hyperplasia of the reticuloendothelial system induced by colloidal carbon or zymosan. *Blood*, **47**, 325–337 (1976)

153 PESCHLE, C., MIGLIACCIO, A. R., MIGLIACCIO, G., LETTIERI, F., MAGUIRE, Y. P., CONDORELLI, M., GIANNI, A. M., OTTOLENGHI, S., GIGLIONI, B., POZZOLI, M. L. and COMI, P. Regulation of Hb synthesis in ontogenesis and erythropoietic differentiation: *in vitro* studies on fetal liver, cord blood, normal adult blood or marrow, and blood from HPFH patients. In *Hemoglobin in Development and Differentiation*, 359–371, edited by G. Stamatoyannopoulos and A. W. Nienhuis. New York, Alan R. Liss, Inc. (1981)

154 PESCHLE, C., MIGLIACCIO, A. R., MIGLIACCIO, G., LETTIERI, F., QUATTRIN, S., RUSSO, G. and MASTROBERARDINO, G. Identification and characterization of three classes of erythroid progenitors in human fetal liver. *Blood*, **58**, 565–572 (1981)

155 PESCHLE, C., MIGLIACCIO, G., LETTIERI, F., MIGLIACCIO, A. R., CECCARELLI, R., BARBA, P., TITTI, F. and ROSSI, G. B. Kinetics of erythroid precursors in mice infected with the anemic or the polycythemic strain of Friend leukemia virus. *Proceedings of the National Academy of Sciences of USA*, **77**, 2054–2058 (1980)

155a PESCHLE, C., MIGLIACCIO, G., MIGLIACCIO, A. R., COVELLI, A., GUILIANI, A., MAVILIO, F. and MASTROBERARDINO, G. Haemoglobin switching in humans. In *Current Concepts in Erythropoiesis*, edited by C. Dunn. London, John Wiley (in press)

156 PRCHAL, J. F., ADAMSON, J. W., STEINMANN, L. and FIALKOW, P. J. The single cell origin of human erythroid colonies. *Journal of Cellular Physiology*, **89,** 489–492 (1976)

157 REMESEN, J. F. and CERUTTI, P. A. Deficiency of gamma-ray excision repair in skin fibroblasts from patients with Fanconi's anemia. *Proceedings of the National Academy of Sciences of USA*, **73,** 2419–2423 (1976)

158 RICH, I. H., HEIT, W. and KUBANEK, B. The release and kinetics of erythropoietin (Ep) from silica-treated macrophages. *Experimental Hematology*, **8,** (Suppl. no. 8), 307–310 (1980)

159 RICKARD, K. A., RENCRICCA, N. J., SHADDUCK, R. K., MONETTE, F. C., HOWARD, D., GARRITY, M. and STOHLMAN, F., Jr. Myeloid stem cell kinetics during erythropoietic stress. *British Journal of Haematology*, **21,** 537–547 (1971)

160 ROBINSON, J., SIEFF, C., DELIA, D., EDWARDS, P. A. W. and GREAVES, M. Expression of cell surface HLA-ABC and glycophorin during erythroid differentiation. *Nature*, **289,** 68–71 (1981)

161 ROSENDAL, M., HODGSON, G. S. and BRADLEY, T. R. Organization of haemopoietic stem cells: the generation age hypothesis. *Cells and Tissue Kinetics*, **12,** 17–29 (1979)

162 ROSSI, G. B., MIGLIACCIO, A. R., MIGLIACCIO, G., LETTIERI, F., Di ROSA, M., MASTROBERARDINO, G. and PESCHLE, C. *In vitro* interactions of PGE and cAMP with murine and human erythroid precursors. *Blood*, **56,** 74–79 (1980)

163 ROWLEY, P. T., OLSSON, W. B. M. and FARELY, B. A. Erythroid colony formation from human fetal liver. *Proceedings of the National Academy of Sciences of USA*, **75,** 984–988 (1978)

164 SASAKI, M. S. Is Fanconi's anaemia defective in a process essential to the repair of DNA cross links? *Nature*, **257,** 501–503 (1975)

165 SCHOFIELD, R. The relationship between the spleen colony-forming cell and the haemopoietic stem cell. *Blood Cells*, **4,** 7–25 (1978)

166 SCHOOLEY, J. C. and MAHLMANN, L. J. Extrarenal erythropoietin production by the liver in the weanling rat. *Proceedings of the Society for Experimental Biology and Medicine*, **145,** 1081–1083 (1974)

167 SCHREIER, M. H. and ISCOVE, N. N. Haematopoietic growth factors are released in cultures of H-2-restricted helper T cells, accessory cells and specific antigen. *Nature*, **287,** 228–230 (1980)

168 SEIDMAN, J. G., LEDER, A., NAA, M., NORMAN, B. and LEDER, P. Antibody diversity. *Science*, **202,** 11–17 (1978)

169 SENSENBRENNER, L. L., STEELE, A. A. and SANTOS, G. W. Recovery of hematologic competence without engraftment following attempted bone marrow transplantation for aplastic anemia: report of a case with diffusion chamber studies. *Experimental Hematology*, **5,** 51–58 (1977)

170 SHARKIS, S. J., COLVIN, M. and SENSENBRENNER, L. L. Characterization of subpopulations of thymocytes which regulate the proliferation of erythroid progenitor cells *in vitro*. *Experimental Hematology*, **9,** (Suppl. no. 9), 196 (Abst.) (1981)

171 SINGER, J. W., BROWN, J. E., JAMES, M. C., DONEY, K., WARREN, R. P., STORB, R. and THOMAS, E. D. Effect of peripheral blood lymphocytes from patients with aplastic anemia on granulocytic colony growth from HLA-matched and mismatched marrows: effect of transfusion sensitization. *Blood*, **52**, 37–46 (1978)

172 SINGER, J. W., DONEY, K. C. and THOMAS, E. D. Coculture studies of 16 untransfused patients with aplastic anemia. *Blood*, **54**, 180–185 (1979)

173 SINGER, J. W., FIALKOW, P. J., DOW, L. W., ERNEST, C. and STEINMANN, L. Unicellular or multicellular origin of human granulocyte-macrophage colonies *in vitro*. *Blood*, **54**, 1395–1399 (1979)

174 SPECK, B., CORNU, P., JEANNET, M., NISSEN, C., BURRI, H. P., GROFF, P., NAGEL, G. A. and BUCKNER, C. D. Autologous marrow recovery following allogenic marrow transplantation in a patient with severe aplastic anemia. *Experimental Hematology*, **4**, 131–136 (1976)

175 STANLEY, F. R. and HEARD, P. M. Factor regulating macrophage production and growth. Purification and some properties of colony-stimulating factor from medium conditioned by mouse L-cells. *Journal of Biological Chemistry*, **252**, 4305–4312 (1977)

176 STOHLMAN, F., Jr. Control mechanisms in erythropoiesis. In *Regulation of Erythropoiesis*, edited by A. S. Gordon, M. Condorelli and C. Peschle, 71–78. Milano, Il Ponte (1971)

177 STORB, R., THOMAS, E. D., BUCKNER, C. D., CLIFT, R. A., DEEG, H. J., FEFER, A., GOODELL, B. W., SALE, G. E., SANDERS, J. E., SINGER, J., STEWART, P. and WEIDEN, P. L. Marrow transplantation in thirty 'untransfused' patients with severe aplastic anemia. *Annals of Internal Medicine*, **92**, 30–36 (1980)

178 STROME, S. E., McLEOD, D. L. and SHREEVE, M. M. Evidence for the clonal nature of erythropoietic bursts: application of an *in situ* method for demonstrating centromeric heterochromatin in plasma cultures. *Experimental Hematology*, **6**, 461–467 (1978)

179 SUDE, T., MIZOGUCHI, H., MIURA, Y., KUBOTA, K. and TAKAKU, F. Suppression of *in vitro* granulocyte-macrophage colony formation by the peripheral mononuclear phagocytic cells of patients with idiopathic aplastic anemia. *British Journal of Haematology*, **47**, 433–442 (1981)

180 SULLIVAN, R., QUESENBERRY, P. J., PARKMAN, R., ZUCKERMAN, K. S., LEVEY, R. H., RAPPEPORT, J. and RYAN, M. Aplastic Anemia: lack of inhibitory effect of bone marrow lymphocytes on *in vitro* granulopoiesis. *Blood*, **56**, 625–632 (1980)

181 SUZUKI, S. and AXELRAD, A. A. FV-2 locus controls the proportion of erythropoietic progenitor cells (BFU-E) synthesizing DNA in normal mice. *Cell*, **19**, 225–236 (1980)

182 SYMANN, M., NINANE, J., ANCKAERT, M. A., HUYBRECHTS, M. and SOKAL, G. In vivo stimulation and inhibition of granulopoiesis. *Experimental Hematology*, **9**, (Suppl. no. 9), 4 (Abst.) (1981)

183 TAKAKU, F., SUDA, T., MIZOGUCHI, H., MIURA, Y., UCHINO, H., NAGAI, K., KARIYONE, S., SHIBATA, A., AKABANE, T., NOMURA, T. and MAEKAWA, T. Effect of peripheral blood mononuclear cells from aplastic anemia patients on the granulocyte-macrophage and erythroid colony formation in samples from normal human bone marrow *in vitro*. A cooperative work. *Blood*, **55**, 937–943 (1980)

184 THOMAS, E. D., STORB, R., GIBLETT, E. R., LONGPRE, B., WEIDEN, P. L., FEFER, A., WHITERSPOON, R., CLIFT, R. A. and BUCKNER, C. D. Recovery from aplastic anemia following attempted marrow transplantation. *Experimental Hematology*, **4**, 97–102 (1976)

185 TILL, J. E. and McCULLOCH, E. A. A direct measurement of the radiation sensitivity of normal mouse bone marrow cells. *Radiation Research*, **14**, 213–222 (1961)

186 TILL, J. E. and McCULLOCH, E. A. Hemopoietic stem cell differentiation. *Biochimica et Biophysica Acta*, **605**, 431–459 (1980)

187 TILL, J. E., McCULLOCH, E. A. and SIMINOVITCH, L. A stochastic model of stem cell proliferation based on the growth of spleen colony-forming cells. *Proceedings of the National Academy of Sciences of USA*, **51**, 29–36 (1964)

187a TOROK-STORB, B., MARTIN, P. J. and HANSEN, J. A. Regulation of *in vitro* erythropoiesis by normal T cells: evidence for two T-cell subsets with opposing functions. *Blood*, **58**, 171–174 (1981)

188 TOROK-STORB, B. J., SIEFF, C., STORB, R., ADAMSON, J. W. and THOMAS, E. D. *In vitro* tests for distinguishing possible immune-mediated aplastic anemia from transfusion-induced sensitization. *Blood*, **55**, 211–215 (1980)

189 TOROK-STORB, B. J., STORB, R., DEEG, H. J., GRAHAM, T. C., WISE, C., WEIDEN, P. L. and ADAMSON, J. W. Growth *in vitro* of donor marrow cultured with recipient lymphocytes predicts the fate of marrow grafts in transfused DLA-identical dogs. *Blood*, **53**, 104–108 (1979)

190 TOROK-STORB, B. J., STORB, R., GRAHAM, T. C., PRENTICE, R. L., WEIDEN, P. L. and ADAMSON, J. W. Erythropoiesis *in vitro*: effect of normal versus 'transfusion-sensitized' mononuclear cells. *Blood*, **52**, 706–711 (1978)

191 TOKSOZ, D., DEXTER, T. M., LORD, B. I., WRIGHT, E. G. and LAJTHA, L. G. The regulation of hemopoiesis in long-term bone marrow cultures. II Stimulation and inhibition of stem cell proliferation. *Blood*, **55**, 931–936 (1980)

192 UDUPA, K. B. and REISSMAN, R. K. *In vivo* erythropoietin requirements of regenerating erythroid progenitors (BFU-E, CFU-E) in bone marrow of mice. *Blood*, **53**, 1164–1171 (1979)

193 VAN DER POLEG, L. H. T. and FLAVELL, R. A. DNA methylation in the human γδβ-globin locus in erythroid and nonerythroid tissues. *Cell*, **19**, 947–958 (1980)

194 VAN ZANT, G. and GOLDWASSER, E. Competition between erythropoietic and colony-stimulating factor for target cells in mouse marrow. *Blood*, **53**, 946–965 (1979)

195 VOS, O., BUURMAN, W. A. and PLOEMACHER, R. E. Mobilization of haemopoietic stem cells (CFU) into the peripheral blood of the mouse; effects of endotoxin and other compounds. *Cell and Tissue Kinetics*, **5**, 467–479 (1972)

196 WAGEMAKER, G. Cellular and soluble factors influencing the differentiation of primitive erythroid progenitor cells (BFU-E) *in vitro*. In *In Vitro Aspects of Erythropoiesis*, edited by M. J. Murphy Jr., C. Peschle, A. S. Gordon and E. A. Mirand, 44–57. New York, Springer (1978)

197 WAGEMAKER, G. Induction of erythropoietin responsiveness *in vitro*. In *Hemopoietic Cell Differentiation*, edited by D. W. Golde, M. J. Cline, D. Metcalf and C. F. Fox, 109–118. New York, Academic (1978)

198 WAGEMAKER, G. Erythropoietin-independent regulation of early erythropoiesis. In *In Vivo and In Vitro Erythropoiesis: The Friend System*, edited by G. B. Rossi, 87–96. Amsterdam, Elsevier (1980)
199 WAGEMAKER, G. and VISSER, T. P. Erythropoietin-independent regeneration of erythroid progenitor cells following multiple injections of hydroxyurea. *Cell and Tissue Kinetics*, **13**, 505–517 (1980)
200 WEINTRAUB, H., LARSEN, A. and GROUDINE, M. α-Globin-gene switching during the development of chicken embryos: expression and chromosome structure. *Cell*, **24**, 333–344 (1981)
201 WEISS, T. L. and GOLDWASSER, E. The biological properties of endotoxin-free human erythropoietin. *Biochemical Journal*, **198**, 17–21 (1981)
202 WIKTOR-JEDRZEJCZAK, W., SHARKIS, S., AHMED, A., SELL, K. W. and SANTOS, G. W. Theta-sensitive cell and erythropoiesis identification of a defect in W/W^v anemic mice. *Science*, **196**, 313–315 (1977)
203 WILLIAMS, N., EGER, R. R., MOORE, M. A. S. and MENDELSOHN, N. Differentiation of mouse bone marrow precursors cells into neutrophil granulocytes by an activity separation from Wehi-3 cell conditioned medium. *Differentiation*, **11**, 59–63 (1978)
204 WILSCHUT, I. J. C., ERKENS-VERSLUIS, M. E., PLOEMACHER, R. E., BENNER, R. and VOS, O. Studies on the mechanism of hemopoietic stem cell (CFUs) mobilization. *Cell and Tissue Kinetics*, **12**, 299–311 (1979)
205 WU, A. M., TILL, J. E., SIMINOVITCH, L. and McCULLOCH, E. A. Cytological evidence for a relationship between normal hematopoietic colony-forming cells of the lymphoid system. *Journal of Experimental Medicine*, **127**, 455–464 (1968)
206 ZUCALI, J. R., STEVENS, V. and MIRAND, E. A. *In vitro* production of erythropoietin by mouse fetal liver. *Blood*, **46**, 85–90 (1975)

Index

Abortion
  mid-tremester, 162, 163, 164, 166–167, 177, 189
  spontaneous, 166
Acid citrate dextrose, 209
Actinomycin D, 33, 34, 37, 38
Acute lymphoblastic leukaemia (ALL), see Leukaemia
Adenoma, thyroid, 43
Adenosine deaminase (ADA), 88
  deficiency, 138, 139
Adjustment to cancer, 14–17
Adriamycin, 34, 104
Adults,
  cancers of, 2–3
  tissue sensitivity, radiotherapy, 30
ALL, see Leukaemia, acute lymphoblastic
Allopurinol, 114
Alveolar capillary block syndrome, 70, 200
Amniocentesis, 162, 164
  in haemophilia, 179, 181
Amniotic fluid cells, 162, 164
Anaemia
  aplastic, see Aplastic anaemia
  Blackfan-Diamond, 140, 236, 281–282
  congenital haemolytic, 140
  Cooley's, see Thalassaemia
  in neonate, 213, 215
  sickle cell, see Sickle cell disease
  transfusional iron overload in, 236, 239
Anaesthetic, 33, 50
Analgesics, 22–23
Anorexia, 20, 49, 71
Anoxia, tumour cells, 45

Antenatal diagnosis, 162–189 (see also Haemoglobinopathy; Haemophilia)
  disorders detectable, 186
  fetal blood sampling, see Fetus
  future perspectives, 189
  mid-tremester abortion, see Abortion
Antibodies, to CALLA, 83, 88, 89
Antimicrobial drugs, 116, 117, 126, 127
Antiplatelet antibody, 224, 226, 228
Anxiety, 15, 16, 18–19
  in haemophilia, 24, 25
Aplastic anaemia,
  acquired,
    aetiology, 278
    pathogenesis, 278–281
  congenital (Fanconi's), 135, 140, 278
  iron overload, 236
  transplantation in, (see also Bone marrow)
    aim of, 118
    gastrointestinal decontamination, 126
    gnotobiotic conditions, 126, 127
    haematological reconstitution, 120, 133
    immunological reconstitution, 121
    infections in, 116, 127–128
    recipient conditioning, 111–113, 125, 138, 281
    rejection in, 128
    results, 133–135, 281
Appetite, 36, 49
Arachnoid veins, 47, 48, 50
Arthropathy, haemophilic, 22, 24
Ascorbic acid, 239, 243
Asparaginase, 53, 57

Ataxia telangiectasia, 140
ATP, see Purpura, thrombocytopenic
Autocytotoxicity, 99
Autogenic treatment, 19
  in haemophilia, 20, 22, 24–26
Autoimmune mechanisms, anaemia, 280
Autoimmune thrombocytopenic purpura
    (ATP), see Purpura, thrombocytopenic
Azathioprine, 230

Bare lymphocyte syndrome, 138
BCNU, 54, 57
Behavioural disorders, haemophilia, 23–24
Behavioural medicine, 14, 19
  in haemophilia, 20, 22, 24–26
Blackfan-Diamond anaemia, 140, 236, 281–282
Bleeding, fetal, 164, 165–166 see also Haemorrhage
Blood,
  cell, antigens, 111, 125
  cells, bone marrow transplants, 118
  cord, 197–198
  exchange, histiocytosis, 103
  product infusion, transplantation, 114
  sampling, fetal, see Fetus
  transfusions, see Transfusion
Blood-testis barrier, 63
Bloom's syndrome, 140
B-lymphocytes, 80
  acute lymphoblastic leukaemia, 84
  after bone marrow grafts, 120, 123
  from myeloid stem cells, 268
Bone,
  exostoses, 41
  lesions, histiocytosis X, 97
  radiation effects, 31, 40-41
Bone marrow,
  aspirations, 18
  depression, radiotherapy, 36–37, 53
  donor, bank, 132
  erythropoiesis in fetus, 197
  hypoplasia, 278, 279
  lymphoblasts, 10
  monocytes, maturation, 95
  retransplantation, 125, 128
  in thrombocytopenic purpura, 226
  transplantation, 88, 89, 110–140 (see also Graft-versus-host)
    anti-CALLA treated, 89
    in aplastic anaemia, see Aplastic anaemia
    autologous, 137
    in congenital haemolytic anaemia, 140

Bone marrow (cont.)
  transplantation (cont.)
    donor selection, 110–111, 138
    early complications, 124–128, 137
    failure, engraftment, 124–125, 127, 137
    follow-up after, 118–124
    in inborn errors, 139
    late complications, 128–130, 137–139
    in leukaemia, see Leukaemia
    procedure, 113
    recipient conditioning, 111–113, 129–130, 138
    results of, 130–137, 281
    supportive care, 113–118, 126
Bowell, radiation reaction, 36
Brain,
  radiotherapy effect, 17, 30, 41–42
  tumours, 41
Burkitt's lymphoma, 84
Burst-forming unit, erythroid (BFU-E), 268–270, 271, 274
  in aplastic anaemia, 278, 279, 280
  in pure red cell aplasia, 282
Burst-promoting factors (BPF), 264, 268, 269, 271, 274
  molecular weight, role, 271, 272
  production, 275

Cancer,
  adjustment to, problems, 14–17
  adults, children, differences, 2–3
  iatrogenic problems, 17–20
  multidisciplinary management, 1–12, 15
  psychosocial aspects, 14–26
Capping defects, 138
Carmustine (BCNU), 54, 57
CCNU, 57
Cell differentiation, haemopoietic, 266
Cell-surface markers,
  haemopoietic stem, progenitors, 266
  lymphocyte, 81–89
Central nervous system (CNS) prophylaxis, 17–18, 35, 41, 46, 47, 53–55
  cranial, 17, 35, 41, 46, 51–55, 114
  craniospinal, 52, 53, 65
  new approaches to, 55–58
  optimum, methods, 54
  spinal, 53
  toxicity, problems, 17–18, 47, 51–52, 54–55, 114
Central nervous system, leukaemia, see under Leukaemia
Cerebrospinal fluid, 48, 49–50, 71
Chediak-Higashi syndrome, 139

Chemotherapy, (*see also specific chemotherapeutic agents*)
  in ALL, 51, 69, 88
  in histiocytosis X, 100, 101, 106
  in malignant histiocytosis, 104, 106
  post-operative, 2, 5, 6
  pre-operative, cancer, 6
  radiation, interaction, 33–34, 37–38, 46, 51, 114
  survival rate improvement, 3
Children's Cancer Study Group, The, 2, 8, 54, 99
Chimerism, 118–120, 126
Chloraphenicol, 278
Christmas disease, 177, 178, 185, 248–259 (*see also* Haemophilia)
Chronic granulomatous disease, 139
Clotting factors, fetal, haemophilia, 177
Coagulation abnormalities, 210
Cognition, iatrogenic effect, 17, 55
Colony-forming units (CFU), 118
  erythroid (CFU-E), 268, 269, 270, 271
    in pure red cell aplasia, 282
  granulocyte (CFU-G), 269, 274
  granulomacrophage (CFU-GM), 265, 269, 271, 272
    in aplastic anaemia, 278, 279, 280
  macrophage (CFU-M), 269, 274
  splenic (CFU-S), 264, 268–271, 279
  factors, 271–273
Colony-stimulating factors (CSF), 264, 265, 269, 270
  GM-CSF, 271, 272, 273, 274
  M-CSF, 271, 274
  molecular weights, 271
  production, 275
  role, 271–273
Common ALL antigen (CALLA, cALL), 81–83, 87
  antiserum to, 83, 89
  in patient management, 88
Communication, disease-related, 15
Cooley's anaemia, *see* Thalassaemia
Corticosteroids, in ATP, 226–228, 231
Co-trimoxazole, 117, 127, 138
CSF, *see* Colony-stimulating factors
Culture techniques, haemopoietic cells, 263–265
Cyclic AMP in erythropoiesis, 274
Cyclophosphamide,
  adverse effects, 114
  in ALL, 66, 88
  in bone marrow transplants, 111, 113, 124
  in thrombocytopenic purpura, 230
Cyclosporin A, 116, 126, 128, 137

Cystitis, haemorrhagic, 114
Cytarabine (cytosine arabinoside), 51, 52, 58, 88

Dactinomycin, *see* Actinomycin D
2'-Deoxycofomycin (DCF), 88
Deoxyhaemoglobin, 203
Deoxynucleotidyl transferase, terminal (TdT), 68, 71, 85
Deoxyribonucleic acid (DNA),
  analysis, gene identification, 180, 189
  globin gene clusters, 167–169, 189, 266
  repair, 278
Desferrioxamine, 170, 236, 238–243
  dosage, administration routes, 240–243
  iron balance and, 239–240
  toxicity, 242
  vitamin C and, 243
Diabetes mellitus, 237
Diazepam, 33
2, 3 Dihydrobenzoic acid (2, 3-DHB), 244
2, 3 Diphosphoglycerate (2,3-DPG), 196, 202
  fetal haemoglobin, effect, 202–204
  'functioning 2,3-DPG fraction', 205
  hypoxia, effect, 203
  levels in fetus, 203
  in neonate, 203, 204–208
Discomfort, iatrogenic, 18–20
Doxorubicin, 53, 104
Duchenne muscular dystrophy, 163

Emesis, 18, 19, 49, 113
Encephalopathy, in ALL, 51, 53, 55, 57
Endocrine radiation effects, 31, 41–44, 68
Endocurie therapy, interstitial, 5
Endothelial cells, 275
Enhancement, chemotherapy, radiation, 34, 37
Enzyme replacement therapy, 139
Eosinophil, histiocytosis X, 96, 97
Eosinophilia, familial reticulosis with, 138
E-rosette, 81, 83
Erythroblast, 268–269, 270, 275
  in pure red cell aplasia, 282
Erythroblastic island, 275
  in aplastic anaemia, 278
  in cord blood, 197
  erythropoietin role, 270–271
  IgG inhibitor, 282
  ontogenic aspects, 276–278

Erythropoiesis,
  in cultures, 265
  IgG inhibitor, 282
  in newborn, fetus, 196–199
    regulation, 197–199
  regualtion, 274, 276
  stress, 270
Erythropoietin, 197–199, 270
  central venous oxygen tension, 215
  erythroid progenitors, 264, 265, 269
    mechanism of action 273
    role, molecular weight, 270–271
  inhibitors, 197, 198
  production, 274–275
  transfusions, effect, 211–212
Exostoses, 41
Eye, in ALL, 71

Factor VIII, 178, 180
  deficiency, 177, 250
  fetal values, 182
  inhibitor, 22, 23, 24
  replacement therapy, 21, 22, 25–26, 248, 257
    concentrates dosage, 257–259
    cryoprecipitates, 248, 257
Factor VIIIC, 178, 180, 182, 183
Factor VIIIRag, 178, 180, 182
Factor IX, 178, 185, 250
  coagulant activity (IXC), 177, 178, 180, 185
  concentrates, dosage, 257–259
  fetal values, 182
Factor XI, deficiency, 249
Familial erythrophagocytic lympho-histiocytosis (FEL), 99, 102–103, 106
Fanconi's anaemia, 135, 140, 278
Fear, of cancer, 15, 16, 18–19
FEL, 99, 102–103, 106
Femoral epiphysis, slipped, 40
Femoral head, shielding of, 41
Ferritin, serum, 239, 243
Fetal calf serum (FCS), 264
Fetoscopy, 165
  in haemophilia, antenatal diagnosis, 179, 181
  pregnancy outcome, 165, 166–187
Fetus,
  blood, oxygen affinity, 196
  blood sampling, 162, 164–166, 173, 181–182, 186 (*see also* Haemoglobinopathy; Haemophilia)
  death, blood sampling, 164, 165

Fetus (*cont.*)
  erythropoiesis in, 196–199
  haemoglobin, *see* Haemoglobin
  liver, 132, 135, 276, 277
  oxygen delivery, transport, 201–204
  tissue transplantation, 130–133, 135
Fibroblasts, 275
Fibroplasia, retrolental, 210–211
Fibrosis,
  hepatic, 237, 243
  testicular relapse, ALL, 63, 68
Fluids, after radiotherapy, 36
Furosemide, 114

Gastrointestinal decontamination, 116, 126, 127, 139
Genes,
  analysis, haemophilia, 180, 189
  globin chains, 167–169, 189, 266
Globin gene clusters, 167–169, 189, 266
Glucose-6-phosphodiesterase (G-6-PD), 264, 267
Gnotobiotic techniques, 116, 126, 127, 128, 139
Gonads,
  radiation effects, 16, 30, 43–44
  relapse in ALL, *see* Leukaemia
Graft,
  bone marrow, *see* Bone marrow
  rejection, 124, 128
Graft-versus-host reaction, 110, 111, 125–126, 137
  chronic, 129
  clinical features, 125, 129
  in Fanconi's anaemia, 135, 278
  granulocyte activity, 123
  immune responses, 123, 129
  infections associated with, 127
  interstitial pneumonia, 128, 135
  mitigation of, 114–116, 126, 137
  in SCID, 130, 132
  types, early, late, 125
Graft-versus leukaemia effect, 137
Granulocyte, 114, 116, 123
Granulocytosis, 274
Granuloma, eosinophilic, 96, 98
  self-limiting process, 100, 101
Granulomacrophage (GM) lineage, 263, 265, 268
  progenitors, 265, 269, 270, 271, 272
  in aplastic anaemia, 278, 279
Granulomatous disease, chronic, 139
Growth hormone deficiency, 41, 42, 55

Haemoglobin,
   fetal, 167, 172, 197–198, 201–204
      2,3-DPG effect, 202–204
      hereditary persistence, 169, 203
      in neonates, levels, 203, 206–207
      synthesis, gestation ages, 203, 213
      transfusion effects, 211–212
   in neonates, 198–200, 205–208, 213–215
   -oxygen dissociation curve, see Oxygen
Haemoglobin A, 172, 174, 203, 204
Haemoglobin C, 167, 172
Haemoglobin E, 167, 170
Haemoglobin S, 167, 172
Haemoglobinopathy, (see also
   β-Thalassaemia)
   antenatal diagnosis, 162–164, 167–177
      acceptance of, at-risk, 175, 177
      laboratory diagnosis, 172
      procedure, 172–173
   molecular basis, 167–169
Haemolytic anaemia, congenital, 140
Haemophilia, 20–26
   adherence to treatment, 25–26
   antenatal diagnosis, 162, 163, 177–189
      acceptance of, at-risk, 187–189
      carrier detection, 179–180, 188
      CRM+, 178, 183–184
      haemophilia A, 177, 178, 180, 183–185
      haemophilia B, 177, 178, 185
      laboratory diagnosis, 181–188
      outcome of pregnancy, 186–187
      steps in, 179
   classification, 177, 249–250
   molecular basis, 177–179
   psychosocial aspects, 23–25, 252
   severity, classification, 250
   therapy, 250–259
      comprehensive care approach, 249, 251–256
      dosages, factors, 258
      education module, 252–256
      factors concentrates, 248, 257–259
      home therapy, 248–259
      pain management, 202–3, 177
Haemophila A, 177, 250–259
Haemophila B, 177, 250–259
Haemophila C, 249
Haemophilia Educational Resource Project, 256
Haemopoiesis, 118, 263
   model, 267–270
Haemopoietic cells, 263 (see also
   Progenitors, Stem cells)
   differentiation, 266–267
   physical interactions, 275

Haemopoietic hormones, see Hormones
Haemopoietic inhibitors, 273–274, 275, 281, 282
Haemorrhage,
   intracerebral, 228, 231
   pain of, 20, 21, 22, 177
   in thrombocytopenic purpura, 225, 228, 231
Haemosiderin, 239, 243
Haemosiderosis, see Iron overload
Hand-Schuller-Christian disease, 96–102
   survival data, 100–101
Headache, 35, 49
Heart,
   in ALL, 70
   rate, oxygen delivery, 215
   transfusional iron overload, 236
Herpes simplex, 116, 127, 129
Herpes zoster, 116, 127, 129
Heterozygotes, antenatal diagnosis, 162–164
Histiocytes, 97, 98, 102, 104
Histiocytosis, 95–106
   characteristic features, 106
Histiocytosis X, 96–102, 106
   acute disseminated, 101
   histopathology, 97–98
   immunology, 98–99
   survival, 100–101
   terminology, classification, 96–97, 105
   therapy, 99–100, 101, 105
Histiocytosis, familial erythrophagocytic (FEL), 99, 102–103, 106
Histiocytosis, malignant, 104, 106
HLA antigens, 110, 111, 124, 130
   graft-vs-host disease, 125
Hodgkin's disease, 43
Hormones, haemopoietic, 263, 269–273
   inhibitors, 273–274
   membrane receptors, 266
   production, 274–275, 278
Hospitalization, 17
Host defence mechanism, 96
Hurler's disease, 139
Hybridoma, 83, 88, 266–267
Hydrocortisona, 51, 242, 265
Hydroxamic acid, 238, 244
5-Hydroxypicolinaldehyde
   thiosemicarbazone (5-HP), 244
Hyperlipidaemia, 99, 102
Hypnosis, 19
Hypogonadism, 237
Hypoxia, 197, 203, 209

Ia-like antigens, 81, 84, 87
Iatrogenic problems, cancer, 17–20
Immune complex, 225, 226, 228, 232
Immunodeficiency disorder,
  in FEL, 102
  severe combined, see Severe combined immunodeficiency
Immunoglobulins,
  after bone marrow grafting, 120, 123
  in graft-vs-host disease, 123
  IgG in thrombocytopenic purpura, 225, 226
Immunological abnormalities,
  in FEL, 99, 102–103
  in histiocytosis X, 98–99
Immunology, lymphoblast, 80–83
Immunosuppression,
  in bone marrow transplantation, 111–113, 124, 129, 138
  occurrence of VAHS, 104–105, 106
Immunosuppressive agents, 230
Infections,
  after bone marrow grafts, 126–128, 129
  after chemotherapy, radiation, 35
  in histiocytosis X, 97
  prevention, bone marrow grafts, 116–118
  virus, in VAHS, 104–106
Inherited haematological disease, 162–189
Inhibitors, haemopoietic, 273–275, 281, 282
Insomnia, chronic, 24–25
Intellectual function, deterioration, 17, 55
Interstitium, 60, 63
Iron, 239
Iron overload, chronic, 170, 236–244
  clinical manifestations, 236–237
  iron balance in, 239
  iron chelation therapy, 238–244 (see also Desferrioxamine)
Isolation, bone marrow transplantation, 116, 126, 127, 128, 139

K-cells, 120, 123
Ketamine, 33, 50
Kidneys,
  in ALL, 71
  erythropoietin production, 274
  radiation damage, chemotherapy, 38
Kostmann's disease, 139
Kupffer cell, 95, 275

Lactoferrin, 274
Laminar cross-flow isolators, 116
Laminar down-flow isolators, 116

Langerhans cell, 95, 98, 120
Langerhans granules, 98
Letterer-Siwe disease, 96–102
  hypertriglyceridaemia, 99
  survival, 100–101
Leukaemia, acute lymphoblastic (ALL), 47
  bone marrow transplantation, 88, 89, 116, 118 (see also Bone marrow)
  immunology, 121, 123
  infections, 116, 127–128
  patient conditioning, 113, 138
  recurrence of leukaemia, 128, 135
  results of, 135–137
  CNS disease, 48–58
    CNS prophylaxis, see Central nervous system
    CSF analysis, 49–50
    incidence, 48
    pathogenesis, 48–49
    predisposing factors, 50–51
    prevention, 55–58
    signs, symptoms, 49
    treatment, 51–53
  extramedullary sites, 70–71
  immunological subtypes, 80–89
    anti-CALLA, 83, 88, 89
    B-cell, 84, 87
    CALLA, 81–83, 85, 87, 88
    non-T, non-B cell, 84–85, 87
    in patient management, 87–89
    pre-B-cell, 84
    T-cell, 48, 50, 70, 83–84
    treatment results, 85–87, 113
  meningeal, 47, 48–49
  parenchymal, 48, 49
  prognostic variables, 6, 8–12, 48, 50, 64, 66, 86–88
  systemic, remission criterion, 71
  testicular relapse, 47, 58–70
    irradiation, 67
    pathogenesis, 60–63
    predisposing factors, 64–69
    presentation, 63–64
    prevention, 64–69
    treatment, 69–70
  treatment,
    behavioural approach, 19–20
    cranial, see Central nervous system
    improvements in, 6–8, 47, 88–89
Leukaemia, acute monocytic, 48
Leukaemia, acute myeloblastic (AML), 48, 49, 58, 83
Leukaemia, acute myelomonocytic, 48
Leukaemia, acute undifferentiated (AUL), 81

Index

Leukaemia, chronic lymphatic (CLL), 84, 282
Leukaemia, chronic myeloid (CML),
 CNS disease in, 48
 common ALL antigen, 81
 G-6-PD in myeloid cells, 268
 treatment, 20, 137
Leukoencephalopathy, 55, 57
Life expectancy, extension, 3–4, 6–8, 14
 adjustment, problems of, 14–17
Lipids, histiocytosis, 99, 102
Liquor, leakage, 165, 166
Liver,
 acute veno-occlusive disease, 114
 anti-platelet antibodies in, 229
 damage, radiotherapy, chemotherapy, 37–38
 erythrocyte production, 274, 275
 fetal, 132, 135, 276, 277
 iron overload, 237, 243
Lomustine (CCNU), 57
Lumbar puncture, ALL, 49, 50
Lungs,
 after bone marrow graft, 130
 infiltration in ALL, 70
 in radiotherapy with chemotherapy, 38
Lymphadenopathy, 50, 64, 65, 70
Lymphoblast,
 antisera against, 89
 bone marrow, classification, 10
 immunology, 80–83
Lymphocyte, 80 (*see also* B-lymphocytes; T-lymphocytes)
 cell surface markers, 81–89
 cytotoxicity in histiocytosis, 99, 102
 null, 269
 proliferation in histiocytosis X, 99, 102, 103
Lymphohistiocytosis, familial erythrophagocytic, 99, 102–103
Lymphoid cell lineage, 263, 267
Lymphomas, 2, 83, 84
Lymphopoiesis, 265
Lyonization, 163, 180

Macrophages, 95–96
 after bone marrow grafting, 120
 CFU-M, CFU-G kinetics, 274
 haemopoietic hormone production, 275, 278
 in histiocytosis X, 98, 99
Major histocompatibility complex (MHC), 110, 111, 138 (*see also* HLA)
Malignancy, secondary, 44, 130

Malignant histiocytosis, 104, 106
Management, cancer, multidisciplinary, 1–12, 15
Markers, cell-surfaces, *see* Cell-surface
Megakaryocytes, 226, 268
Membrane transport defects, 138
Meningeal leukaemia, 47, 48–49 (*see also* Leukaemia)
Menses, thrombocytopenic purpura, 229, 231
2-Mercaptoethane sulphonate sodium, 114
6-Mercaptopurine, 88
Methotrexate,
 in ALL,
  CNS relapse, 17, 50, 51–57
  in T-cell disease, 88
  testicular relapse, 66, 70
 cytocidal concentration, 56
 in graft-vs-host disease, 114–116, 126
Microenvironment, stem cells, 265, 275, 276
Mikulicz syndrome, 71
Misonidazole, 45
Mixed lymphocyte culture-relative response index (MLC-RRI), 124
Monocytes, 95–96, 274, 275
Mucosal reaction to radiation, 35, 36
Multidisciplinary management, cancer, 1–12, 15
Mycosis fungoides, 84
Myelofibrosis, 198
Myeloid cell lineage, 263, 267–268 (*see also* Erythroid progenitors; Granulomacrophage lineage)
 stem cell, 264, 268–270, 271
 in aplastic anaemia, 278
Myelopoiesis, 267–268

Nalidixic acid, 117
National Hemophilia Foundation, USA, 249, 256
Natural killer (NK) cells, 120, 123, 124, 125
Nausea, 18, 19, 35, 113
Neomycin, 116, 117
Neonate,
 erythropoiesis in, 196–199
 haemoglobin, *see* Haemoglobin
 oxygen delivery, transport, *see* Oxygen
 transfusions in, 209–219
Nephritis, radiation, 38
Nephroblastoma, 38, 44
Neutropenia, cyclic, 272
Nezelof's disease, 138
Nitrosoureas, 57

Nucleoside phosphorylase (NP) deficiency, 138, 139
Nucleotidyltransferase, terminal (TdT), 68, 71, 85
Nutrition, parenteral, 114

Omenn's disease, 138
Ommaya reservoir, 53, 57
Operant reinforcement, 19, 20
Orchidectomy, 69
Oropharyngeal reaction, radiation, 35–36
Osteopetrosis, malignant, 139
Ovaries,
 radiation effects, 43–44
 relapse in ALL, 59
Oxygen,
 affinity, of haemoglobin,
  2,3-DPG effect, 202, 205
  factors affecting, 202, 208
  fetal blood, 196, 201–204
  in newborn, 204–208, 210
  transfusions, see Transfusion
 arterial, 200–201
 available, 213–215
 carrying capacity, 205–208
 delivery, transport, 200–219
  in fetus, 201–204
  in newborn, 204–208
  nomogram for, 216–218
  transfusion effect, see Transfusion
  variables in, 210, 212, 216–219
 dissociation curve, 201–202, 204, 209
 P_{50}, 202, 204–208, 215, 217
 tension, 201
  central venous, 215, 218
Oxygenation, tumour cells, 45

Pain, 18–20
 chronic arthritic, 21–22
 in haemophilia, 20–23, 177
 perception, 20
  self-regulation, 21, 22
Pancreas, iron overload, 237
Papilloedema, 49
Parenchymal leukaemia, 48, 49
Perceptual function, 17, 55
Phenothiazines, 19
Philadelphia chromosome, 81, 83
Phosphates, organic, 196, 201 (see also 2,3 Diphosphoglycerate)
Pituitary-hypothalamic region, radiation, 41–42
Placenta, haemopoietic hormones, 278

Platelet,
 antibody, 224, 225, 226, 228
 counts, 37
  in ATP, 228, 230, 231
  testicular relapse of ALL, 65
 transfusion, 47, 50
Pluripotent stem cells, 266, 267, 268, 270
Pneumocystis carinii, 116, 127, 138
Pneumonia,
 interstitial, 127–128, 135, 137, 138
 Pneumocystis carinii, 127, 138
Pneumonitis, 34, 38, 70
Polycythaemia vera, 198, 268
Polymyxin B/E, 116, 117
Prednisolone, 50, 53, 66
Prednisone, 227, 230–231
Proerythroblasts, 269
Progenitor cells, 267–282 (see also Colony-forming units)
 clonogenic cultures, 263–264
 erythroid, see Erythroid
 granulomacrophage, see Granulomacrophage
 haemopoietic hormones, see Hormones
 long-term cultures, 264–265
Prognosis, individual variability, 15
Prostaglandins, 167, 274
Prothymocytes, 85
Psychosocial aspects, 14–26, 45, 55
 in bone marrow transplantation, 118
 in haemophilia, 23–25, 252
Pure red cell aplasia (PRCA), 281–282
Purpura, autoimmune thrombocytopenic (AIP), 224–232
 clinical presentation, 225–226
 idiopathic, (ITP), 224
 immune aetiology, 224–225
 management, 226–231
  corticosteroids, 226–228, 231
  immunosuppressive, 230
  splenectomy, 228–230, 231
 platelet counts, 228, 230, 231
 prognosis, 231–232
 'severe' classification, 228
 transient, in neonates, 224

Quantal mitosis, 276

Radiation reaction, 35, 37
Radiotherapy, 30–46
 changes, advances in, 5–6, 33
 in CNS prophylaxis, see Central nervous system

Index 305

Radiotherapy (*cont.*)
  future of, 45–46
  limitations of, 45
  pre-operative, 6
  problems, paediatric, 30–34
    chemotherapy, interaction, 33–34, 37–38, 46, 51, 114
    child handling, restraint, 31–33
    tissue sensitivity, 30–31, 45
  sequelae of, 34–45
    immediate, 34–37, 52, 54, 114
    late, 39–44, 114, 130
    psychological, 45
    second malignancies, 44, 130
  survival rate, improvement, 3–4
  in testicular relapse, ALL, 69–70
  total body irradiation, 111, 113, 114, 124
'Recall' reactions, 33, 37
Red blood cell, (*see also* Erythropoiesis)
  after bone marrow grafting, 118–120
  antigens, 111, 125
  in FEL, 102
  in fetus, 196
  function, 201
  pure, aplasia (PRCA), 281–282
Rejection, transplantation, 124, 128
Relaxation training, 19
Respiratory distress syndrome, 208, 209, 210
Restraining devices, radiotherapy, 33
Reticulocyte index, transfusions, 211
Reticulosis, familial, 138
Rhabdomyosarcoma, 6, 46
Rhodotorulic acid (RA), 244

School re-integration, cancer, 15–16
Sedation, radiotherapy, 33
Severe combined immunodeficiency (SCID), 99, 110, 111, 138–139 (*see also* Bone marrow)
  disorders in, 111, 138
  fetal tissue trnasplantation, 130–133, 138
  graft-vs-host disease, 132
  immunological reconstitution, 118, 120, 127, 133, 139
  infections in, 116, 126–127
  MHC genotypically non-identical donor, 139
  results transplantation, 130–133, 138
  thymic factors, 133, 138
Sex-linked inheritance, 163
Sexual functioning, 16–17
Sezary syndrome, 83, 84
Sibling, reactions of, to cancer, 16

Sickle cell disease, 169, 170–171
  antenatal diagnosis, 172, 173, 174, 176
  iron overload, 236
Skeleton, late radiation effects, 40–41
Skin, late radiation effects, 39
Sleep, self-regulation, 24–25
Soft tissue, late radiation effects, 39
Somnolence syndrome, 'benign', 54
Spleen, 226, 228, 232
Splenectomy, 228–230, 231
Staphylococcus aureus, 116, 117
Stem cells, haemopoietic, 266–282 (*see also* Colony-forming units)
  in aplastic anaemia, 278, 279
  cultures, 263–265
  depletion, 279
  differentiation, 266, 270, 276
  haemopoietic hormones, *see* Hormones
  intrinsic, extrinsic defect, 279
  marker, 267
  myeloid, *see* Myeloid
  number, circulating, 269
  pluripotent, 266, 267, 268, 270
  transformation *in vivo*, 266
Steroids, 226–228, 231
Streptomyces pilosus, 238
Stress,
  after cancer diagnosis, 15
  erythropoiesis, 270
  in haemophilia, 24, 25
Stromal factors, aplastic anaemia, 279
Surgery, cancer, 3–5
Survival rate, cancer, 3–4, 6–8, 14

Terminal DNA nucleotidyltransferase (TdT), 68, 71, 85
Testis,
  radiation effects, 16, 44, 67
  relapse in ALL, *see* Leukaemia
Tetrahydrocannabinol (THC), 19
Tetrahydrouridine, 58
β-Thalassaemia,
  antenatal diagnosis, 162, 164, 170, 172–177
  in Cypriots, Asians, 175–176
  haemoglobin E, 167, 170, 174
  intermedia, 170
  major, 169, 172, 174
    iron overload, 236, 240, 243
  molecular basis, 167–169, 170
  treatment, 170
Therapeutic Ratio, 30, 45

Therapy, cancer, (see also Chemotherapy; Radiotherapy)
  milestones in, 3–4
  multi-modality, 2, 3–4, 12
Thrombocythaemia, essential, 268
Thrombocytopenic purpura, see Purpura
Thrombotic disease, factor IX, 258
Thymic factors, in SCID, 133, 138
Thymocyte, 84, 132
Thymus abnormalities, 97
Thyroid, radiation effects, 43
T-lymphocytes, 80, 84
  in ALL, 48, 50, 70, 83–84
  bone marrow grafts,
    elimination in, 116, 137
    reconstitution, 120–124, 138
  colony-stimulating factors production, 265, 275
  deficiency, 138
  in graft-vs-host disease, 123, 137
  haemopoietic hormone production, 265, 275, 278
  helper, 275
  inhibitor, in pure red cell aplasia, 282
  lineage, 263, 267, 268
  in SCID, 133
  TG+ inhibitors, aplastic anaemia, 275, 281
Total body irradiation, 111, 113, 114, 124
  risks, 130
Total lymphoid irradiation (TLI), 116, 124, 126
Transfusion,
  dependent anaemia, iron overolad, 236, 239 (see also Iron overload)
  exchange in FEL, 103
  extrauterine, 209–212
  graft failures, 124
  granulocyte, 114, 116
  intrauterine, 208–209

Transfusion (cont.)
  need for, factors influencing, 212–219
    clinical approach, 213–216
    practical approach, nomogram, 216–219
  platelet, 47, 50
  thalassaemia, 170
Transplantation, bone marrow, see Bone marrow
Triglycerides, 99, 102
Trimeprazine (Vallergan), 33

VAHS, 104–105, 106
Vincristine,
  in ALL, relapses, 53, 66
  in thrombocytopenic purpura, 230, 231
  with radiotherapy, 34, 37, 38
Virus-associated haemophagocytic syndrome (VAHS), 104–105, 106
Virus infections, 225
Vitamin C, 243
Vitamin K, 178
Von Willebrand's disease (vWd), 177, 178, 186

White blood cell (WBC),
  after bone marrow grafting, 116, 118–120
  in ALL, 8, 10, 50, 64
  in radiotherapy, 37
Willebrand factor (WF), 178
Wilms' tumour, 6, 34, 37, 38
Wiskott-Aldrich syndrome, 139

X chromosome, 189, 267

Yolk sac, 196